Advances in Rapid Sex-Steroid Action

Gabriella Castoria · Antimo Migliaccio
Editors

Advances in Rapid Sex-Steroid Action

New Challenges and New Chances in Breast and Prostate Cancers

Springer

Gabriella Castoria
Department of General Pathology
II University of Naples
Naples
Italy
e-mail: gabriella.castoria@unina2.it

Antimo Migliaccio
Department of Pathology
II University of Naples
Naples
Italy
e-mail: antimo.migliaccio@unina2.it

ISBN 978-1-4614-1763-7 e-ISBN 978-1-4614-1764-4
DOI 10.1007/978-1-4614-1764-4
Springer New York Dordrecht Heidelberg London

Library of Congress Control Number: 2011941855

Cover design: eStudio Calamar

Printed on acid-free paper

Springer is part of Springer Science+Business Media (www.springer.com)

To Rosario Castoria, Giuseppe Migliaccio,
and our families

Preface

For many years, those of us working in the field of steroid hormones were used to looking at the steroidal receptor as ligand inducible transcriptional factors. In the late 1960s, a lone voice (the mind goes to the pioneering work of C. Szego) began to raise the hypothesis that estrogens could act through different ways. Nowadays, after more than 40 years, no one has any doubts that steroids through their receptors, in addition to regulating gene transcription, activate outside from the nucleus a plenty of signaling pathways involved in the most important hormone actions, such as the cell growth, differentiation and motility.

Nevertheless, despite the large amount of information about steroid signaling gained in the last years, the definite understanding of the mechanism of action of the steroid hormones appears as a puzzle that challenges our mind. In particular, a drawing of the interplay between the different signaling cascades and receptor dependent transcriptional activation is still far from being exhaustive.

Of course, this book does not pretend to address this issue but is rather aimed to provide up to date information about some exciting new insights into the cooperative interaction between the c-Src, other tyrosine kinases, PI3-K and steroid receptors. The molecular events are analyzed in two different settings: breast and prostate cancer. Furthermore, a small section of this book is dedicated to new tools for steroid receptor analysis and regulatory networks.

The simple message that this book conveys is that the dissection of these networks could definitely change our understanding of the role of steroid hormones in biology and disease. The combinatory targeting of all hormone signaling effectors could dramatically change the outcome of breast and prostate cancers.

Gabriella Castoria
Antimo Migliaccio

Contents

Contributors

Rebecca A. Alyea Department of Biochemistry and Molecular Biology, University of Texas Medical Branch, Galveston, TX, 77555 -0645, USA, e-mail: rebecca.alyea@gmail.com

Ferdinando Auricchio Dipartimento di Patologia Generale-II Università di Napoli, Via L. De Crecchio, 7, 80138, Naples, Italy,e-mail: ferdinando.auricchio@unina2.it

Elisabetta Baldi Department of Clinical Physiopathology, Andrology Unit and Center for Research, Transfer and High Education DeNothe, University of Florence, Viale Pieraccini, 6, 50139, Florence, Italy, e-mail: e.baldi@dfc.unifi.it

Cecilia Ballaré Chromatin and Gene Expression Laboratory, Gene Regulation Programme, Centre for Genomic Regulation (CRG) and UPF, Barcelona, Spain, e-mail: cecilia.ballare@crg.eu

Anannya Banga Department of Biochemistry and Molecular Biology, University of Texas Medical Branch, Galveston, TX, 77555 -0645, USA, e-mail: banga007@umn.edu

Silvère Baron Génétique des Eucaryotes et Endocrinologie Moléculaire, UMR 6547 CNRS, Equipe Physiologie Comparée et Endocrinologie Moléculaire, Université Blaise Pascal, Campus Universitaire des Cézeaux, 24, Avenue des Landais, 80026, 63171, Aubiere Cedex, France, e-mail: silvere.baron@univ-bpclermont.fr

Miguel Beato Chromatin and Gene Expression Laboratory, Gene Regulation Programme, Centre for Genomic Regulation (CRG) and UPF, Barcelona, Spain, e-mail: miguel.beato@crg.eu

Antonino Belfiore Department of Clinical and Experimental Medicine, University of Catanzaro, 88100, Catanzaro, Italy, e-mail: belfiore@unicz.it

Antonio Bilancio Dipartimento di Patologia Generale-II Università di Napoli, Via L. De Crecchio, 7, 80138, Naples, Italy, e-mail: antonio.bilancio@unina2.it

Michael J. Bolt Department of Molecular and Cellular Biology and Medicine, Baylor College of Medicine, Houston, TX, USA, e-mail: bolt@bcm.edu

Lorella Bonaccorsi Department of Clinical Physiopathology, Andrology Unit and Center for Research, Transfer and High Education DeNothe, University of Florence, Viale Pieraccini, 6, 50139, Florence, Italy, e-mail: lorella.bonaccorsi@unifi.it

Giancarlo Castellano Chromatin and Gene Expression Laboratory, Gene Regulation Programme, Centre for Genomic Regulation (CRG) and UPF, Barcelona, Spain, e-mail: giancarlo.castellano@crg.eu

Gabriella Castoria Dipartimento di Patologia Generale-II Università di Napoli, Via L. De Crecchio, 7, 80138, Naples, Italy, e-mail: gabriella.castoria@unina2.it

Andrew C.B. Cato Institute of Toxicology and Genetics, Karlsruhe Institute of Technology, Hermann-von-Helmholtz-Platz 1, 76344, Eggenstein-Leopoldshafen, Germany, e-mail: andrew.cato@kit.edu

C. Chang Department of Urology and Pathology, George Whipple Laboratory for Cancer Research, University of Rochester, Rochester, NY, USA, e-mail: chang@urmc.rochester.edu

Laura Corbo Equipe Labellisée "La Ligue", U590 INSERM, Centre Léon Bérard, 28 rue Laennec, 69008, Lyon, FrançeUniversité de Lyon 1, ISPB and IFR62, , 69003, Lyon, France, e-mail: laura.corbo@lyon.unicancer.fr

Marzia Di Donato Dipartimento di Patologia Generale-II Università di Napoli, Via L. De Crecchio, 7, 80138, Naples, Italy, e-mail: marziadd@hotmail.it

Karim Fizazi Department of Medicine, Institut Gustave Roussy, 39 rue Camille Desmoulins, 94805, Villejuif, France, e-mail: fizazi@igr.fr

Marina Ines Flamini Molecular and Cellular Gynecological Endocrinology Laboratory (MCGEL), Department of Reproductive Medicine and Child Development, Division of Obstetrics and Gynecology, University of Pisa, Via Roma 57, 56100, Pisa, Italy, e-mail: flaminimarinaines@hotmail.com

Jofre Font-Mateu Chromatin and Gene Expression Laboratory, Gene Regulation Programme, Centre for Genomic Regulation (CRG) and UPF, Barcelona, Spain, e-mail: jofre.font@crg.eu

Gianni Forti Endocrine Unit, Department of Clinical Physiopathology, University of Florence, Viale Pieraccini, 6, 50139, Florence, Italy, e-mail: g.forti@dfc.unifi.it

Xiao-Dong Fu Department of Physiology, Zhongshan School of Medicine, Sun Yat-Sen University, 510080, Guangzhou, People's Republic of China, e-mail: mcgel@obgyn.med.unipi.it

Pia Giovannelli Dipartimento di Patologia Generale-II Università di Napoli, Via L. De Crecchio, 7, 80138, Naples, Italy, e-mail: pia.giovannelli@unina2.it

Randall Goldblum Department of Pediatrics, University of Texas Medical School Branch, Galveston, TX, 77555, USA, e-mail: rmgoldbl@utmb.edu

Sean M. Hartig Department of Molecular and Cellular Biology and Medicine, Baylor College of Medicine, Houston, TX, USA, e-mail: hartig@bcm.edu

Yow-Jiun Jeng Department of Biochemistry and Molecular Biology, University of Texas Medical Branch, Galveston, TX, 77555-0645, USA, e-mail: yjeng@utmb.edu

Kuo-Pao Lai Department of Urology and Pathology, George Whipple Laboratory for Cancer Research, University of Rochester, Rochester, NY, USA, e-mail: kuopao_lai@urmc.rochester.edu

Rosamaria Lappano Department of Pharmaco-Biology, University of Calabria, Rende, CS, Italy, e-mail: rosamaria3@interfree.it

Francois Le Dily Chromatin and Gene Expression Laboratory, Gene Regulation Programme, Centre for Genomic Regulation (CRG) and UPF, Barcelona, Spain, e-mail: francois.ledily@crg.eu

S. O. Lee Department of Urology and Pathology, George Whipple Laboratory for Cancer Research, University of Rochester, Rochester, NY, USA, e-mail: soook_lee@urmc.rochester.edu

Muriel Le Romancer Equipe Labellisée "La Ligue", U590 INSERM, Centre Léon Bérard, 28 rue Laennec, 69008, Lyon, France, Université de Lyon 1, ISPB and IFR62, 69003, Lyon, France, e-mail: muriel.leromancer@lyon.unicancer.fr

Marcello Maggiolini Department of Pharmaco-Biology, University of Calabria, Rende, CS, Italy, e-mail: marcellomaggiolini@yahoo.it

Michael A. Mancini Department of Molecular and Cellular Biology and Medicine, Baylor College of Medicine, Houston, TX, USA, e-mail: mancini@bcm.edu

Marco Marcelli Department of Molecular and Cellular Biology and Medicine, Baylor College of Medicine, Houston, TX, USA, The Michael E. DeBakey VA Medical Center, Baylor College of Medicine, Houston, TX, USA, e-mail: mediwala@bcm.edu

Sara Marchiani Department of Clinical Physiopathology, Andrology Unit and Center for Research, Transfer and High Education DeNothe, University of Florence, Viale Pieraccini, 6, 50139, Florence, Italy, e-mail: sara.marchiani@unifi.it

Christophe Massard Department of Medicine, Institut Gustave Roussy, 39 rue Camille Desmoulins, 94805, Villejuif, France, e-mail: christophe.massard@igr.fr

Terumi Midoro-Horiuti Department of Pediatrics, University of Texas Medical Branch, Galveston, TX, 77555, USA, e-mail: tmidoro@utmb.edu

Sanjay N. Mediwala The Michael E. DeBakey VA Medical Center, Baylor College of Medicine, Houston, TX, USA, e-mail: mediwala@bcm.edu

Antimo Migliaccio Dipartimento di Patologia Generale-II Università di Napoli, Via L. De Crecchio, 7, 80138, Naples, Italy, e-mail: antimo.migliaccio@unina2.it

Laurent Morel Génétique des Eucaryotes et Endocrinologie Moléculaire, UMR 6547 CNRS, Equipe Physiologie Comparée et Endocrinologie Moléculaire, Université Blaise Pascal, Campus Universitaire des Cézeaux, 24, Avenue des Landais, 80026, 63171, Aubiere Cedex, France, e-mail: laurent.morel@univ-bpclermont.fr

Monica Muratori Department of Clinical Physiopathology, Andrology Unit and Center for Research, Transfer and High Education DeNothe, University of Florence, Viale Pieraccini, 6, 50139, Florence, Italy, e-mail: monica@muratori@dfc.unifi.it

A. Silvina Nacht Chromatin and Gene Expression Laboratory, Gene Regulation Programme, Centre for Genomic Regulation (CRG) and UPF, Barcelona, Spain, e-mail: silvina.nacht@crg.eu

Zafar Nawaz Braman Family Breast Cancer Institute, University of Miami, Sylvester Comprehensive Cancer Center, Miami, FL 33136, USA, Department of Biochemistry and Molecular Biology, University of Miami, Miller School of Medicine, Miami, FL 33136, USA, e-mail: znawaz@med.miami.edu

Emmanuel Oppong Institute of Toxicology and Genetics, Karlsruhe Institute of Technology, Hermann-von-Helmholtz-Platz 1, 76344, Eggenstein-Leopoldshafen, Germany, e-mail: emmanuel.oppong@kit.edu

Sarah J. Parsons Department of Microbiology and Endocrinology, University of Virginia Cancer Center, Charlottesville, VA 22908, USA, e-mail: sap@virginia.edu or MAS3X@hscmail.mcc.virginia.edu

Coralie Poulard Equipe Labellisée “La Ligue”, U590 INSERM, Centre Léon Bérard, 28 rue Laennec, 69008, Lyon, France, Université de Lyon 1, ISPB and IFR62, 69003, Lyon, France, e-mail: coralie.poulard@lyon.unicancer.fr

Angel Matias Sanchez Molecular and Cellular Gynecological Endocrinology Laboratory (MCGEL), Department of Reproductive Medicine and Child Development, Division of Obstetrics and Gynecology, University of Pisa, Via Roma 57, 56100, Pisa, Italy, e-mail: angelsanchez2001@hotmail.com

Sylwia Sekula-Neuner, Forschungszentrum Karlsruhe Institute fur Nanotechnologie, 3640-76021, Karlsruhes, Germany, e-mail: sekula@int.fzk.de

Stéphanie Sentis Equipe Labellisée “La Ligue”, U590 INSERM, Centre Léon Bérard, 28 rue Laennec, 69008, Lyon, France, Université de Lyon 1, ISPB and IFR62, 69003, Lyon, France, e-mail: stephanie.sentis@lyon.unicancer.fr

Margaret A. Shupnik Division of Endocrinology, Department of Medicine, University of Virginia Cancer Center, Charlottesville, VA 22908, USA, e-mail: mas3x@virginia.edu

Tommaso Simoncini Molecular and Cellular Gynecological Endocrinology Laboratory (MCGEL), Department of Reproductive Medicine and Child Development, Division of Obstetrics and Gynecology, University of Pisa, Via Roma 57, 56100, Pisa, Italy, e-mail: t.simoncini@med.unipi.it

Joyce M. Slingerland Braman Family Breast Cancer Institute, Department of Medicine, University of Miami-Miller, Miami, FL 33136, USA, e-mail: jslingerland@med.miami.edu

Jun Sun Braman Family Breast Cancer Institute, University of Miami Sylvester Comprehensive Cancer Center, Miami, FL 33136, USA, e-mail: jsun@med.miami.edu

Lara Tamburrino Department of Clinical Physiopathology, Andrology Unit and Center for Research, Transfer and High Education DeNothe, University of Florence, Viale Pieraccini, 6, 50139, Florence, Italy, e-mail: lara.tamburrino@unifi.it

Guillermo P. Vicent Chromatin and Gene Expression Laboratory, Gene Regulation Programme, Centre for Genomic Regulation (CRG) and UPF, Barcelona, Spain, e-mail: guillermo.vicent@crg.eu

Cheryl S. Watson Department of Biochemistry and Molecular Biology, University of Texas Medical Branch, Galveston, TX, 77555 -0645, USA, e-mail: cswatson@utmb.edu

Roni H. G. Wright Chromatin and Gene Expression Laboratory, Gene Regulation Programme, Centre for Genomic Regulation (CRG) and UPF, Barcelona, Spain, e-mail: roni.wright@crg.eu

S. Yeh Department of Urology and Pathology, George Whipple Laboratory for Cancer Research, University of Rochester, Rochester, NY, USA, e-mail: shuyuan_yeh@urmc.rochester.edu

Roser Zaurin Chromatin and Gene Expression Laboratory, Gene Regulation Programme, Centre for Genomic Regulation (CRG) and UPF, Barcelona, Spain, e-mail: roser.zaurin@crg.eu

Dragoslava Zivadinovic Department of Biochemistry and Molecular Biology, University of Texas Medical Branch, Galveston, TX, 77555 -0645, USA, e-mail: ddzivadi@utmb.edu

Wen Zhou Braman Family Breast Cancer Institute, University of Miami, Sylvester Comprehensive Cancer Center, Miami, FL 33136, USA, Department of Biochemistry and Molecular Biology, University of Miami, Miller School of Medicine, Miami, FL 33136, USA, e-mail: wzhou@med.miami.edu

Non-genomic Action of Steroid Hormones: More Questions than Answers

Antimo Migliaccio, Gabriella Castoria, Antonio Bilancio, Pia Giovannelli, Marzia Di Donato and Ferdinando Auricchio

Abstract In this chapter we aim to draw the attention of potential readers to several aspects of our research on non-genomic action of sex steroid hormones that have not as yet been fully investigated and might offer interesting developments in future studies. The first aspect concerns the dependence of phenotype on hormone concentration. The second, regards the analysis of mechanisms responsible for the simultaneous stimulation of cell migration and inhibition of proliferation. Besides its physiological relevance, the migration-proliferation dichotomy might also be involved in the intermediate stages of progression from hormone dependency to hormone independency in breast and prostate cancers. Thirdly, the increasing number of non-reproductive cells that

A. Migliaccio · G. Castoria · A. Bilancio · P. Giovannelli · M. Di Donato · F. Auricchio (✉)
Dipartimento di Patologia Generale - II Università di Napoli,
Via L. De Crecchio, 7, 80138 Naples, Italy
e-mail: ferdinando.auricchio@unina2.it

A. Migliaccio
e-mail: antimo.migliaccio@unina2.it

G. Castoria
e-mail: gabriella.castoria@unina2.it

A. Bilancio
e-mail: antonio.bilancio@unina2.it

P. Giovannelli
e-mail: pia.giovannelli@unina2.it

M. Di Donato
e-mail: marziadd@hotmail.it

G. Castoria and A. Migliaccio (eds.), *Advances in Rapid Sex-Steroid Action*,
DOI: 10.1007/978-1-4614-1764-4_1, © Springer Science+Business Media, LLC 2012

respond to steroid hormones through receptor-mediated non-genomic action in the absence of receptor-dependent transcription challenges the classic model of steroid hormone action as restricted to classic cell types rather than valid for all steroid target cells. Cross talk between membrane receptors and nuclear steroid receptors regulates nuclear steroid receptor action. An additional cross talk occurring between membrane receptors and extra-nuclear steroid receptors modulates to a great extent the intensity of growth factor signaling. The observed convergence of steroid-stimulated steroid receptor heterodimers on signaling pathways enhances signaling and offers new flexibility in the use of steroid antagonists. Surprisingly, steroid receptor nuclear export is a crucial step in the proliferative response mediated by non-genomic action of steroid receptors. Finally, receptor association with signaling effectors and scaffold proteins is the key event that initiates non-genomic proliferative, anti-apoptotic and migratory programs. It is therefore a promising target for novel anti-cancer therapy. Each of these aspects has been analyzed in several cell types and in relation to different biological effects. Much more work is required to fully evaluate their role in hormone action and their application in cancer therapy.

Keywords Steroids · Growth factors · Non-genomic action · Protein/protein interaction · Proliferation/migration · Steroid receptor trafficking

Abbreviations

AR	androgen receptor
Crm1	chromosome region maintenance 1
EGF	epidermal growth factor
EGF-R	epidermal growth factor receptor
ER	estradiol receptor
Fln	filamin
FKHR	forkhead in rhabdomyosarcoma
GR	glucocorticoids receptor
MAPK	mitogen activated protein kinase
MEK-1	mitogen-activated kinase kinase
NES	nuclear export signal
NLS	nuclear localization signal
PDGF	platelet-derived growth factor
PDGF-R	PDGF receptor
PI3-K	phosphatidylinositol-3-kinase
PKC	protein kinase C
PR	progesterone receptor

Contents

1 Introduction

Studies investigating the non-genomic action of steroid hormones began many years ago and initial findings were published randomly. The group headed by Szego pioneered this field with their report on specific plasma membrane binding sites for estrogen [1], preceded by the observation of acute stimulation of cAMP and rapid calcium mobilization by estrogen [2, 3]. Several groups, including our own, have contributed to identifying classic steroid receptors (SRs) as responsible for many rapid hormonal effects (proliferation, migration, protection from apoptosis). A number of different approaches have been used, including ectopic expression of SRs in cells devoid of these receptors, siRNA knockdown of SRs, use of specific antagonist inhibitors and mouse models, as well as genetic and pharmacological tools. SRs interact with signaling effectors or signaling effector-associated scaffold proteins in response to steroids or growth factors. These interactions are the keys that open up complex signaling networks to receptor action. Recent findings also confirm the central role of receptor/effector association in rapid hormonal action [4].

The present chapter is not aimed at giving an overall view of the rapid actions of steroid hormones, since many general reviews on this subject have been published [5–8]. Its intention is rather to provide a critical analysis of issues that are not yet fully understood. Focusing interest on these aspects might lead to new insights into our knowledge of hormone action and thus new options for a more tailored therapeutic approach in human breast and prostate cancers.

2 Phenotype Dependence on Hormone Concentration: An Isolated Case or a General Rule?

Growth factors, such as EGF [9–11], VEGF [12], and PDGF [13], can trigger motility or proliferation. Cell type, ligand concentrations, abundance and distribution of the cognate receptors influence whether cells migrate, differentiate or divide. In NIH3T3 cells, low PDGF concentration induces migration whereas high concentration triggers proliferation and this decision depends on the different endocytic routes (clathrin- and non-clathrin-mediated) taken by PDGF receptor (PDGF-R) [13]. Using the same cells, we observed that different concentrations of androgens trigger different phenotypes ([14, 15] and manuscript in preparation). In fact, picomolar concentration of this steroid induces a proliferative response, whereas higher (nanomolar) concentration activates migration and inhibits proliferation in NIH3T3 fibroblasts (migration/proliferation dichotomy). Analysis of the pathways activated by the two androgen concentrations revealed some interesting aspects. Low androgen concentration induces proliferation as a consequence of androgen receptor (AR) association with Src and p85, the regulatory subunit of PI3-kinase [14]. Association of the tripartite complex was previously detected in MCF-7 cells stimulated by estradiol [16] and association of AR with Src was also detected in prostate cancer-derived LNCaP cells treated with androgen [17]. Association of steroid receptors with Src and p85 triggers activation of a complex network targeting the G1-S phase of cell cycle and induces cell proliferation [14, 16]. In contrast, fibroblast stimulation with nanomolar androgen concentration does not induce AR association with Src and p85, confirming the mitogenic role of this association. These findings also raise the question of how nanomolar androgen concentration triggers the migratory phenotype. The key event is association of AR with filamin A (FlnA) [15]. Members of the Fln family cross-link cortical cytoplasmic actin and contribute to anchor plasma membrane proteins, such as integrins, to the cortical actin. FlnA is a scaffold protein, which under basal conditions or in response to microenvironmental signals, interacts with a variety of proteins, some of which regulate Rac activity and cell migration [18]. Mutations in FlnA and B are associated with human genetic diseases due to altered migration or abnormal development of different organs. In periventricular heterotopia, an X-chromosome–linked brain malformation, neurons fail to migrate to the correct cortical site, suggesting that FlnA is required for neuronal migration [19]. Androgen stabilizes AR/FlnA co-localization at intermediate cytoskeletal filaments and induces a complex including AR/FlnA/integrin beta1 in NIH3T3 fibroblasts. This ternary complex activates Rac and induces tyrosine phosphorylation of both FAK and paxillin. As a consequence, the migration speed of fibroblasts is significantly increased ([15] and Fig. 1).

The observation that assembly of the tripartite AR/Src/PI3-K complex generates a proliferative phenotype whereas association of AR with FlnA produces a migratory phenotype supports the view that receptor-associated partners dictate the type of activated pathway and the type of biological outcome upon hormonal

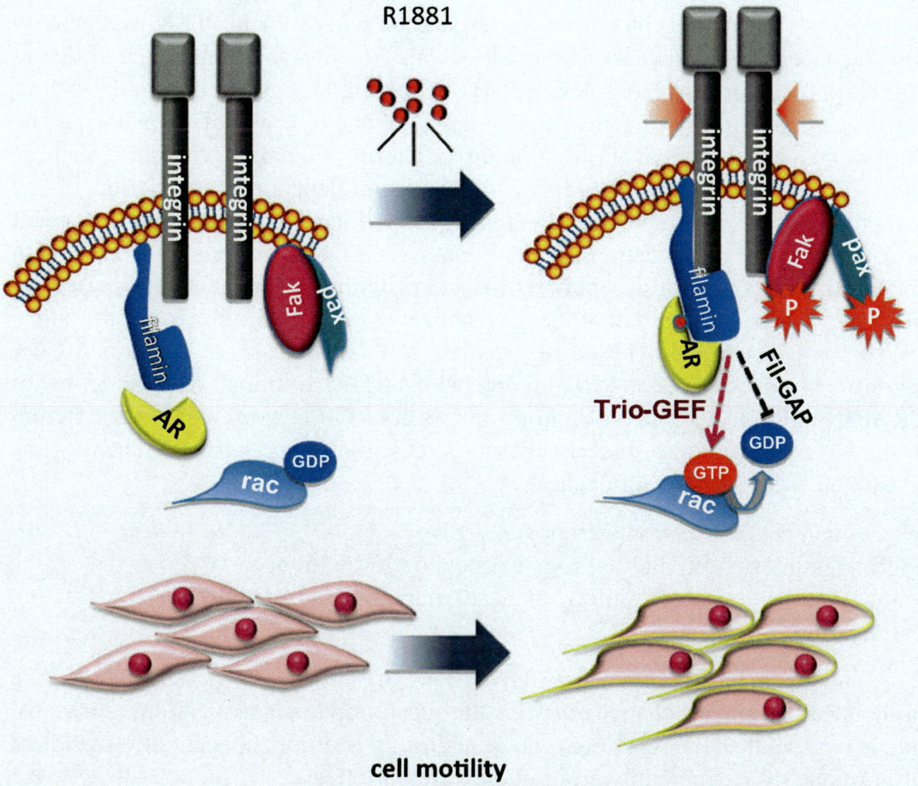

Fig. 1 Mechanism of androgen-induced cell motility. Androgens stabilize AR/FlnA co-localization at intermediate cytoskeleton filaments and induce a tripartite complex including AR/FlnA/integrin beta1 in fibroblasts NIH3T3 (Castoria et al. 2011). This complex, most likely through the Trio-GEF, activates Rac on the hand. Rac activity could be switched-off by the filamin-associated GTPase activating protein (*Fil-GAP*). On the other hand, the AR/FlnA/integrin beta 1 complex also triggers FAK activation and tyrosine phosphorylation of the scaffold paxillin. Once activated, this machinery leads to cell motility of target cells

stimulation of target cells. In addition to receptor-protein interactions other factors can regulate the type of hormonal responses. Differences in receptor number and small changes in ligand concentration markedly affect the duration of MAPK activation and the hormonal effects [20]. The rate of internalization of receptors and whether they are down-regulated as a result of activation of downstream signaling pathways may also affect the type of signaling. Different androgen concentrations, for instance, may affect phosphorylation and internalization rate of AR. Again, different activation kinetics could be generated by differential usage of signaling pathways downstream of the receptors [20]. Thus, there are potentially different ways for AR to signal proliferation, migration or other processes. Different hormone concentrations might favor specific association of the receptor with signaling effectors on the basis of their reciprocal affinity and signaling effector levels. In NIH3T3 fibroblasts, for example, higher androgen concentrations might shift the receptor from its association with Src and PI3-K triggered by lower concentration towards association with FlnA. Accordingly, the different affinity of receptors or other intermediary factors might regulate the availability of cellular subdomain components, such as caveolin and rafts associated with specific effectors, to receptors. Scaffold proteins anchoring signaling effectors, such as FlnA or p130Cas, might also mediate the ligand-dependent association of the receptor with a set of specific effectors. Lastly, ligand concentration-dependent post-translational modifications of SRs, which facilitate or induce association with specific partners, could also play a role in regulating different receptor associations. This type of regulation has been proposed for estradiol receptor alpha (ER alpha), whose methylation at arginine 260 facilitates Src, PI3-K and FAK recruitment to the receptor ([21] and "Post-Transcriptional Modifications of ER alpha in Rapid Estrogen's Action" in this book). It is worth noting that steroid hormone concentrations undergo blood fluctuations or permanent changes, as illustrated by the following examples:

- circadian rhythm of testosterone;
- changes in estrogen and androgen concentration with age;
- low androgen concentration in testicular disorders, with acute reduction following castration.

Although in most cases these fluctuations are mild, it is possible that more pronounced hormonal changes modify the receptor/partner association and signal intensity as well as the resulting type of action. In addition, concentration gradient of hormone inside the cells might elicit different effects.

3 Migration and Proliferation Dichotomy Regulated by Rapid Hormonal Actions: A Step Towards Hormone Resistance?

Migration and differentiation rarely occur in actively proliferating cells and, in turn, signals stimulating migration or differentiation inhibit proliferation [22]. The migration/differentiation dichotomy is regulated by molecular switches. A G-alpha i-GIV complex binds EGF-R and decides whether cancer cells migrate or proliferate [11]. Our recent work identified the switch regulating this dichotomy in NIH3T3 cells in androgen-activated Rac [14, 15]. Preliminary findings also suggest that a similar mechanism operates in other cell types, such as fibrosarcoma and prostate cancer-derived cells, when they transit from a hormone-dependent to a hormone-independent phenotype. In fact, some of these cell types exhibit androgen-independent growth and androgen-dependent migration (manuscript in preparation).

In the previous section, we described how physiological concentration of androgens stimulates NIH3T3 cell migration through association of AR with FlnA and integrin beta1. This complex activates Rac and induces tyrosine phosphorylation of FAK and paxillin [15]. Interestingly, activation of Rac simultaneously leads to cell migration and cell cycle arrest. Analysis of the mechanism responsible for this arrest is currently under investigation in our lab. However, our preliminary findings indicate that cells stimulated by androgens make decisions about migration versus proliferation through Rac and its dependent pathways leading to cell cycle regulation.

The observation that AR mediates cell cycle arrest is not unexpected (see also "Differential Functions of Stromal and Epithelial Androgen Receptor in Prostate Cancer Before and After Castration Resistant Stage" in this book) and requires further comment. AR inhibits proliferation of normal prostate epithelia while it stimulates proliferation of prostate cancer cells. Although this switch has not been investigated in terms of cell motility and invasiveness, it involves molecular changes that confer novel activities to AR expressed in prostate cancer cells. Experimental findings indicate that AR acts as a licensing factor for DNA replication in cancer cells. It undergoes proteasomal degradation during each cell cycle to allow re-initiation of DNA replication in the next. The lack of mitotic AR degradation inhibits the next round of cell division and halts cell cycle in normal prostate epithelial cells [23]. An obvious corollary of these reports is that not only ligand concentration, but also AR level fluctuations within the various phases of cell cycle ensure DNA duplication in target cells. Again, findings in tissue recombinants of human prostate stromal cell lines with human prostate cancer epithelial cell lines also showed that AR might function as a suppressor in epithelial cells and a proliferator in stromal cells ([24] and "Differential Functions of Stromal and Epithelial Androgen Receptor in Prostate Cancer Before and After Castration Resistant Stage" in this book). The arguments put forward here propose that AR might play a dual and opposite role in controlling proliferation of target cells.

4 Non-Reproductive Cells Express Very Low Amounts of Steroid Receptors: A Model of 'Pure' Non-Genomic Receptor Action?

Our considerations in the previous sections of this chapter highlight the importance of SR levels and ligand concentration in target cells. Reproductive hormone-responsive cells respond to steroids with increased receptor-dependent transcriptional activity or increased receptor-dependent co-activation of transcription factors [25]. SRs also trigger rapid actions in the extra-nuclear compartment. Only a small fraction of the total receptor molecules expressed in reproductive cells is involved in this rapid action (roughly evaluated at about 10%). This receptor sub-population resides in the cytoplasm and/or at cell membrane. Use of receptor detection methods with increased sensitivity (Western blot, Northern blot, confocal microscopy analysis, mass spectrometry) is revealing that an increasing number of untransformed or transformed non-reproductive cells harbor very low receptor levels. This is the case of NIH3T3 cells, which express low amount of AR (about 10-20% of that detected in human prostate cancer-derived LNCaP cells). This receptor is constitutively poised in cytoplasm and at membrane, where it mediates rapid responses in the absence of receptor-dependent transcriptional action [14, 15] and unpublished data). Similarly, rat uterine stromal cells express classic PR, which is incompetent in transcriptional activity. This receptor, however, mediates transient activation and nuclear translocation of MAPKs, thus leading to cell cycle entry upon progestin stimulation of these cells [26]. The ligand-bound PR most likely clusters MAPKs in the active nuclear compartment, where MAPKs drive expression of genes involved in cell cycle.

In Cos cells ectopically expressing increasing amounts of human AR (hAR), we observed that at low hormone receptor levels, the cells respond to physiological concentrations of hormone with signaling activation in the absence of receptor nuclear translocation. This finding was validated by the absence of receptor-dependent transcriptional action. In contrast, Cos cells expressing higher receptor levels respond to hormone in terms of both rapid action and receptor transcriptional action. This different behavior suggests that higher receptor concentration is required for receptor-dependent transcriptional to occur [14].

Rapid hormonal action in newly discovered hormone-responsive cells expressing low steroid receptor levels triggers stimulation of migration, cell cycle progression and likely other processes. All these effects are independent of SR transcriptional activity. This new group of hormone-responsive cells is expected to raise more interest in the future, since the number of non-reproductive cells expressing low levels of steroid receptors is increasing at an unexpected rate, as a result of both the improved sensitivity of receptor assays as well as the increased attention focused on rapid steroid action. This will broaden our current understanding of hormone responsiveness and probably extend the application of hormonal therapy to other human diseases.

5 Growth Factor Signaling Depends on Extra-Nuclear Steroid Receptors: Are Other Partners Implicated?

We previously reported that EGF signaling depends on extra-nuclear AR and ER alpha in breast cancer MCF-7 cells, and on AR as well as ER beta in prostate cancer LNCaP cells [27]. In these cells, growth factor effects leading to proliferation and motility are drastically reduced by steroid antagonists or silencing of ERs or AR. Both these conditions reduce the Src- and steroid receptor-dependent phosphorylation of EGF-R, thereby inhibiting EGF signaling and signaling-dependent proliferation and migration. Mechanistic approaches showed that challenging of MCF-7 and LNCaP cells with EGF triggers association of EGF-R with a tripartite complex made up of ER, AR and Src. This complex directs Src activity on EGF-R and induces EGF-R phosphorylation [27]. Thus, it appears that growth factor receptor-mediated signals are regulated by steroid receptors in different cell types (see also "Cooperative Interactions Between c-Src, Estrogen Receptors and Receptor Tyrosine Kinases in Breast Cancer" in this book). The obvious corollary of this observation is the validation of both classic and new steroid receptor antagonists in pathological processes of cells expressing SRs that depend on sustained activation of growth factor receptors (e.g. EGF-R, Erb-B2). These findings raise the intriguing question of whether in the absence of steroid receptors other partners of growth factor receptors are needed for strong signaling elicited by growth factors. Answering this question could reveal new insights into growth factor biology.

Recent papers on prostate cancer-derived cells have shown that androgens and estrogens up-regulate insulin-like growth factor-1 receptor (IGF-1R) expression through non-genomic pathways ([28, 29] and "The IGF-I Axis in Prostate Cancer: The Role of Rapid Steroid Actions" in this book). Again, estradiol-dependent increase in pancreatic insulin content requires ER alpha-dependent MAPK activation [30]. These latter findings have been recently highlighted by a report focused on the role of estradiol-activated Src/MAPK pathway in insulin synthesis in vivo [4]. In sum, different findings illustrate our current understanding of the molecular mechanisms of reciprocal cross talk between sex steroid receptor and growth factor signaling. We now appreciate that steroid receptor and growth factor signaling pathways intersect and directly interact at multiple levels of signal transduction. This synergism has been documented in normal development of target tissues as well as in cancer progression and endocrine therapy resistance (see also "Cooperative Interactions Between c-Src, Estrogen Receptors and Receptor Tyrosine Kinases in Breast Cancer" in this book).

6 Hetero-Association Between Steroid Receptors: A Tool to Enhance Hormone Signaling?

In the course of our studies on rapid steroid action, we observed physical and functional associations between different types of sex steroid receptors depending on cell types. Progesterone receptor B (PR-B) is associated with ER alpha in T47D cells, which are derived from human mammary cancer cells and express PR-B under basal conditions [31]. Findings in these cells show that anti-estrogens inhibit signaling activation and progestin-stimulated DNA synthesis [32]. Furthermore, PR-B and ER alpha are associated in co-immunoprecipitation experiments in T47D cells. Again, Cos cells ectopically expressing both receptors respond to progestins with Src activation much more vigorously than cells expressing PR-B alone. The same cross talk between PR-B and ER alpha was observed in rat uterine stromal cells [26]. Thus, it appears that in cells expressing PR-B and ER alpha, progestin activates a PR-B/ER alpha complex and induces association of ER alpha with

Src [32]. PR-B is also able to directly associate with Src [33]. These associations foster Src-dependent signaling activation. Subsequent studies further clarified the molecular mechanism underlying progesterone activation of the Src-dependent pathway by cross talk between PR-B and ER alpha. This activation depends on the association of unliganded ER alpha with PR-B via two domains of PR [34].

Steroid receptor hetero-association also occurs between ER alpha and AR in MCF-7 cells and between ER beta and AR in prostate cancer-derived LNCaP cells [17]. In both these cell lines, androgen- or estradiol-induced signaling activation and G1-S progression can be equally prevented by either estradiol or androgen antagonists, implying that either steroid activates the ER/AR complex. Cos cells ectopically expressing only one of the two receptors respond to the cognate ligand with a much weaker Src activation than cells expressing both receptors [17]. These findings suggest that steroid receptor hetero-association enhances signaling activation triggered by a steroid hormone. In the presence of either estradiol or androgen the ternary ER/AR/Src complex is assembled. Within the complex, phosphotyrosine 537 of ER alpha and most likely phosphotyrosine 442 of ER beta interacts with the Src-SH2 domain, whereas a proline stretch of AR binds to the Src-SH3 domains. Each of these associations removes one of two inhibitory intramolecular bindings of Src. Therefore, in cells expressing one receptor, either ER or AR, it should be expected that only one inhibitory loop of Src is removed and Src is partially activated in response to the cognate hormone. Expression of both receptors, ER and AR, releases the two inhibitory interactions of Src, thus fully enabling Src activation.

The discovery of an ER/AR/Src complex in target (breast and prostate cancer) cells also implies that either steroid antagonist (anti-estrogen or anti-androgen) may simultaneously reduce the action of both the cognate receptor and the associated receptor. On the basis of these observations, the use of antagonists might find broader therapeutic application.

7 The Proliferative Role of Steroid Receptor Nuclear Export: A Paradox of Classic Receptor Transcriptional Action?

It is largely accepted that steroid receptor-dependent transcriptional activity drives hormone-directed cell proliferation [35]. An exception to this view is provided by the findings that receptor nuclear export triggers DNA synthesis. Rapid action of steroid hormones induces nuclear translocation of signaling effectors endowed with kinase activity [26, 36, 37]. In turn, these signaling effectors phosphorylate transcription factors, including steroid receptors [38] or receptor co-activators [39], with consequent modulation of their activity.

Recently, we observed that the PI3-K pathway activated by ER alpha in estradiol-treated MCF-7 cells triggers nuclear phosphorylation of FKHR. Under quiescence conditions, FKHR negatively regulates cyclin D1 transcription, thus repressing cell cycle and initiation of DNA synthesis [40]. In MCF-7 cells stimulated with estradiol, once phosphorylated, FKHR binds with ER alpha and the ER alpha/FKHR complex is subsequently exported from nuclei by a Crm1-dependent process. Export of this complex enhances cyclin D1 transcription and initiates G1-S phase progression [41] and submitted).

One of the questions raised by these findings is why ER alpha and FKHR need to be exported in association. At least two explanations could be envisaged. Firstly, both proteins exhibit a weak NES [41, 42] and their assembly enhances export of the complex. Alternatively, complexation of the two proteins masks an export inhibitory sequence (i.e. NLS) of one of the two partners. In both cases interaction with Crm1 could be facilitated and the complex released into the cytoplasm.

In breast cancer T47D cells, progestin triggers MAPK-dependent phosphorylation of nuclear PR-B at serine 294, thus facilitating the export of PR-B, which undergoes degradation in the cytoplasm. This event switches off transcriptional activity of PR. The observation that leptomycin B inhibits this process suggests that release of PR-B into the cytoplasm occurs through a Crm1-dependent mechanism [43]. Recent findings show that a constitutively active orphan nuclear receptor, ERR alpha, binds with a member of the MAP kinase family, ERK8, thus inducing Crm1-dependent export of the complex. The role of this translocation into cytoplasm has not yet been investigated, although it can be hypothesized that the orphan nuclear receptor released into cytoplasm through its association with signaling effectors drives their activation [44].

Altogether, these findings indicate that interference in steroid and orphan nuclear receptor export machinery might represent a therapeutic tool to redirect steroid and orphan receptors in nuclei or cytoplasm and alter receptor action, including cell proliferation. The following section of the chapter addresses this issue.

8 Receptor/Protein Associations: A Promising Target for Cancer Therapy?

AR and ER (alpha or beta) play a central role in the progression of prostate and mammary cancer. Inhibiting the action of these receptors is, therefore, the most widely used approach in the treatment of these diseases. Both classic and new hormone antagonists, such as second-generation anti-androgens [45] as well as inhibitors of steroid synthesis, have been developed and exploited. More recently, interest has been focused on molecules targeting other sites in pathways involving steroid receptors [46]. Inhibition of AR and ER alpha binding to co-regulators interferes in different ways in the transcriptional action of the receptors. Again, the binding of SRs to DNA has been targeted. A reassessment of the rapid action of steroid receptors in cell proliferation and cell migration may offer new approaches in the therapy of prostate and mammary cancers.

Association of ER or AR with signaling effectors, scaffold proteins or cargo proteins, which in different ways are necessary for triggering the hormonal effects initiated by steroid receptors, represents a potential target of this therapy. The molecular basis of ER and AR associations with Src triggered by either steroid hormones or EGF has been discussed in previous sections of this chapter together with their role in hormone- or growth factor-dependent growth. ER alpha or ER beta association with Src occurs in mammary cancer and prostate cancer cells, respectively. This association can be suppressed by nanomolar concentration of a small peptide mimicking the sequence surrounding ER alpha phosphotyrosine 537, which interacts with Src-SH2 domain [47]. The finding that this peptide interferes in ER alpha-dependent (MCF-7 cells) or ER beta-dependent (LNCaP cells) signaling suggests that the latter receptor exhibits a phosphotyrosine residue homologous to phosphotyrosine 537 of ER alpha, most likely at position 442. In turn, a small peptide interfering in the association of AR with Src, which occurs between a proline-rich sequence of AR and Src-SH3, also abolishes the AR-dependent activation of Src and its dependent mitogenic route at nanomolar concentration [48]. The inhibitory effect of these peptides on the growth of mammary or prostate cancer cells in vitro and in xenografts is dramatic and underlines the role of AR/ER/Src association in the progression of these human cancer cells.

ER alpha nuclear export requires interaction of an ER-NES with Crm1. Inhibition of this export also prevents the export of FKHR and initiation of DNA synthesis [41], thus offering a novel tool to interfere in mammary cancer cell proliferation. An ER alpha mutant, mutated in NES, permanently resides in the nucleus and is unable to mediate both FKHR export and DNA synthesis. In addition, small peptides mimicking the ER alpha-NES retain the receptor in nuclei of cells stimulated with hormone and prevent DNA duplication [41]. Other hormone-regulated interactions of ER alpha with signaling effectors or scaffolds have been reported. Interference in these protein/protein interactions regulating different functions could likely offer the possibility of controlling steroid receptor-dependent cancer progression.

Predictably, further development of protein/protein interaction analysis [49] will stimulate the design and synthesis of new molecules interfering in the association of partners with steroid receptors or their downstream effectors, thus inhibiting specific receptor functions (e.g. proliferation, apoptosis, migration, differentiation and others) without modifying other useful functions.

Acknowledgements The work presented in this article was funded by a grant from the Associazione Italiana per la Ricerca sul Cancro (A.I.R.C. - Grant No. IG 5389). Pia Giovannelli was supported by a fellowship from A.I.R.C. (ITALY). The funders had no role in study design, data collection and analysis, decision to publish, or preparation of the manuscript. The authors declare that no competing interests exist.

References

1. Pietras RJ, Szego CM (1977) Specific binding sites for oestrogen at the outer surfaces of isolated endometrial cells. Nature 265:69–72
2. Szego CM, Davis JS (1967) Adenosine 3′, 5′-monophosphate in rat uterus: acute elevation by estrogen. Proc Natl Acad Sci USA 58:1711–1718

3. Pietras RJ, Szego CM (1975) Surface modifications evoked by estradiol and diethylstilbestrol in isolated endometrial cells: evidence from lectin probes and extracellular release of lysosomal protease. Endocrinology 97:1445–1454
4. Wong WP, Tiano JP, Liu S, Hewitt SC, Le May C, Dalle S, Katzenellenbogen JA, Katzenellenbogen BS, Korach KS, Mauvais-Jarvis F (2010) Extranuclear estrogen receptor-alpha stimulates NeuroD1 binding to the insulin promoter and favors insulin synthesis. Proc Natl Acad Sci 107:13057–13062
5. Cato AC, Nestl A, Mink S (2002) Rapid actions of steroid receptors in cellular signaling pathways. Sci STKE 138:re9
6. Song RX, Santen RJ (2006) Membrane initiated estrogen signaling in breast cancer. Biol Reprod 75:9–16
7. Foradori CD, Weiser MJ, Handa RJ (2008) Non-genomic actions of androgens. Front Neuroendocrinol 29:169–181
8. Levin ER (2011) Extranuclear steroid receptors: roles in modulation of cell functions. Mol Endocrinol 25:377–384
9. Chen P, Gupta K, Wells A (1994) Cell movement elicited by epidermal growth factor receptor requires kinase and autophosphorylation but is separable from mitogenesis. J Cell Biol 124:547–555
10. Chen P, Xie H, Sekar MC, Gupta K, Wells A (1994) Epidermal growth factor receptor-mediated cell motility: phospholipase C activity is required, but mitogen-activated protein kinase activity is not sufficient for induced cell movement. J Cell Biol 127:847–857
11. Ghosh P, Beas AO, Bornheimer SJ, Garcia-Marcos M, Forry EP, Johannson C, Ear J, Jung BH, Cabrera B, Carethers JM, Farquhar MG (2010) A G{alpha}i-GIV molecular complex binds epidermal growth factor receptor and determines whether cells migrate or proliferate. Mol Biol Cell 21:2338–2354
12. Gerhardt H, et al. (2003) VEGF guides angiogenic sprouting utilizing endothelial tip cell filopodia. J Cell Biol 161:1163–1177
13. De Donatis A, Comito G, Buricchi F, Vinci MC, Parenti A, Caselli A, Camici G, Manao G, Ramponi G, Cirri P (2008) Proliferation versus migration in platelet-derived growth factor signaling: the key role of endocytosis. J Biol Chem 283:19948–19956
14. Castoria G, Lombardi M, Barone MV, Bilancio A, Di Domenico M, Bottero D, Vitale F, Migliaccio A, Auricchio F (2003) Androgen stimulated DNA synthesis and cytoskeletal changes in fibroblasts by a non transcriptional receptor action. J Cell Biol 161:547–556
15. Castoria G, D'Amato L, Ciociola A, Giovannelli P, Giraldi T, Sepe L, Paolella G, Barone MV, Migliaccio A, Auricchio F (2011) Androgen-induced cell migration: role of androgen receptor/filamin a association. PLoS One 6:e17218
16. Castoria G, Migliaccio A, Bilancio A, Di Domenico M, de Falco A, Lombardi M, Fiorentino R, Varricchio L, Barone MV, Auricchio F (2001) PI3-kinase in concert with Src promotes the S-phase entry of estradiol-stimulated MCF-7 cells. EMBO J 20:6050–6059
17. Migliaccio A, Castoria G, Di Domenico M, de Falco A, Bilancio A, Lombardi M, Barone MV, Ametrano D, Zannini MS, Abbondanza C, Auricchio F (2000) Steroid-induced androgen receptor-oestradiol receptor beta/Src complex triggers prostate cancer cell proliferation. EMBO J 19:5406–5417
18. Stossel TP, Condeelis J, Cooley L, Hartwig JH, Noegel A, Schleicher M, Shapiro SS (2001) Filamins as integrators of cell mechanics and signalling. Nat Rev Mol Cell Biol 2:138–145
19. Feng Y, Walsh CA (2004) The many faces of filamin: a versatile molecular scaffold for cell motility and signalling. Nat Cell Biol 6:1034–1038
20. Marshall CJ (1995) Specificity of receptor tyrosine kinase signaling: transient versus sustained extracellular signal-regulated kinase activation. Cell 80:179–185
21. Le Romancer M, Treilleux I, Leconte N, Robin-Lespinasse Y, Sentis S, Bouchekioua-Bouzaghou K, Goddard S, Gobert-Gosse S, Corbo L (2008) Regulation of estrogen rapid signaling through arginine methylation by PRMT1. Mol Cell 31:212–221
22. Fedotov S, Iomin A (2007) Migration and proliferation dichotomy in tumor-cell invasion. Phys Rev Lett 98:118101

23. Vander Griend DJ, Litvinov IV, Isaacs JT (2007) Stabilizing androgen receptor in mitosis inhibits prostate cancer proliferation. Cell Cycle 6:647–651
24. Niu Y, Chang TM, Yeh S, Ma WL, Wang YZ, Chang C (2010) Differential androgen receptor signals in different cells explain why androgen-deprivation therapy of prostate cancer fails. Oncogene 29:3593–3604
25. Beato M, Herrlich P, Schütz G (1995) Steroid hormone receptors: many actors in search of a plot. Cell 83:851–857
26. Vallejo G, Ballaré C, Barañao JL, Beato M, Saragüeta P (2005) Progestin activation of nongenomic pathways via cross talk of progesterone receptor with estrogen receptor ß induces proliferation of endometrial stromal cells. Mol Endocrinol 19:3023–3037
27. Migliaccio A, Di Domenico M, Castoria G, Nanayakkara M, Lombardi M, de Falco A, Bilancio A, Varricchio L, Ciociola A, Auricchio F (2005) Steroid receptor regulation of epidermal growth factor signaling through Src in breast and prostate cancer cells: steroid antagonist action. Cancer Res 65:10585–10593
28. Pandini G, Mineo R, Frasca F, Roberts CT Jr, Marcelli M, Vigneri R, Belfiore A (2005) Androgens up-regulate the insulin-like growth factor-I receptor in prostate cancer cells. Cancer Res 65:1849–1857
29. Pandini G, Genua M, Frasca F, Squatrito S, Vigneri R, Belfiore A (2007) 17beta-estradiol up-regulates the insulin-like growth factor receptor through a nongenotropic pathway in prostate cancer cells. Cancer Res 67:8932–8941
30. Alonso-Magdalena P, Ropero AB, Carrera MP, Cederroth CR, Baquié M, Gauthier BR, Nef S, Stefani E, Nadal A (2008) Pancreatic insulin content regulation by the estrogen receptor ER alpha. PLoS ONE 3:e2069
31. Chalbos D, Vignon F, Keydar I, Rochefort H (1982) Estrogens stimulate cell proliferation and induce secretory proteins in a human breast cancer cell line (T47D). J Clin Endocrinol Metab 55:276–283
32. Migliaccio A, Piccolo D, Castoria G, Di Domenico M, Bilancio A, Lombardi M, Gong W, Beato M, Auricchio F (1998) Activation of the Src/p21ras/Erk pathway by progesterone receptor receptor via cross-talk with estrogen receptor. EMBO J 17:2008–2018
33. Boonyaratanakornkit V, Scott MP, Ribon V, Sherman L, Anderson SM, Maller JL, Miller WT, Edwards DP (2001) Progesterone receptor contains a proline-rich motif that directly interacts with SH3 domains and activates c-Srcc-Src family tyrosine kinases. Molecular Cell 8:269–280
34. Ballaré C, Uhrig M, Bechtold T, Sancho E, Di Domenico M, Migliaccio A, Auricchio F, Beato M (2003) Two domains of the progesterone receptor interact with the estrogen receptor and are required for progesterone activation of the c-Srcc-Src/Erk pathway in mammalian cells. Mol Cell Biol 23:1994–2008
35. Brisken C, O'Malley B (2010) Hormone action in the mammary gland. Cold Spring Harb Perspect Biol 2:a003178
36. Nilsen J, Brinton RD (2003) Divergent impact of progesterone and medroxyprogesterone acetate (Provera) on nuclear mitogen-activated protein kinase signaling. Proc Natl Acad Sci U S A. 100:10506–10511
37. Castoria G, Migliaccio A, Di Domenico M, Lombardi M, de Falco A, Varricchio L, Bilancio A, Barone MV, Auricchio F (2004) Role of atypical PKC in estradiol-triggered G1/S progression of MCF-7 cells. Mol Cell Biol 24:7643–7653
38. Levin ER (2005) Integration of the extranuclear and nuclear actions of estrogen. Mol Endocrinol 19:1951–1959
39. O'Malley BW (2005) A life-long search for the molecular pathways of steroid hormone action. Mol Endocrinol 19:1402–1411
40. Schmidt M, Fernandez de Mattos S, van der Horst A, Klompmaker R, Kops GJ, Lam EW, Burgering BM, Medema RH (2002) Cell cycle inhibition by FoxO forkhead transcription factors involves downregulation of cyclin D. Mol Cell Biol 22:7842–7852
41. Lombardi M, Castoria G, Migliaccio A, Barone MV, Di Stasio R, Ciociola A, Bottero D, Yamaguchi H, Appella E, Auricchio F (2008) Hormone-dependent nuclear export of estradiol receptor and DNA synthesis in breast cancerbreast cancer cells. J Cell Biol 182:327–340

42. Birkenkamp KU, Coffer PJ (2003) Regulation of cell survival and proliferation by the FOXO (forkhead box, class O) subfamily of forkhead transcription factors. Biochem Soc Trans 31:292–297
43. Qiu M, Olsen A, Faivre E, Horwitz KB, Lange CA (2003) Mitogen-activated protein kinase regulates nuclear association of human progesterone receptor. Mol Endocrinol 17:628–642
44. Rossi M, Colecchia D, Iavarone C, Strambi A, Piccioni F, Verrotti di Pianella A, Chiariello M (2011) Extracellular signal-regulated kinase 8 (ERK8) controls estrogen-related receptor alpha; (ERR alpha) cellular localization and inhibits its transcriptional activity. J Biol Chem 286:8507–8522
45. Tran C, Ouk S, Clegg NJ, Chen Y, Watson PA, Arora V, Wongvipat J, Smith-Jones PM, Yoo D, Kwon A, Wasielewska T, Welsbie D, Chen CD, Higano CS, Beer TM, Hung DT, Scher HI, Jung ME, Sawyers CL (2009) Development of a second-generation antiandrogen for treatment of advanced prostate cancer. Science 324:787–790
46. Shapiro DJ, Mao C, Cherian MT (2011) Small molecule inhibitors as probes for estrogen and androgen receptor action. J Biol Chem 286:4043–4048
47. Varricchio L, Migliaccio A, Castoria G, Yamaguchi H, de Falco A, Di Domenico M, Giovannelli P, Farrar W, Appella E, Auricchio F (2007) Inhibition of estradiol receptor/Src association and cell growth by an estradiol receptor alpha tyrosine-phosphorylated peptide. Mol Cancer Res 11:1213–1221
48. Migliaccio A, Varricchio L, de Falco A, Castoria G, Arra C, Yamaguchi H, Ciociola A, Lombardi M, Di Stasio R, Barbieri A, Baldi A, Barone MV, Appella E, Auricchio F (2007) Inhibition of the SH3 domain-mediated binding of Src to the androgen receptor and its effect on tumor growth. Oncogene 26:6619–6629
49. Bonetta L (2010) Protein-protein interactions: interactome under construction. Nature 468:851–854

Part I
Breast Cancer

Progesterone Signaling to Chromatin in Breast Cancer Cells. Two Initial Cycles of Remodeling

Guillermo P. Vicent, Roser Zaurin, Cecilia Ballaré, A. Silvina Nacht, Roni H. G. Wright, Francois Le Dily, Giancarlo Castellano, Jofre Font-Mateu and Miguel Beato

Abstract Steroid hormones control gene activity by direct interaction of their intracellular receptors with hormone responsive elements on DNA but they can also crosstalk to kinase cascades activated by signals impinging on membrane receptors. Progesterone treatment of cells in culture leads to the rapid activation of several kinases and in particular the Src/Ras/Erk/Msk1 cascade, by activating a small population of membrane-anchored progesterone receptors (PR). One to five minutes after hormone treatment, activated Erk enters the nucleus and causes the

G. P. Vicent · R. Zaurin · C. Ballaré · A. Silvina Nacht · R. H. G. Wright · F. Le Dily · G. Castellano · J. Font-Mateu · M. Beato (✉)
Chromatin and Gene Expression Lab, Gene Regulation Programme, Centre for Genomic Regulation (CRG) and UPF, Barcelona, Spain
e-mail: miguel.beato@crg.eu

G. P. Vicent
e-mail: guillermo.vicent@crg.eu

R. Zaurin
e-mail: roser.zaurin@crg.eu

C. Ballaré
e-mail: cecilia.ballare@crg.eu

A. Silvina Nacht
e-mail: silvina.nacht@crg.eu

R. H. G. Wright
e-mail: roni.wright@crg.eu

F. Le Dily
e-mail: francois.ledily@crg.eu

G. Castellano
e-mail: giancarlo.castellano@crg.eu

J. Font-Mateu
e-mail: jofre.font@crg.eu

G. Castoria and A. Migliaccio (eds.), *Advances in Rapid Sex-Steroid Action*,
DOI: 10.1007/978-1-4614-1764-4_2, © Springer Science+Business Media, LLC 2012

recruitment of the activated ternary complex of pPR, pERK and pMSK1 to target chromatin, leading to phosphoacetylation of histone H3 and displacement of an HP1γ containing repressive complex. Thus, progestin activation of the Src/Ras/Erk/Msk1 cascade directly impacts chromatin. Within one minute of adding synthetic progesterone analogues to breast cancer cells, PR recruits to the target genes an ATP-dependent chromatin remodeling complex, NURF, a histone methyltransferase complex, ASCOM, which trimethylates histone H3 at lysine 4, and an activated Cyclin A/CDK2 complex, that phosphorylates histone H1 and facilitates its displacement. This first cycle of chromatin remodeling is a prerequisite for a second cycle starting 5 min after hormone addition, in which a different ATP-dependent chromatin remodeling complex, BAF, and a histone acetyltransferase, PCAF, cooperate to promote the displacement of core histones H2A and H2B, that facilitates access to the promoter of additional receptor complexes and other transcription factors necessary for gene induction. Thus, at both phases in activation of target promoters, a histone tail modification stabilizes the binding of an ATP-dependent chromatin remodeler to target promoters. These findings highlight the concept of transcription initiation as a process involving consecutive cycles of enzymatic chromatin remodeling, where each enzyme complex is necessary at a given time point and catalyzes a particular remodeling step.

Keywords Progesterone · Chromatin · MMTV · BRCA1 · Nucleosome · Progesterone responsive elements · Gene regulation

Contents

1 Introduction

The physiological action of steroid hormones in their target cells is mediated by intracellular receptors, which are members of the nuclear receptor family. The steroid hormone receptors (SHR) were originally considered as ligand-regulated transcription factors that upon binding to specific hormone regulatory element (HREs) regulate the transcription rate of their target genes. In the last years, this simplistic view has been abandoned and replaced by a more complex vision, involving at least two subpopulations of SHR: a minor one anchored in the cell membrane via a palmitoyl residue [1], and a major one shuffling between the cytoplasm and the cell nucleus. The majority of the available data supporting this complex view have been obtained using ligands synthetic analogues of the physiological hormones, which are not efficiently metabolized in the target tissues and exhibit higher affinity for SHR than the natural ligands. The situation may be even more complex when considering the physiological hormones, which are heavily metabolized and give rise to products with the potential to interact with a larger number of receptors.

In breast cancer cells the membrane attached SHR are part of an ill-defined complex that includes estrogen receptor alpha (ERα), progesterone receptor (PR), and possibly androgen receptor (AR), as well as members of the growth factor receptor family, such as the EGF receptor (EGFR), and likely caveolin. When activated by synthetic ligands the membrane attached receptors interact with c-SRC via de SH2 domain, in the case of ERα or via de SH3 domain in the case of PR and AR, and activate an interconnected network of kinase signaling pathways to coordinate the cell response at various levels. There are also interactions of SHRs with CDK2, PI3K/AKT, JAK/STAT, and likely other kinases. Several of these kinase pathways converge in the cell nucleus, where they act on the nuclear population of SHRs, on protein components of chromatin and on nuclear enzymes, which all together orchestrate the regulation of various gene networks by mechanisms that are not fully understood.

In the following we will describe our present knowledge of the signaling network used by the synthetic progesterone analogue R5020 in the breast cancer cell line T47D. We will place these results in the context of the genome-wide interactions of PR with nuclear genome and their consequences for gene expression. While we will mainly summarize our own experimental findings with a model promoter, the mouse mammary tumor virus (MMTV), and at the whole genome level, we will also report findings by other labs to complete the global vision and to indicate debated points.

2 Nucleosome Organization is Required for Efficient PR Binding and Gene Regulation

Elucidating the global function of a transcription factor in a particular cell type implies the identification of its binding sites in the genome of the cell. The possible role of chromatin structure in defining effective binding sites is still an unresolved question. The dominant view assumes that nucleosomes are an obstacle for transcription factor binding and that factors bind preferentially to nucleosome depleted regions, but there are reports on binding of transcription factors to nucleosomally organized sequences. Apart from the MMTV promoter that we will describe in more detail below, a good example is p53. Using the 5′-upsream region of the p21 gene that contains two p53 binding sites, a better binding has been reported in vitro to chromatin organized sequences when compared to free DNA [2]. A genome wide study with MCF7 breast cancer cells has yielded similar results [3], suggesting that the particular topology of the nucleosomally organized p53 target sites favors DNA binding and regulation of transcription. Upon activation of p53 by DNA damage, the region around p53 binding sites becomes depleted of nucleosome reads. However, these studies detect nucleosomal occupancy of a large chromatin region, over 2 kb, and probably reflect a transition from heterochromatin to euchromatin, rather than localized changes of individual nucleosomes.

The hormone responsive region of the MMTV promoter contains a cluster of five imperfect HREs upstream of a NF1 binding site [4]. In nucleosomes assembled in vitro as well as when integrated as a single copy transgene in breast cancer cells, the HREs are precisely positioned on the surface of a histone octamer particle with a rotational orientation that exposes the major grooves of the two halves of the HRE1 palindrome and of the HRE4 half palindrome, while masking the major grooves of HRE2 and HRE3 [5]. Purified PR binds to nucleosomally organized HRE1 with similar affinity as to the same sequence in naked DNA, while it cannot access the central HREs2 and 3 in nucleosomes [5]. Access to these central HREs requires ATP-dependent remodeling of the nucleosome core particle [6], which leads to displacement of histone H2A/H2B dimers [7]. On the surface of the resulting histones H3/H4 tetramer particle we observed a synergistic binding of PR and NF1 [8]. We also found that the linker histone H1 contributes to the basal repression of the MMTV promoter but is necessary for optimal induction by promoting a nucleosome position that facilitates the synergism between PR and NF1 [9, 10]. Thus, it seems that the organization of the MMTV promoter in chromatin plays an essential role in regulating the promoter activity in response to progesterone. The question was whether this is a peculiarity of the proviral promoter or a general property of PR target genes.

We have approached this issue in breast cancer cells treated with progestins by performing ChIP-seq experiments with antibodies against PR and RNA polymerase II. Under the same experimental conditions we have performed global gene expression analysis and nucleosome mapping experiments (Ballaré et al. unpublished). Our data indicate that before hormone addition, there are only 844 PR binding sites (PRbs), while upon hormone treatment over 25,000 PRbs are found, most of them already detected 5 min after hormone addition and persisting for up to 6 h. Although PRbs are mainly found within 100 kb of hormone responsive genes and in introns, there is a significative enrichment within 1 kb distance from the transcription start sites. Only a small percentage of these PRbs contain the classic palindromic progesterone responsive element (PRE), while around 80% of the PRbs encompass several copies of a half PRE, often as direct repeats at variable distances. In contrast with the dominant view, the sites where PR will bind exhibit high nucleosome occupancy prior to hormone treatment, suggesting that the organization in nucleosomes favors PR binding. The nucleosomes encompassing the PRbs become sensitive to MNase digestion upon addition of hormone correlating with the recruitment of NURF and BAF complexes. In most cases, the enhanced nuclease sensitivity is accompanied by a hormone-dependent depletion of histones H1 and H2A. PR binding to nucleosomally organized sequences and hormone induced nucleosome remodeling are more pronounced around the transcription start sites of upregulated genes, correlating with the strongest PRbs. Predicted PREs that do not bind PR do not show an enrichment of nucleosomes, supporting the notion that nucleosome occupancy is important for PR binding and hormonal gene regulation in living cells and confirming our findings with the MMTV promoter.

3 Preparing the Chromatin for Gene Regulation

A central requisite for the genomic action of hormones is their ability to facilitate access to the genetic information stored in the compacted DNA in chromatin, a process that requires extensive chromatin remodeling. Here we summarize our present knowledge of this process based on the action of synthetic progesterone analogue R5020 in the breast cancer cell line T47D.

The large majority of the PR molecules in T47D cells are shuttling between the cytoplasm and the cell nucleus, while a small fraction is attached to the cell membrane in a complex with estrogen receptor (ER) [11]. Upon hormone addition, the membrane-attached PR activates c-SRC and downstream RAS/RAF/MEK/ERK/MSK1 pathway, partly via ER, leading to ERK-mediated phosphorylation of PR and formation of complexes of pPR with the activated kinases ERK and MSK1. This activated ternary complex is targeted by PR to PRbs in chromatin [12]. Progestins also activate the PI3K/AKT pathway, the Cyclin A/CDK2 pathway, the JAK/STAT pathway, and possibly several other kinase pathways. Many of these kinases are also targeted to PR binding sites in chromatin, but except for CDK2 we do not know their targets and their function in hormonal gene regulation.

Prior to hormone induction the sites where PR will bind are organized in nucleosomes with progesterone responsive elements (PRE) partly exposed in the surface. We have shown that hormone receptors can bind to a PRE within nucleosomes provided the major groove of the palindromic sequences TGTYCt is not oriented towards the histone octamer but facing outwards [5]. This is a property that hormone receptors share with other factors that recognize relatively short sequences of DNA. On the contrary transcription factors, like NF1, that establish contacts with 10 or more DNA base pairs and completely embrace the DNA double helix cannot recognize their sites when they are wrapped around nucleosomes, no matter their rotational orientation [13].

When the activated ternary complex of pPR, pERK and pMSK1 reaches the MMTV promoter in chromatin, it binds to the exposed HRE1, leading to the MSK1-dependent phosphorylation of N-terminal tail of histone H3 at serine 10 [12]. This phosphorylation leads to the displacement of a repressive complex that is anchored at the trimethylated lysine 9 of the H3 tail via the chromodomain of

HP1γ [12]. We do not know yet the exact composition of this complex but it includes HDACs and histone demethylases. We also do not know whether acetylation of lysine 14 of the histone H3, which is observed after hormone treatment, is also required for displacement of the repressive complex.

We have identified two consecutive cycles of chromatin remodeling during the initial 5–10 min of hormone action, during which protein kinases, histone modifying enzymes and ATP-dependent chromatin remodeling complexes cooperate to facilitate access of transcription factors to previously hidden information. All these factors are recruited to the PR target sites by direct or indirect interaction with the hormone-activated PR. Although the precise order of events in individual target sites is no known, we can establish a sequence for target sites at the level of whole cell population based on the global effect of inhibiting individual steps. What follows has to be interpreted with some caution, as it may be the average result of more stochastic processes taking place at individual target sites in individual cells.

The first cycle takes place within 1–2 min after hormone addition and involves PR-mediated recruitment of the ATP-dependent chromatin remodeling complex NURF, the histone methylase complex ASCOM, CyclinA/CDK2 and the poly (ADP-ribose) polymerase PARP1, along with the displacement of the histone demethylases KDM5B, also known as PLU1 or JARID1B. The outcome of the coordinated action of these five enzymes is an increase in the trimethylation of lysine 4 of histone H3, which stabilizes the binding of NURF and the phosphorylation and likely the parylation of histone H1, which is displaced from the target site ([14]; Wright et al., unpublished).

The second cycle, that takes place in the subsequent 5–10 min, involves the PR-mediate recruitment of complexes with the histone acetyl transferase PCAF and the ATP-dependent chromatin remodeling complex BAF [12]. PCAF acetylates K14 of histone H3, a modification that anchors the BAF complex. The outcome of this second cycle is the ATP-dependent displacement of H2A/H2B dimers. The two cycles are connected since blocking the first cycle precludes the second. After these two cycles, previously hidden binding sites for NF1 and PR become accessible and the two factors bind synergistically to the MMTV promoter on the surface of tetramer of histone H3 and H4 [8].

A summary of the PR-interactors highlighted in the present chapter is shown in Fig. 1. Most of the partners of PR are functionally connected with chromatin either because they remodeled/modified directly the target chromatin or because they stabilized the binding of the remodeler, as described above for the MMTV promoter.

Using expression arrays and ChIPseq we found that a similar mechanism operates in a large number of cellular progesterone target genes ([14]; Ballaré et al. unpublished), although activation of other kinase pathways, such as JAK/STAT and PI3K/AKT, as well as parylation play important roles in progesterone action of different sets of genes.

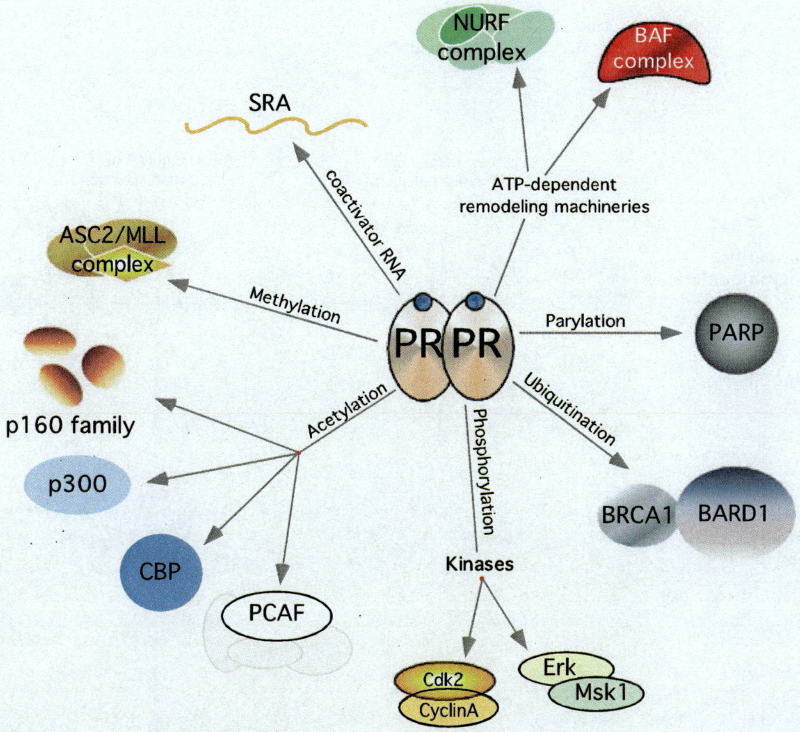

Fig. 1 PR interactors. The indicated interactors illustrate the diversity of structural and enzymatic factors that PR recruits to target promoters. The interactors are involved in different nuclear events: (1) Opening of the local chromatin structure through ATP-dependent remodeling or histone acetyltransferase (HAT) activity (BAF, NURF, p160, CBP/P300, PCAF); (2) Stabilization of chromatin remodelers by histone tail modifications (ASCOM, PCAF); (3) Downstream effectors of signaling pathways whose kinase activity impact either on chromatin or on PR itself (Erk, Msk1, Cdk2). The SRA, or steroid receptor RNA activator, serves as a specific coactivator of steroid receptors and, as such, brings a new level of complexity to nuclear receptor-mediated transcription [21]

4 BRCA1 as a Physiological Brake for Hormone Action

Germ-line mutations in the BRCA1 gene strongly increase the risk of developing breast cancer in women. One popular hypothesis to explain this tissue specificity postulates a link between BRCA1 and the action of ovarian hormones, estrogen and progesterone. Indeed it has been shown that BRCA1 counteracts the effect of estrogens and possibly progesterone in breast cancer cells [15–17]. Given the relevance of progesterone for normal mammary development and breast cancer formation, we searched for a functional relationship between BRCA1 and PR in the PR-positive breast cancer cell line T47D. We found that BRCA1 inhibits the transcriptional activity of PR by at least two mechanisms involving its E3

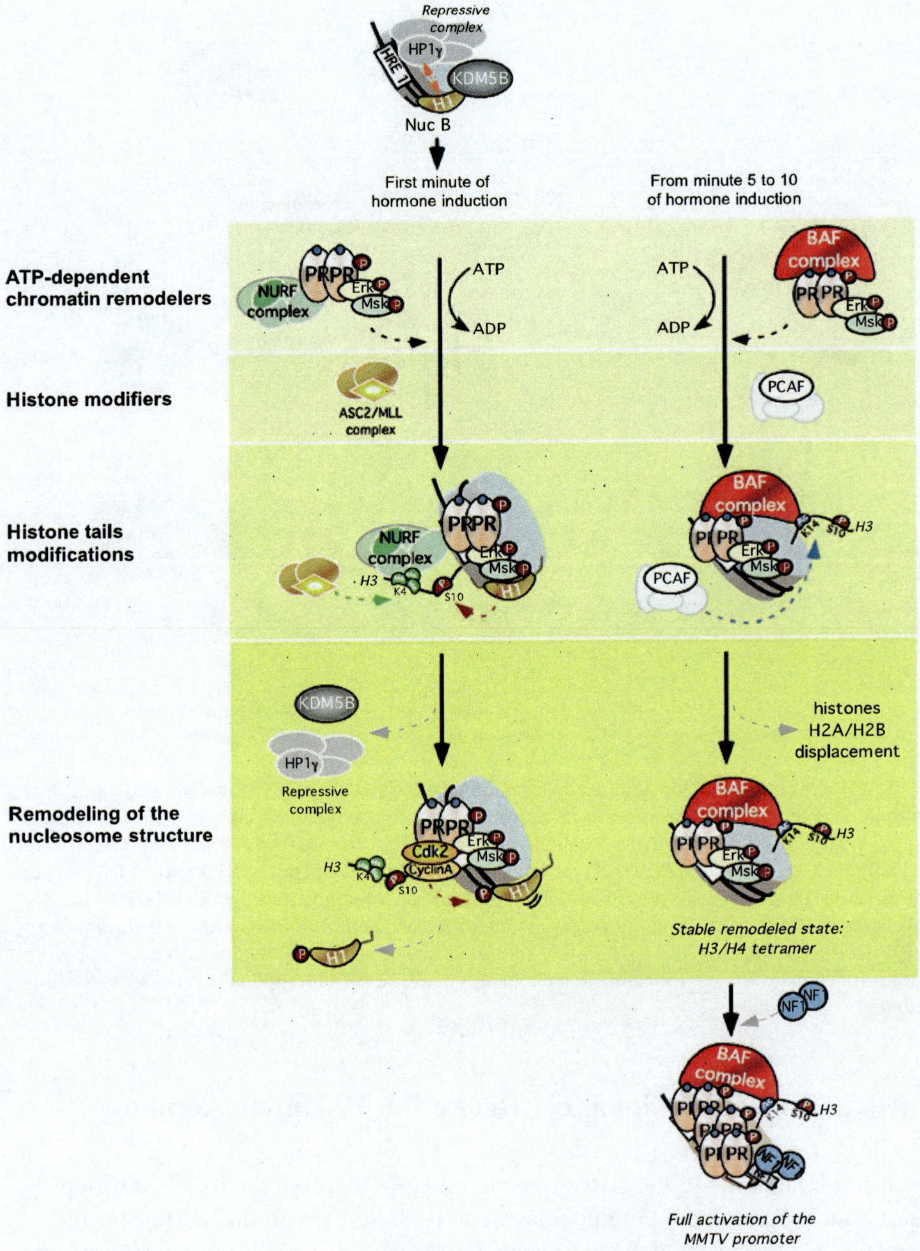
Repressive complex
HP1γ
HRE 1
KDM5B
H1
Nuc B
First minute of hormone induction
From minute 5 to 10 of hormone induction
ATP-dependent chromatin remodelers
NURF complex
PR PR
Erk
Msk
ATP
ADP
BAF complex
Histone modifiers
ASC2/MLL complex
PCAF
Histone tails modifications
H3
K4
S10
K14
Remodeling of the nucleosome structure
Repressive complex
Cdk2
CyclinA
histones H2A/H2B displacement
Stable remodeled state: H3/H4 tetramer
NF1
Full activation of the MMTV promoter

◀ **Fig. 2** Initial steps in PR activation of the MMTV promoter. One minute after hormone addition the activated complexes of pPR, pErk, pMsk1 with either the NURF complex or the methyltransferase ASCOM complex are recruited to the promoter, which is occuppied by a repressive complex containing HP1γ and KDM5B, among other factors. Msk1 phosporylates H3 at serine 10 promoting the displacement of the repressive complex. The combined action of the ASCOM complex and the displaced KDM5B increases histone H3 in K4 trimethylation, stabilizing NURF at the promoter. NURF remodeling facilitates access of the Cdk2-CyclinA kinase, which phosphorylates histone H1 and promotes its displacement, which also requires activation of PARP1. This first cycle of chromatin remodeling is a prerequisite for a second cycle starting 5 min after hormone addition; activated PR complexes bind BAF and PCAF and recruit them to the target chromatin. The BAF complex, stabilized by PCAF-dependent H3K14 acetylation, catalyzes ATP-dependent H2A/H2B displacement. Opening of the nucleosome core particle facilitates NF1 binding generating a stable $(H3/H4)_2$ platform that exposes previously hidden HREs for the recruitment of additional PR and BAF complexes, facilitating interaction with other coactivators and assemble of the transcription initiation complex. At both phases in activation of the promoter, a histone tail modification stabilizes the binding of an ATP-dependent chromatin remodeling complex to the target promoter followed by a nucleosome remodeling step. Thus, transcription initiation is a complex process including connected cycles of enzymatic chromatin remodeling, where each enzyme complex is crucial at a given time point

ubiquitin ligase activity. First, BRCA1 has a direct effect on the cellular level of PR and, hence, on the extent of PR recruitment to target promoters through the promotion of ligand-independent and -dependent degradation of PR [18]. We demonstrated by in vitro and in vivo assays that BRCA1/BARD1 might be the main E3 ubiquitin ligase responsible for the ubiquitination and degradation of PR in the absence of hormone. Second, following hormone treatment the BRCA1/BARD1 complex is recruited via interaction with PR to the hormone-responsive regions of PR target genes and affects the local levels of monoubiquitinated histone H2A, contributing to the epigenetic silencing of these promoters [18]. This connection between BRCA1/BARD1 and progesterone receptor activity may contribute to explain the particular tissue specificity of BRCA1-related tumours. Given the relationship of BRCA1 with DNA repair, it is interesting to note that breast cancers with mutations in BRCA1 or 2 are particularly responsive to chemotherapies involving inhibition of PARP1, which is also involved in DNA repair [19, 20].

5 Conclusions

Our focus on the initial events of the hormone signaling to chromatin has unraveled an unexpected complexity that integrates several kinases, tumor suppressor genes, histone modifying enzymes and ATP-dependent chromatin remodeling complexes in a coordinate sequence of enzymatic activities aimed at controlling the extent of hormone action and the preparation of the chromatin for access of the RNA polymerase II and other basic factors of the transcriptional machinery. A schematic model that attempts to include our present knowledge of these multiples steps is shown in Fig. 2. We are aware that this scheme represents only a part of the numerous steps involved in gene regulation and that many more PR partners will have to be incorporated in the model, even if we limit ourselves to the very initial 10 min of hormone action.

Acknowledgments The experimental work summarized in this review was supported by grants from the Departament d'Innovació Universitat i Empresa (DIUiE), Ministerio de Educación y Ciencia (MEC) BFU2010-15313 and BFU2006-10693, Consolider (CSD2006-00049), and EU IP HEROIC. G.P.V. is a recipient of a fellowship of the I3 Programme.

References

1. Pedram A, Razandi M, Sainson RC, Kim JK, Hughes CC, Levin ER (2007) A conserved mechanism for steroid receptor translocation to the plasma membrane. J Biol Chem 282:22278–22288
2. Espinosa JM, Emerson BM (2001) Transcriptional regulation by p53 through intrinsic DNA/chromatin binding and site-directed cofactor recruitment. Mol Cell 8:57–69
3. Lidor Nili E, Field Y, Lubling Y, Widom J, Oren M, Segal E (2010) p53 binds preferentially to genomic regions with high DNA-encoded nucleosome occupancy. Genome Res 20:1361–1368
4. Beato M, Herrlich P, Schütz G (1995) Steroid hormone receptors: many actors in search of a plot. Cell 83:851–857
5. Piña B, Brüggemeier U, Beato M (1990) Nucleosome positioning modulates accessibility of regulatory proteins to the mouse mammary tumor virus promoter. Cell 60:719–731
6. Di Croce L, Koop R, Venditti P, Westphal HM, Nightingale K, Becker P, Beato M (1999) Two-steps synegism between progesterone receptor and the DNA binding domain of NF1 on MMTV minichromosomes. Mol Cell 4:45–54
7. Vicent GP, Nacht AS, Smith CL, Peterson CL, Dimitrov S, Beato M (2004) DNA instructed displacement of H2A and H2B at an inducible promoter. Mol Cell 16:439–452
8. Vicent GP, Zaurin R, Nacht AS, Font-Mateu J, Le Dily F, Beato M (2010) Nuclear factor 1 synergizes with progesterone receptor on the mouse mammary tumor virus promoter wrapped around a histone H3/H4 tetramer by facilitating access to the central hormone-responsive elements. J Biol Chem 285:2622–2631
9. Koop R, Di Croce L, Beato M (2003) Histone H1 enhances synergistic activation of the MMTV promoter in chromatin. EMBO J 22:588–599
10. Vicent GP, Meliá MJ, Beato M (2002) Asymmetric binding of histone H1 stabilizes MMTV nucleosomes and the interaction of progesterone receptor with the exposed HRE. J Mol Biol 324:501–517
11. Ballaré C, Uhrig M, Bechtold T, Sancho E, Di Domenico M, Migliaccio A, Auricchio F, Beato M (2003) Two domains of the progesterone receptor interact with the estrogen receptor and are required for progesterone activation of the c-Srcc-Src/Erk pathway in mammalian cells. Mol Cell Biol 23:1994–2008
12. Vicent GP, Ballaré C, Nacht AS, Clausell J, Subtil-Rodríguez A, Jordan A, Beato M (2006) Induction of progesterone target genes requires activation of Erk and Msk kinases and phosphorylation of histone H3. Mol Cell 24:367–381

13. Eisfeld K, Candau R, Truss M, Beato M (1997) Binding of NF1 to the MMTV promoter in nucleosomes: Influence of rotational phasing, translational positioning and histone H1. Nucleic Acids Res 25:3733–3742
14. Vicent GP, Nacht AS, Font-Mateu J, Castellano G, Gaveglia L, Ballare C, Beato M (2011) Four enzymes cooperate to displace histone H1 during the first minute of hormonal gene activation. Genes Dev 25:845–862
15. Fan S, Wang J, Yuan R, Ma Y, Meng Q, Erdos MR, Pestell RG, Yuan F, Auborn KJ, Goldberg ID, Rosen EM (1999) BRCA1BRCA1 inhibition of estrogen receptor signaling in transfected cells. Science 284:1354–1356
16. Ma Y, Katiyar P, Jones LP, Fan S, Zhang Y, Furth PA, Rosen EM (2006) The breast cancer susceptibility gene BRCA1BRCA1 regulates progesterone receptor signaling in mammary epithelial cells. Mol Endocrinol 20:14–34
17. Zheng L, Annab LA, Afshari CA, Lee WH, Boyer TG (2001) BRCA1 mediates ligand-independent transcriptional repression of the estrogen receptor. Proc Natl Acad Sci U S A 98:9587–9592
18. Calvo V, Beato M (2011) BRCA1 Counteracts Progesterone Action by Ubiquitination Leading to Progesterone Receptor Degradation and Epigenetic Silencing of Target Promoters. Cancer Res 71:3422–3431
19. Bryant HE, Schultz N, Thomas HD, Parker KM, Flower D, Lopez E, Kyle S, Meuth M, Curtin NJ, Helleday T (2005) Specific killing of BRCA2-deficient tumours with inhibitors of poly(ADP-ribose) polymerase. Nature 434:913–917
20. Farmer H, McCabe N, Lord CJ, Tutt AN, Johnson DA, Richardson TB, Santarosa M, Dillon KJ, Hickson I, Knights C, Martin NM, Jackson SP, Smith GC, Ashworth A (2005) Targeting the DNA repair defect in BRCA mutant cells as a therapeutic strategy. Nature 434:917–921
21. Lanz RB, McKenna NJ, Onate SA, Albrecht U, Wong J, Tsai SY, Tsai MJ, O'Malley BW (1999) A steroid receptor coactivator, SRA, functions as an RNA and is present in an SRC-1 complex. Cell 97:17–27

Cooperative Interactions Between c-Src, Estrogen Receptors and Receptor Tyrosine Kinases in Breast Cancer

Sarah J. Parsons, Jessica E. Pritchard, Emily M. Fox and Margaret A. Shupnik

Abstract Estrogen predominantly mediates its effects through the estrogen receptors, ER-α and ER-β, which directly modulate gene expression and participate in rapid cytoplasmic signaling. Within minutes of estrogen stimulation, the ER interacts with and signals through the non-receptor tyrosine kinase, c-Src, and HER family of receptor tyrosine kinases to promote biological outcomes. In addition, these proteins have been shown to cooperate with one another to facilitate growth factor and progesterone signaling in the absence of estrogen. Because of their involvement in estrogen-dependent and independent signaling, cancer progression, and resistance to hormonal and cytotoxic therapies, the c-Src and HER family proteins have been identified as targets for the treatment of breast cancer, as well as other malignancies. Several small-molecule inhibitors and monoclonal antibodies are currently being tested or used in the clinic for the treatment of these tumors.

Keywords Estrogen receptor · Progesterone receptor · Androgen receptor · c-Src · HER family receptors · Therapeutic resistance

---

S. J. Parsons (✉)
Department of Microbiology, University of Virginia Cancer Center,
Charlottesville, VA 22908, USA
e-mail: sap@virginia.edu

J. E. Pritchard
Department of Microbiology, University of Virginia Cancer Center,
Charlottesville, VA 22908, USA

E. M. Fox
Hematology/Oncology Division, Ingram Cancer Center,
Vanderbilt University, Nashville, TN 37240, USA

M. A. Shupnik
Department of Medicine, Division of Endocrinology,
University of Virginia Cancer Center,
Charlottesville, VA 22908, USA

G. Castoria and A. Migliaccio (eds.), *Advances in Rapid Sex-Steroid Action*,
DOI: 10.1007/978-1-4614-1764-4_3,

Abbreviations

4ICD	HER4 intracellular domain
AF	activation function
AIB1	amplified in Breast Cancer-1
AR	androgen receptor
CHK-A	choline kinase-α
Cox II	cytochrome c oxidase subunit II
DBD	DNA-binding domain
DOC-2/DAB2	differentially expressed in ovarian cancer/disabled 2
EGFR	epidermal growth factor receptor
ER	estrogen receptor
ERE	estrogen-responsive element
GPCR	G protein-coupled receptor
HER	Human EGFR family
HR	hormone receptor (i.e. ER or PR)
HRG	heregulin
IGF-1	insulin-like growth factor-1
LBD	ligand-binding domain
MNAR	modulator of non-genomic action of estrogen receptor
MMP	Matrix metallo-proteinase
NSCLC	non-small cell lung cancer
PI3K	PI3-kinase
PR	progesterone receptor
Ser	serine
SFK	Src family kinase
SH3	Src homology 3
SRC-1	steroid coactivator-1
TGF	transforming growth factor
TKI	tyrosine kinase inhibitor
Tyr	tyrosine

Contents

1 Introduction

Breast cancer is a hormone-dependent malignancy that accounts for more than one in four cancers diagnosed in American women and is the second leading cause of female cancer-related deaths [1, 2]. The steroid hormone 17β-estradiol plays a critical role in the development and progression of breast cancer, and increased exposure to estrogen (such as early menarche and late menopause) is associated with many of the epidemiological risk factors for breast cancer. Removal of estrogen via ovariectomy or cessation of hormone-replacement therapy correlates with reduced risk [1, 2], consistent with estrogen being required for the development and growth of the mammary gland during puberty, pregnancy, and lactation [3], as well as cell proliferation under both physiological and patho-physiological states [4].

Biological effects of estrogen are mediated through the estrogen receptors, ER-α or ER-β. Normal human mammary tissue expresses both ER subtypes, although, surprisingly, both are expressed primarily in non-proliferating cells [5]. In early breast cancers, ER-α is highly over-expressed and ER-β expression is decreased compared to normal breast tissue, whereas expression of both receptors declines in more invasive cancers [4, 6, 7]. The predominant role of ER-α in breast tumors has allowed its expression, alone or with the estrogen-stimulated progesterone receptor (PR), to be used as a criterion for treatment of patients with adjuvant endocrine therapy such as tamoxifen or aromatase inhibitors. Several studies examined ER-β expression to assess if there is any benefit in determining its status to predict responses to endocrine therapy. The majority concluded that ER-β together with ER-α favors positive responses to endocrine therapy, but it is unclear if there is any further benefit than measuring ER-α alone. In contrast, the positive association between ER-β and HER2 expression in high-grade ER-α-negative breast cancer does not favor positive responses to endocrine therapy, which may be due to interactions of ER-β and HER2 in these tumors, as well as development of such tumors from a different type of mammary cell, such as a myoepithelial cell [4].

In general, declining expression of ER in breast tumors is associated with increased expression of growth factor receptors, particularly of the human EGFR, or HER family [8]. Over-expression of HER2 occurs more frequently in the early stages of breast cancer, and is therefore thought to be involved in tumor initiation and early stages of progression. HER2 is amplified in 10-35% of human breast carcinomas, an event associated with a poor disease prognosis. Approximately 30% of human breast tumors over-express EGFR and this is correlated with a loss of ER expression, estrogen responsiveness, and a poorer prognosis. EGFR also plays a role in normal breast development and is found in ductal epithelial cells of normal breast tissue. c-Src, a non-receptor tyrosine kinase that is localized to intracellular membranes of the cell, has also been found to be over-expressed or highly activated in human breast tumor specimens and cell lines, with estimates that 70% of tumors have c-Src tyrosine kinase activity from 2-to-50-fold greater than those found in normal breast epithelium or immortalized mammary epithelial cells [8]. Such increases in a high percentage of human breast neoplasias provide correlative evidence that c-Src is involved in some facet of breast cancer development. Increasing evidence suggests that the estrogen-mediated and growth factor-mediated pathways regulating tumor progression may require common downstream signaling pathways, providing nodes of cross talk between the two types of receptors [9]. This review concentrates on the interactions between the ER, c-Src, and members of the HER family and how these interactions may impact breast cancer proliferation.

2 Canonical vs Rapid Signaling of Estrogen and the ERs

The ERs, along with PRs and androgen receptors (ARs), are members of the nuclear receptor family of transcription factors. Nuclear receptors contain a central zinc finger DNA-binding domain (DBD) and a C-terminal ligand-binding domain (LBD). Full transcriptional activity of nuclear receptors requires cooperation between the N-terminal ligand-independent activation function-1 (AF-1) domain and a C-terminal ligand-dependent activation function-2 (AF-2) domain in the LBD. AF-1 associates with coactivators and is the site of several phosphorylations that modulate receptor activity, whereas the AF-2 domain contains helix 12, which facilitates the recruitment and interaction of coactivators. Ligand binding induces an activating conformational change that reorganizes the LBD and displaces the receptor from chaperones such as heat shock proteins, promotes dimerization, and facilitates the recruitment and binding of coactivator proteins such as steroid coactivator-1 (SRC-1), SRC-2 (GRIP1), and SRC-3, also called Amplified in

Breast Cancer-1 (AIB1). Coactivators, alone or with coregulators such as CBP and p300, contain intrinsic histone acetyltransferase activity that modifies lysines and increases chromatin accessibility and ultimately transcription of target genes. In contrast, binding of antagonists like tamoxifen and raloxifene to the ER displaces helix 12 and increases association of corepressors such as NCoR, SMRT, Sin3, and REA with histone deacetylases, resulting in a more condensed chromatin structure that represses gene transcription [10]. ERs bind directly to DNA at estrogen response elements (EREs) but also associate with other transcription factors, such as Sp1 or AP1, to regulate gene activity. Many proliferative and survival genes are regulated by such "tethered" transcription factor mechanisms [11]. Both ER subtypes bind similarly to EREs, but can differentially regulate genes, particularly via tethered factors; ER-β generally has less transcriptional activity compared to ER-α and has been proposed to act as a brake for ER-α activity, either directly or indirectly [10].

ER function can also be modified by extracellular signals. Growth factors such as EGF and insulin-like growth factor-1 (IGF-1) activate protein kinase pathways leading to phosphorylation and activation of ER and coactivators [12]. For example, in MCF-7 cells EGF stimulates ER-α activity and coactivator binding via phosphorylation of Ser118 on ER-α by ERK and over-expression of the EGF receptor family member HER2 or constitutive activation of the PI3 kinase (PI3K) pathway [12]. Resulting increases in ER activity can then lead to the activation of proliferative pathways, even in the absence of estrogen.

In addition to direct modulation of gene expression, estrogen/ER can rapidly stimulate cytoplasmic signaling pathways, including many of those shared by growth factors such as MAPK, PI3K and Akt [12]. Although most ER-α and ER-β proteins reside in the nucleus, a population of ER is localized to the cytosolic and membrane compartments. This population is especially important in ER+ breast cancers (40-70% of tumors), where ER-α protein is over-expressed up to 10-fold over levels in normal breast tissue. ER can become associated directly with the cytoplasmic membrane via a palmitic acid covalently associated with a specific cysteine in the ligand binding domain (C447 in hER-α) [13]. In this situation, more ER is available for crosstalk with membrane and cytoplasmic signaling molecules and may thus have additional impact on modulating the rate of proliferation. The recently described GPR30, a bona fide estrogen-binding G-protein coupled receptor (GPCR), acts via G protein $\beta\gamma$ subunits and also has the potential to modulate estrogen-stimulated changes in PKA or ERK activity, but estrogen-stimulated proliferation of breast cancer cells has not been associated with this protein [14]. Most rapid actions of estrogen in breast cancer cells, and ultimately cell proliferation, appear to be associated with the cognate nuclear ERs. Estrogen stimulation of ERK in breast cancer cells occurs within 3-15 min, and can be inhibited with antiestrogens such as ICI 182,780, or knockdown of ER-α [15]. Cells from ER-α/ER-β-KO mice cannot support rapid estrogen cytoplasmic signaling, and introduction of siRNAs for ER-α and/or ER-β abrogates rapid estrogen signaling and cell proliferation in breast cancer cells, whereas introduction of GPR30 siRNA and knockdown of this protein does not [16–18]. In addition to effects on enzyme signaling, ligand-bound cytoplasmic ERs can also induce rapid phosphorylation of cytoplasmic transcription factors such as Stat3 and Stat5, which are then translocated to the nucleus and linked to estrogen-dependent proliferation of breast cancer cells [4, 19]. Such pathways likely cooperate with nuclear actions of ER [19, 20].

3 Rapid Estrogen Signaling Involving ER, c-Src and HER Family Members

3.1 Estrogen-Dependent c-Src-ER Interactions: Complexes, Physiological Role, Mechanism of Action, and Regulation

One of the key cytoplasmic proteins that mediates rapid estrogen signaling via the ER is c-Src [15, 21–23]. c-Src is the founding member of the Src family kinases (SFKs) of intracellular, membrane-localized non-receptor tyrosine kinases [24–26], and its substrates include many known estrogen effector proteins, including ER-α [27], PI3K [28], AR [29] and EGFR [30–32]. c-Src has been implicated in colorectal, breast, melanoma, ovarian, gastric, head and neck, pancreatic, lung, brain, and blood cancer development/progression [8], though it is poorly oncogenic on its own. However, mice expressing endogenous c-Src and the polyomavirus middle T antigen transgene under the control of a mammary-specific promoter form more tumors at a faster rate than those expressing polyomavirus middle T on a c-Src null background [24], indicating that c-Src can cooperate with other oncogenic factors to enhance tumorigenicity.

c-Src's oncogenic role in breast cancer is consistent with its function as an estrogen effector. In MCF-7 cells, estrogen rapidly enhances c-Src activity and ER-α Tyr537 phosphorylation [33]. A report by Kumar and colleagues [34] suggests that this activation may result from direct association of c-Src with ER-α and myristoylated, GDP-bound $G_{\alpha i}$ (Fig. 1a, #1), but other mechanisms of activation have also been described (see below). Phosphorylation of ER-α Tyr537 by activated c-Src enhances ER-α binding to EREs in vitro and in vivo [22, 35]. In contrast, inhibition of c-Src in ER+ BT-474 cells by a SFK-targeted tyrosine kinase inhibitor (TKI) results in increased ER-α protein levels and ER-mediated transcription [36, 37]. Together, these results suggest that SFKs can stimulate or inhibit ER transcription, depending upon the cell line and treatment.

Modulator of non-genomic action of estrogen receptor (MNAR/PELP-1), a scaffolding protein, associates with ligand-bound ER-α, ER-β, AR, and glucocorticoid receptor through LXXLL motifs, similar to those of nuclear receptor coactivators, and also binds to the c-Src SH3 domain via a proline-rich region [22]. Its association with ER-α and c-Src have been shown to increase within minutes of estrogen stimulation (Fig. 1a, #4) [22, 27, 33, 38–40]. These interactions lead to stimulation of c-Src

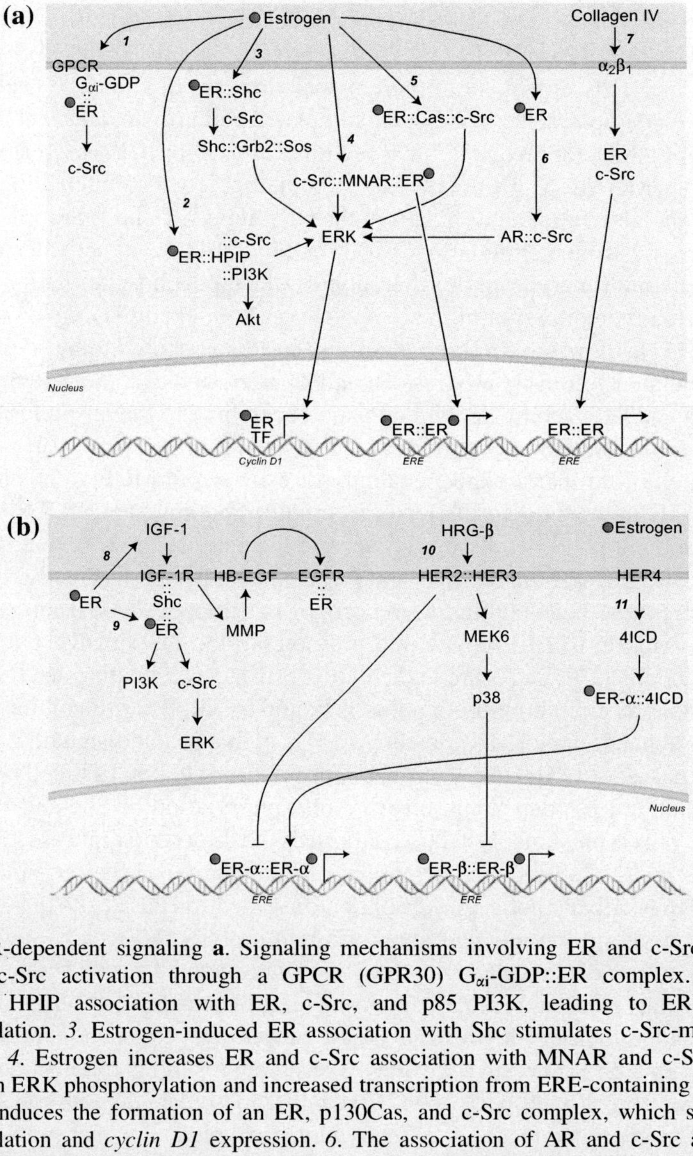

Fig. 1 ER-dependent signaling **a**. Signaling mechanisms involving ER and c-Src *1*. Estrogen mediates c-Src activation through a GPCR (GPR30) $G_{\alpha i}$-GDP::ER complex. *2*. Estrogen stimulates HPIP association with ER, c-Src, and p85 PI3K, leading to ERK and AKT phosphorylation. *3*. Estrogen-induced ER association with Shc stimulates c-Src-mediated ERK activation. *4*. Estrogen increases ER and c-Src association with MNAR and c-Src activation, resulting in ERK phosphorylation and increased transcription from ERE-containing promoters. *5*. Estrogen induces the formation of an ER, p130Cas, and c-Src complex, which supports ERK phosphorylation and *cyclin D1* expression. *6*. The association of AR and c-Src activate ERK through an estrogen and ER-dependent mechanism. *7*. Type IV collagen signals through integrins, ER, and c-Src to induce transcription from ERE-containing promoters. **b.** HER family members modulate estrogen-induced signaling and transcription. *8*. Estrogen signals through the ER to elevate IGF-1 levels, resulting in IGF-1R-dependent EGFR activation. *9*. Estrogen rapidly stimulates the association of ER, Shc, and IFG-1R, causing ERK and PI3K activation. *10*. HRG-β signaling via HER2 and HER3 inhibits estrogen-induced transcription from ERE-containing promoters through different mechanisms. *11*. The truncated form of HER4 (*4ICD*) associates with ER-α at ERE-containing promoters and facilitates estrogen-induced gene transcription

enzymatic activity and activation of the MAPK pathway. It is proposed that MNAR enhances activation of c-Src by providing more effective interaction between ER and c-Src as well as by relieving c-Src inhibition through binding to the SH3 domain. Although the hierarchy among all of these associations is not known, it is clear that c-Src plays a fundamental role in estrogen-stimulated cell growth, an event that may also require growth factor receptors, such as those for EGF or IGF-1 [4, 41].

In addition to MNAR, p130Cas (BCAR-1), hematopoietic Pbx interacting protein (HPIP), and Shc also function as adaptors that facilitate ER and c-Src interaction. Within 3 min of estrogen stimulation, p130Cas binds ER-α and activates c-Src to form a transient, multimeric complex that supports the rapid phosphorylation of ERK 1/2 and, eventually, expression of the cell cycle protein, cyclin D1, in T47-D cells (Fig. 1a, #5) [21]. In fact, c-Src kinase activity has been shown to be required for estrogen-stimulated cell-cycle progression and proliferation in some systems [6, 24, 28, 42]. ER-α and ER-β compete with one another to bind to the adaptor, HPIP. Of interest, estrogen stimulation is required for ER-α to associate with HPIP, whereas ER-β and the scaffold interact independently of estrogen in MCF-7 cells [43, 44]. Estrogen quickly induces the formation of a complex containing HPIP, ER-α, c-Src, and the p85 subunit of PI3K; these proteins and the activity of c-Src and PI3K are required for estrogen-stimulated ERK and AKT phosphorylation (Fig. 1a, #2) [43]. However, there have been conflicting reports of the impact of HPIP on estrogen-induced transcription of ERE-containing promoters [43, 44]. Finally, two studies have implicated Shc, ER, and c-Src in mediating estrogenic signaling and biological outcomes. Shc is a scaffolding protein that is bound by Grb2, a protein that recruits the guanine exchange factor, Sos, leading to Ras activation and signaling through the MAPK cascade [45]. The estrogen stimulation of MCF-7 cells triggers SFK-dependant and ER-dependent tyrosine phosphorylation of Shc and ERK 1/2 (Fig. 1a, #3). This is presumably achieved through the direct and rapid association of Shc with ER-α as well as the formation of the Shc-Grb2-Sos complex [15]. In addition, Kousteni and colleagues [46] demonstrated in HeLa cells that estrogen protection from etoposide-induced apoptosis requires ER, c-Src, Shc, and MEK, suggesting that Shc-dependent rapid signaling may mediate resistance to chemotherapeutic agents. Further evidence supporting an ER-mediated cell survival role for c-Src is the finding that in ER+ MCF-7 breast cancer cells estrogen increases ER-α association with c-Src, Shc, and the IGF-1 receptor, resulting in ER-α-dependent PI3K activation (Fig. 1b, #9) [15, 16, 47]. Together these data demonstrate that, not only is c-Src an important mediator of many biological responses that support breast cancer progression, it can do so through its participation in estrogen signaling.

3.2 Estrogen-Dependent HER Family and ER Interactions

The HER family of transmembrane receptor tyrosine kinases contains four members (HER1 (EGFR), HER2, HER3, and HER4) that homo- and heterodimerize and become activated upon ligand-binding. The extracellular domain mediates ligand binding and receptor dimerization, while the intracellular portion contains the catalytic domain and phosphorylation sites that provide docking sites for adaptor proteins and substrates with SH2 domains [48–50]. In addition to EGFR activation by its own ligands, cytokines, sex hormones, and GPCR ligands have been shown to signal through the EGFR [51] and to promote MAPK, PI3K, c-Src, and Stat signaling [8].

EGFR overexpression in breast cancer correlates strongly with a loss of differentiation, advanced clinical stage, enhanced tumor proliferation, resistance to endocrine therapy, and poor prognosis [52], suggesting that the EGFR is an important player in breast cancer progression. Additionally, overexpression of the EGFR in cell culture models can result in morphological transformation and in vivo tumorigenesis [52, 53], and targeted overexpression of its ligand, transforming growth factor-α (TGF-α), in the mouse mammary gland causes hyperplasia and adenomas following multiple pregnancies and lactation [54]. Aberrant EGFR activation results from gene amplification, transcriptional overexpression, and/or autocrine stimulation of the receptor [55].

HER2 is amplified in 20-30% of all breast tumors; however, its expression is often inversely correlated with that of the ER [56, 57]. In several cancers, including breast, HER2 expression is a poor prognostic marker [58], and its ectopic overexpression in cell models enhances tumorigenicity, possibly through the basal autophosphorylation of HER2 [53]. Trastuzumab, a HER2-targeted monoclonal antibody, has been used successfully in the treatment of HER2+ breast cancers, and its effects are independent of ER status [59]. However, chemotherapeutic treatment of breast cancers with high HER2 levels demonstrates poor clinical outcomes [60, 61], with ER+ or PR+ (hormone receptor-positive, HR+) cancers showing better responses [62–66] than HR- cancers, suggesting that HER2 sensitizes ER+ breast cancers to chemotherapy. Thus, while HER2 has clearly been shown to promote certain breast cancers, it appears to have some divergent functions in ER+ and ER− tumors.

The roles of HER3 and HER4 in breast cancer have been less extensively studied, particularly in relationship to the ER and estrogen signaling. Two studies on HR+ breast cancers have shown that increased HER3 levels [67] or HER3 pTyr1289 [68] in tumors portends a poor prognosis. In contrast, both studies demonstrated that higher levels of HER4 within the HR+ population correlated with increased overall survival [67, 68].

HER family members are often misregulated in estrogen-responsive breast tumors. Though ER-α and EGFR/HER2 expression in cancerous cells is inversely correlated, they are dually expressed in adjacent normal cells [69–72]. Estrogen causes the downregulation of both EGFR and HER2 mRNA in ER+ breast cancer cell lines, and evidence suggests that this occurs through an ER-mediated mechanism [73, 74]. In contrast, HER4 and ER-α are recruited to the ERBB4 promoter within an hour of estrogen exposure and prolonged stimulation increases HER4 expression in T47-D cells [75].

Estrogen can rapidly transactivate the EGFR to achieve effector-molecule activation and biological responses. For example, estrogen-activated ER leads to increased IGF-1 levels and IGF-1R-, MMP-, and HB-EGF-dependent EGFR activation in MCF-7 cells and association of the IGF-1R with ER-α (Fig. 1b, #8) [76, 77]. This pathway is necessary for estrogen-induced ERK 1/2 phosphorylation, net growth, and decreased apoptosis, possibly through Shc and c-Src [77–79]. Elevated IGF-1 levels may result from post-translational regulation of IGF-1 turnover or from ER-mediated transcription [77, 80].

In contrast to this ER-dependent mechanism, GPR30 also signals through the EGFR independently of the ER. GPR30 stimulates HB-EGF cleavage through a c-Src-dependent mechanism, thereby stimulating EGFR-mediated ERK and PI3K activation to support estrogen-stimulated DNA synthesis and survival [81]. GPR30 can also associate with ER-α in an EGFR-independent manner in ER+ endometrial cancer cells [82–84] but the implications of this association have yet to be demonstrated.

Though HER2 and HER3 have not been explicitly implicated in estrogen signaling, their heterodimerization with EGFR suggests that they may also participate in downstream estrogen signaling [50]. Studies on HER4 have focused predominately on HER4's soluble, cleaved form, the intracellular domain (4ICD). 4ICD was shown to associate with ER-α [85] and occupy the promoters of estrogen-regulated genes (e.g. ERBB4, SDF-1, PGR) within an hour of estrogen stimulation [75], suggesting that the ER-α4ICD complex can regulate the expression of estrogen target genes (Fig. 1b, #11). ER-α, ER-β and 4ICD are also present in the mitochondria of ER+ breast cancer cells, and their localization to this organelle is differentially regulated by estrogen [86–88]. (Localization of ER is increased but that of 4ICD is decreased.) Data suggest that 4ICD promotes rapid tamoxifen-induced apoptosis in ER+ breast cancer cell lines, though it is unclear if interaction with the ER is necessary and, if so, if the interaction occurs in the mitochondria [85].

3.3 Estrogen-Independent Interactions Between ER, c-Src, and HER Family Members

Little experimental evidence supports the existence of a trimeric complex consisting of ER, c-Src, and any HER family member either in the absence or presence of estrogen. However, c-Src and some HER family members have been shown to individually associate with and participate in signaling with the ER in the absence of estrogen.

For example, in ER-α expressing cells EGF can stimulate the interaction of ER-α with EGFR, induce proliferation, and decrease apoptosis. These events are preceded by rapid serine and tyrosine phosphorylation of ER-α [89–91]. A role for ER-α in EGF signaling is further supported by the inability of mice lacking ER-α or treated with anti-estrogens to support EGF-stimulated DNA synthesis and growth [91–93].

Heregulin (HRG, neuregulin-1), a ligand for HER3 and HER4, has been shown to modulate ER transcriptional activity through the HER family. This ligand stimulates rapid HER3/HER4 heterodimerization with HER2 and activation of all

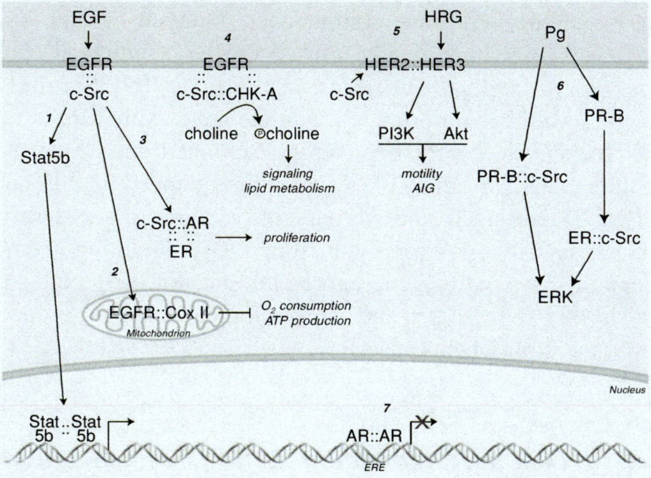

Fig. 2 Estrogen-independent actions of HER family members, PR, and AR. *1*. EGF-induces c-Src and EGFR association, c-Src-mediated phosphorylation of EGFR Tyr845, and the subsequent activation of Stat5b. *2*. EGF promotes c-Src-dependent EGFR translocation to the mitochondria, pTyr845 EGFR-dependent association with Cox II, and inhibition of Cox activity. *3*. EGF causes the formation of a pro-proliferative complex of c-Src, AR, and ER. *4*. Over-expressed EGFR and c-Src bind and stabilize CHK-A, thereby increasing total cellular CHK-A activity. *5*. C-Src regulates HRG-induced PI3K and AKT phosphorylation and biological outcomes by promoting HER2-HER3 hetero-dimerization. *6*. Progesterone (Pg) induces ERK phosphorylation through ER-dependent and -independent mechanisms. *7*. AR occupancy of ERE-containing promoters inhibits estrogen-induced transcription

three receptors in breast cancer cell lines [94–96] and, in the case of the HRG-β isoform, inhibits estrogen-induced occupancy and transcription of ERE-containing promoters in a HER2- and HER3-dependent manner [96] (Fig. 1b, #10). Of note, HRG-β suppresses ER-α- and ER-β-mediated gene transcription in MCF-7 cells by unique mechanisms: ER-β requires phosphorylation of its AF-1 domain (or A/B domain), MEK6, and p38 for inhibition, whereas ER-α needs none of these (Fig. 1b, #10) [96]. A recent study in T47-D cells showed that overexpression of ER-β suppresses HRG-induced HER2 tyrosine phosphorylation [97], suggesting multiple levels of regulation and crosstalk between HER family members and the ERs.

Interactions and signaling between c-Src and ER in the absence of estrogen has not been widely reported in the literature, though a few studies have shown both progestins and basement membrane proteins stimulate such signaling. In T47-D cells PR-B and ER-α basally associate in a direct interaction that was shown in a yeast two-hybrid system to occur independently of ER-α Tyr537 phosphorylation by c-Src [35, 98]. Yet, ER-α binds c-Src in a PR-dependent manner within 2 min of exposure to a synthetic progestin (R5020) (Fig. 2, #6). However, ER and PR are both necessary for R5020-induced c-Src activation and c-Src-mediated ERK 1/2 phosphorylation and cell growth [35, 98], suggesting that the physical interaction of ER-α with c-Src may mediate signaling and biological outcomes in response to progestin. The basement membrane components, collagen-IV and laminin-1, can increase ER-α levels in primary and cultured murine mammary epithelial cells through binding of $\alpha_2\beta_1$ and $\alpha_6\beta_1$ integrins, respectively [99]. Similarly, collagen-IV and fibronectin have been reported to modulate gene expression through the ER and c-Src (Fig. 1a, #7). In contrast to estrogen-induced classical gene transcription, which requires the C-terminus of ER-α and is enhanced by, but not dependent upon, c-Src, type IV collagen and fibronectin, requires the N-terminal portion of ER-α and c-Src activity for expression from ERE-containing promoters [100]. The implications of this type of gene expression are not fully elucidated, though one possibility is that it regulates the morphological changes induced by these basement membrane components.

3.4 Estrogen Receptor-Independent Actions of c-Src and HER Family Members in Breast Cancer

In addition to their interactions with the ER, c-Src and HER family members participate independently of the ER in signaling pathways that regulate a plethora of processes driving the progression of breast cancer. Several of these pathways are mediated by synergistic interactions of HER family members with c-Src [101, 102]. For example, activation of the EGFR (through direct binding of ligand or transactivation by GPCRs, cytokine receptors, or estrogen) recruits c-Src or related cytoplasmic tyrosine kinases to the receptor [101, 103, 104], which in turn phosphorylate the receptor at specific tyrosine sites, most notably EGFR Tyr 845. Phosphorylation of this site by c-Src is required for EGFR-mediated DNA synthesis and results in activation of the transcription factor, Stat5b, (Fig. 2, #1) and association of the EGFR with cytochrome c oxidase subunit II (Cox II), a component of the ATP-generating oxidative phosphorylation pathway (Fig. 2, #2) [105, 106]. Translocation of the EGFR and c-Src to the mitochondria results in tyrosine phosphorylation of Cox II, a reduction in Cox II activity, and reduced ATP generation, suggestive of a Warburg-like effect [106]. The vIII variant of EGFR, found frequently in glioblastomas and less frequently in breast cancers, has also been localized to the mitochondria, where it is reported to regulate cell survival [107].

Independently of pTyr 845, EGFR and c-Src also activate Stat3 [101, 108]. The Stat family regulates transcription of multiple genes that contribute to breast cancer cell proliferation, survival and migration, in the latter case through transcriptional as well as cytoplasmic events [109]. In addition to transcription and energy metabolism, the synergism between EGFR and c-Src can regulate phospholipid synthesis, specifically through recruitment and stabilization of choline kinase-α (CHK-A), a key enzyme in the production of phosphatidylcholine, the major phospholipid of cellular membranes [110] (Fig. 2, #4). In addition to its role in membrane biogenesis, phosphocholine, the product of CHK-A catalysis has been implicated as a second messenger, regulating cell survival through PI3-kinase [111, 112].

c-Src and EGFR also participate in numerous other signaling pathways that regulate cell adhesion/migration, survival, proliferation, cell–cell interactions, and angiogenesis, all processes critical to tumorigenesis. The downstream substrates of EGFR and c-Src that regulate these processes are frequently shared, including members of the integrin/FAK/paxillin pathway, the PI-3 kinase/Akt pathway, the Shc/Ras/ERK pathway, the cadherin/catenin pathway, and the VEGF/HIF-α pathway. These and other pathways regulated by c-Src and/or EGFR have been reviewed extensively elsewhere [113–117].

c-Src also plays an important role in regulating HER2 activation. A 2001 study showed that c-Src and HER2/HER3 formed a complex in breast cancer cells that was independent of ligand stimulation by HRG, but inhibition of c-Src kinase activity reduced or ablated HRG-dependent soft-agar colony growth, indicating that c-Src played a critical role in HER2/3-mediated anchorage-independent proliferative function [118]. Subsequent studies demonstrated that c-Src positively regulates HER2/3 hetero-complex formation by an upstream mechanism, which results in regulation of downstream intracellular effectors of the complex, including PI3K and FAK, thereby regulating cell motility and anchorage-independent growth induced by HRG (Fig. 2, #5) [119]. c-Src is also involved in transactivation of HER2 by the GPCR, CXCR4. The ligand for CXCR4, stromal cell-derived factor-1α, binds CXCR4 to induce migration of breast cancer cells, and inhibition of c-Src kinase activity ablates this activity [120]. Similarly, TGF-β induces clustering of HER2 and integrins through a c-Src/FAK-dependent mechanism that is postulated to play a role in regulating breast cancer cell migration and survival [121]. Together, these studies provide substantial evidence of cooperativity between c-Src and HER family members that can function to promote breast cancer formation and progression.

4 AR in Breast Cancer and Possible Interactions With ER, c-Src, and HER Family Members

The critical role of the AR in the development and potential treatment of prostate cancer has long been appreciated, but now emerging evidence suggests that the balance between ER-α and AR signaling is also a critical determinant of growth in the normal and malignant breast. Several recent studies indicate that AR status is a positive prognostic indicator in ER+ breast cancer [122–124]. Consistent with a positive role for the AR in breast cancer outcome, the AR can potently inhibit ER-α transactivation activity and estrogen-stimulated growth of breast cancer cells [122]. These inhibitory actions are suggested to occur in part by AR association with EREs on chromatin and direct inhibition of ER's genomic actions (Fig. 2, #7). However, in addition, AR participates in rapid "non-genomic" signaling cascades, which may also influence breast cancer proliferation.

In both human mammary and prostate cancer cells, steroid hormones or EGF trigger association of an AR-ER complex with c-Src (Fig. 2, #3) [125]. This interaction activates c-Src and affects the G1 to S cell cycle progression. Androgens also activate ERK via EGFR/IGF-1R in prostate cancer cells [126]. Unlike the ER, but similar to the PR, the AR associates directly with c-Src via a polyproline-rich sequence in its N-terminus [127]. A 10 amino acid synthetic peptide specifically inhibits the AR/c-Src interaction. Importantly, treatment of MCF-7 breast cancer cells with nanomolar concentrations of this peptide inhibits the estrogen-induced association between the AR, ER, and c-Src, c-Src/Erk pathway activation, cyclin D1 expression, and DNA synthesis, without interfering in receptor-dependent transcriptional activity, and can also inhibit EGF-stimulated proliferation in these cells (Fig. 1a, #6) [127]. Interestingly, disruption of the AR/c-Src complex by either this peptide, or a protein termed DOC-2/DAB2 (differentially expressed in ovarian cancer/disabled 2) was also shown to antagonize AR-mediated prostate cancer cell growth [127, 128], suggesting common AR-dependent mechanisms in both systems.

Progesterone can inhibit AR signaling, and the increased risk of breast cancer associated with hormone replacement therapy containing estrogens plus progestins has been suggested to be associated with these anti-androgenic actions and the reduction of the protective effects of the AR [129, 130].

Finally, the AR may serve a very different role in ER-negative breast cancers, and expression of functional ARs occurs in a subset of HR- cancers expressing several HER family members [131]. A recent study demonstrated both in vitro and in vivo synergies between AR and MEK inhibitors in molecular apocrine breast cancer [132]. Furthermore, combination therapy with these inhibitors overcame trastuzumab resistance in molecular apocrine cells. Therefore, a combination therapy strategy with AR and MEK inhibitors may provide an attractive therapeutic option for the ER−/AR+ subtype of breast cancer. Overall, understanding the role of androgen signaling in different subtypes of breast cancer and how this is modulated by other steroids and growth factors will increase our understanding of breast cancer risk and inform the development of optimal preventive and treatment strategies for this disease.

5 Progesterone Receptor Interactions With ER, c-Src and HER Family Members

PRs consist of two proteins that are expressed from a single gene via transcription from two alternative promoters. The larger protein is termed PR-B, but the N terminus-truncated PR-A lacks the first 164 amino acids of PR-B; the two isoforms are typically both expressed in cells [133]. The two proteins can have distinct responses on specific genes, and PR-A can antagonize effects of PR-B [134]. In breast cancer cells, progestins both stimulate and inhibit cell cycle progression while increasing expression of TF, EGFR, c-fos, and c-myc genes. Progestin treatment can also potentiate effects of EGF by upregulating levels of HER family members (presumably by genomic mechanisms) and by enhancing phosphorylation of signaling molecules associated with activated receptors, including ERK, Stats and Shc [133].

Both PR-A and PR-B are phosphorylated at equivalent sites under basal conditions and in response to ligand binding and growth factor signaling cascades [133, 135]. Progestin induces EGFR-, c-Src-, and ERK-dependent phosphorylation of PR-B on the MAPK consensus site, Ser345. Ser345-phosphorylated PR-B receptors strongly associate with specificity protein 1 (Sp1) transcription factors to regulate PR cell cycle (p21) and growth-promoting (EGFR) target genes whose promoters lack canonical progesterone response element sequences [136]. In response to growth factors such as EGF, Ser294 of PR-B is rapidly (3-5 min) phosphorylated via a MAPK-dependent pathway. PR Ser294 is a key site for direct regulation of PR subcellular location, activity, and turnover in response to phosphorylation events, and phosphorylated PR has increased sensitivity to lower levels of ligand [137]. Additional post-translational modifications of PR can also regulate activity. For example, sumoylation of the PR is hormone-dependent and has a suppressive effect on transcription [138]. Recently, EGF-induced phosphorylation of PR Ser-294 via MEK or Cdk2 was shown to block PR Lys-388 sumoylation of PR-B but not PR-A, thereby derepressing receptor activity and contributing to transcription of several proliferation genes [139]. Together, these data suggest therapeutic potential for PR-targeted breast cancer treatment by exploiting multiple nodes along the PR signaling pathway, including PR-B, EGFR, c-Src, ERK, or Sp1.

Unlike ERs, the PRs were not originally found in a wide variety of complexes with intracellular signaling molecules and were proposed to exert their extranuclear actions primarily by direct association with c-Src, alone or in conjunction with ER-α. Human PR-B stimulation of ERK activity was shown to require functional and physical association with c-Src [140, 141] (Fig. 2, #6). The amino terminus of PR contains a polyproline SH3 recognition motif (aa 421–428) that is necessary and sufficient for mediating direct interaction of PR with SH3 domains of c-Src and related tyrosine kinases in a ligand-dependent manner in vitro and in breast cancer cells. Mutation of the PXXP sequence in the PR or addition of a minimal synthetic peptide containing the PR polyproline motif abolished the ability of progestins to bind c-Src and activate both c-Src (or HcK) and p42/p44 ERKs, whereas mutation of the DNA binding domain had no effect. Transient stimulation of ERK was associated with transient effects on cell proliferation [140]. Other investigators have also found that PR-induced S-phase cell cycle entry is ERK-dependent and mediated by the PR-B interaction with the SH3 domain of c-Src kinase in breast cancer cells [142].

In contrast, studies by other investigators suggested that progestin activation of ERK in breast cancer cells requires PR association with both the ER and c-Src (Fig. 2, #6) [35]. In T47-D breast cancer cells, treatment with R5020 activated c-Src and ERK2 within 2–5 min. Surprisingly, this ERK activation was blocked following treatment with anti-estrogens. Further protein–protein interaction experiments using endogenous (in T47-D cells) or exogenous (transfected into COS-7; monkey kidney fibroblast cells) proteins showed that there was an interaction between c-Src, the PR and the ER. In subsequent studies, it was proposed that activation of c-Src and the MAPK pathway by progestins depends upon the presence of the unliganded ER-α phosphorylated at tyrosine 537, which interacts with PR-B via two domains termed ER-interacting domains I (aa 165-345) and II (aa 456-546) that flank, but do not include, PR's proline-rich sequence [98]. It is possible that some of the differences in results between these two groups are because overexpression of steroid receptors in COS-7 cells leads to concentration-dependent formation of different signaling complexes that require other signaling and adaptor molecules. Finally, additional PR sequences have been defined, including a proline-rich CD domain that can associate with MEK [143]. These data suggest that the PR may serve as a scaffold protein and associate with more signaling molecules than previously thought, thus providing docking interactions to coordinate the activation of downstream signaling pathways upon PR trans-activation. These properties may be relevant to breast cancer progression characterized by high protein kinase activities, and therapies targeted to block only the transcriptional activity would fail to target other relevant (non-nuclear) biological actions.

6 Cancers Other Than Breast Cancer Whose Etiology is Influenced by the Estrogen Receptor, c-Src, and HER Family Members

The role of the ER in the genesis and development of cancers in non-reproductive organs is complex (when studied) or altogether unexplored. The existence of two major isoforms of the ER, ER-α and ER-β, as well as related steroid receptors, and their different responses to steroid hormones adds to the difficulty in defining a clear role for this class of receptors in non-reproductive tissue cancers.

For example, ERs (mostly ER-β) are expressed in a subset of gliomas, which are inhibited and even undergo apoptosis in response to both agonists and antagonists of the ER in experimental animals [144], raising the question as to whether the ER plays an oncogenic or tumor suppressive role. Esophageal cancers can also express ER-α and -β, but the relationship between expression of these receptors and clinical outcome remains controversial [145].

However, in colon cancer ER expression is reduced or absent, both in tumors themselves and in a subpopulation of cells in the normal colonic mucosa that accumulate as a function of age, suggesting that in younger colonic mucosa the ER may be protective against the disease. Reduced expression of the ER is associated with methylation of CpG islands in the ER gene [146] and may represent one of the earliest events in disease formation. A meta-analysis done by Grodstein and colleagues [147] showed that a reduced incidence of the disease is associated with women undergoing postmenopausal hormone replacement therapy. Together these findings provide some evidence that estrogen has protective, pro-survival effects in the colon. A similar methylation of the ER gene locus was found in prostate cancer, which increased in frequency with disease progression [148]. Tanaka et al. [149] also reported the existence of polymorphisms within the ER gene, one of which (in codon 10) may be a risk factor for developing prostate cancer. The mechanistic role of this polymorphism is unknown.

In thyroid cancers, a recent study by Kavanagh et al. [150] in which 111 thyroid tumor samples were analyzed showed that ER-α co-localization with its coactivator, SRC-1, in the nucleus strongly correlated with non-anaplastic tumors and reduced disease-free survival, while co-localization with its corepressor, NCoR, was associated with anaplastic tumors and predicted increased survival. These findings suggest that coregulators of the ER-α can contribute to disease outcome.

Multiple studies have reported the presence of ERs in pancreatic and non-small cell lung cancer (NSCLC) cell lines and tumor samples, but the responses of these cells to anti-hormonal therapies have been variable. Konduri and Schwarz [151] and Kawai et al. [152] concluded that variations in the ratio of ER-β/ER-α may help to explain the inconsistencies among studies and may highlight the complexities involved in anti-hormonal therapies for these cancers.

In summary, the role of the ER in the etiology and progression of cancers in non-reproductive tissues is quite well substantiated by evidence in a number of disease sites. However, whether the ER plays a pro-tumorigenic or anti-tumorigenic role appears to differ from tissue to tissue and regulated by the ratio of the two ER isoforms, the predominance of coactivators vs. corepressors, and the other prognostic indicators of disease that are unique or dominant in those organs.

7 Role of c-Src/HER Family in Resistance to Hormone, Cytotoxic, or Targeted Therapies in Breast Cancer

7.1 c-Src as a Resistance Factor in Hormone, Cytotoxic, and Targeted Therapies in Breast Cancer

Because c-Src is overexpressed and hyperactivated in the majority of breast cancers [101, 153, 154] and plays a crucial role in orchestrating signaling pathways controlling a wide range of cellular functions in breast cancer (see above), it is being more closely examined as a factor in resistance to multiple therapeutic strategies, including those that use hormonal, cytotoxic, or molecularly targeted agents. Its biologically synergistic partners, HER family members, which are co-overexpressed with c-Src in ~70% of breast cancers can also play a role in resistance.

7.2 c-Src as a Resistance Factor to Hormonal Therapy in Breast Cancer

Several preclinical studies have tested the anti-tumor effect of a combination of c-Src inhibitors and anti-estrogen agents. Vallabhaneni and colleagues [155] tested the combination of tamoxifen and dasatinib (c-Src inhibitor) in mouse xenografts of MCF-7 breast cancer cells engineered to be resistant to tamoxifen treatment by deregulation of MNAR (PELP-1, an ER transcriptional coregulator and scaffold) or HER2. They found that treatment with dasatinib alone had significant anti-tumor activity on both cell lines but that combined treatment exhibited greater anti-tumor activity in the MCF-7-PELP1 resistant cells. Riggins and collaborators [41] showed that MCF-7 cells overexpressing the c-Src substrate and activator, p130Cas, exhibited tamoxifen-resistant cell growth in response to estrogen, and that this resistance was dependent upon the c-Src/EGFR Tyr 845/Stat5b axis. Together, these studies provide strong evidence for c-Src as a resistance factor in hormonal therapy and rationale for clinical trials in breast cancer combining anti-estrogens with c-Src-targeted inhibitors.

7.3 c-Src and EGFR as Resistance Factors to Cytotoxic Therapies in Breast Cancer

Studies in pancreatic, ovarian and colon cancer cell lines support the idea of c-Src as a resistance factor, reporting c-Src-mediated insensitivities to gemcitabine and 5-fluorouracil [116, 156], paclitaxel [157] and oxaliplatin [158], respectively. In MCF-7 breast cancer cells, c-Src has been shown to mediate resistance to adriamycin [159] and doxorubicin [160].

EGFR has also been implicated in resistance to capecitabine + lapatinib in patients [161] and doxorubicin in MCF-7 cells [160]. An intriguing study by Chang and colleagues [162] that focused on an intrinsically docetaxel- or doxorubicin/cyclophosphamide-resistant subpopulation of breast cancer cells that were termed "breast cancer stem cells" (CD44+/CD24-/HER2-) found that co-treatment of patients with lapatinib (a dual EGFR/HER2 inhibitor) decreased the frequency of these cells, suggesting that EGFR may play a role in the survival or renewal of this stem cell-like population that harbors intrinsic resistance to chemotherapeutic agents.

7.4 c-Src and EGFR as Resistance Factors to Inhibitors of EGFR Family Members

Trastuzumab is a monoclonal antibody used extensively to treat HER2+ breast tumors, but the majority of the patients inevitably experience recurrence of their tumors. This resistance has been linked to formation of EGFR/Met receptor (hepatocyte growth factor receptor) complexes [163] and elevated levels of HB-EGF, an alternative ligand of the EGFR [164]. Zhang and colleagues [165] recently identified c-Src as a major resistance factor to trastuzumab in breast cancer xenografts. Resistant cells showed increased levels of EGFR, HER2, and IGF-1R as well as hyperactivated c-Src, a known coactivator and signaling partner to these receptors. Treatment with c-Src inhibitors reduced tumor size, indicating that active c-Src was critical to the resistant phenotype. C-Src was also linked to lapatinib resistance in a study utilizing lapatinib-resistant breast cancer cell lines [166].

8 c-Src/HER Family Targeted Therapies in Single Agent or Combinatorial Studies

Based on a preponderance of evidence (some of which is described in this chapter), efforts are underway from all sectors of the scientific community to develop inhibitors for c-Src and HER family members. Many of them have been or are being tested in animals, and a select few have moved to the clinical setting. Below are representative examples of therapeutic agents that are available to target these two families of tyrosine kinases. More complete listings of c-Src/HER family inhibitors can be found in more extensive reviews on the subject [58, 167–169].

8.1 c-Src Targeted Therapies

Two small molecule c-Src inhibitors are currently being tested in the clinic. Dasatinib (BMS-354825, Sprycel), an ATP-competitive inhibitor [170, 171] of SFKs, Bcr-Abl, c-Kit, PDGFR, c-FMS, and EphA2 [170], is approved for treatment of imatinib-resistant chronic myelogenous leukemia and Philadelphia chromosome-positive acute lymphoblastic leukemia [171]. Based on studies in breast cancer cell lines [170, 171], dasatinib was tested in triple negative disease and shown to have only a very modest effect as a single agent [172]. Similar results were observed in patients with advanced HR+ or HER+ disease. However, results from a phase I trial evaluating dasatinib and capecitabine demonstrated a 22% partial response rate and 33% who had stable disease [171], indicating that combinatorial treatment was more effective than single agents. Ongoing trials are testing the efficacy of dasatinib with estrogen antagonists [171, 173].

Saracatinib (ADZ0530) is a selective, potent, orally-available competitive ATP-inhibitor that targets both SFKs and Abl tyrosine kinase. It inhibits the in vitro proliferation, migration and invasion of breast, leukemia, prostate, colon, ovarian, or NSCLC cell lines and shows mixed ability to inhibit growth of pancreatic and ER+ breast cancer xenografts [174]. This inhibitor is currently being evaluated with the aromatase inhibitor, anastrozole, in a phase I/II trial in postmenopausal advanced/metastatic HR+ breast cancer patients [175].

8.2 EGFR and HER2 Inhibitors

Perhaps the best known EGFR inhibitor is gefitinib (Iressa, ZD1839), an orally-active, reversible ATP-competitive TKI [174], approved for NSCLC that is refractory to chemotherapy [176]. Studies indicate that gefitinib and endocrine therapy co-treatment of endocrine-resistant cell lines restores sensitivity to the hormonal treatment [177], and results from multiple phase II trials show that while gefitinib may be advantageous to some HR+ breast cancer populations, those subsets need to be more clearly defined [178]. To this end, several phase II trials assessing its use as a monotherapy or in conjunction with ER-targeted drugs are currently being carried out in metastatic HR+ breast cancer patients [179].

Erlotinib (Tarceva) is another orally active, reversible EGFR TKI [174] that has been approved both for the treatment of selected NSCLC and pancreatic cancers [176]. This drug is currently being evaluated in phase II trials in HR+ breast cancers in conjunction with letrozole or fulvestrant, which inhibit estrogen production and ER function, respectively [177].

Trastuzumab (Herceptin) is a humanized monoclonal antibody that targets the HER2 extracellular domain [174] and is approved for the treatment of HER2+ breast cancer as a monotherapy or in conjunction with chemotherapeutic or hormonal agents [180]. Results of multiple preclinical and clinical studies have demonstrated that combinatorial treatments significantly improved disease-free survival, response rate, time to progression, and clinical benefit as compared to single treatments. Given the efficacy of trastuzumab, a monoclonal antibody that inhibits HER2 and HER3 dimerization, pertuzumab, has been developed and is being evaluated in phase III clinical trials [178].

Lapatinib ditosylate (Tykerb) is an orally-active, reversible, ATP competitor that targets EGFR and HER2 [180] and is approved for use with capecitabine or letrozole in certain populations of HER2+ advanced or metastatic breast cancer [176, 180). Phase II and III studies are currently underway testing lapatinib in combination with tamoxifen in patients who had previously failed tamoxifen treatment or with fulvestrant in postmenopausal women with stage III or IV HR+ breast cancer. Additionally, lapatinib is being evaluated as a monotherapy for metastatic breast cancer resistant to hormone therapy in a phase II study [179].

Acknowledgments This work was generously supported by the National Cancer Institute (P30-CA44579) (M.A.S., S.J.P.), Womens' Oncology Fund of the University of Virginia Cancer Center (M.A.S, S.J.P.), National Cancer Institute (RO1CA123037) (S.J.P), National Cancer Institute Institutional Training Grant (T32 CA009109) (J.E.P), and the Wagner Fellowship Fund (J.E.P.).

References

1. Clemons M, Goss P (2010) Mechanisms of Disease: estrogen and the risk of breast cancer. N Engl J Med 344:276–285
2. Gompel A, Plu-Bureau G (2010) Is the decrease in breast cancer incidence related to a decrease in postmenopausal hormone therapy? Ann N Y Acad Sci 1205:268–276
3. Brisken C, O'Malley B (2010) Hormone action in the mammary gland. Cold Spring Harb Perspect Biol 2:a003178
4. Fox EM, Davis RJ, Shupnik MA (2008) ERbeta in breast cancer–onlooker, passive player, or active protector? Steroids 73:1039–1051

5. Clarke RB, Howell A, Potten CS, Anderson E (1997) Dissociation between steroid receptor expression and cell proliferation in the human breast. Cancer Res 57:4987–4991
6. Fox EM, Bernaciak TM, Wen J, Weaver AM, Shupnik MA, Silva CM (2008) Signal transducer and activator of transcription 5b, c-Src, and epidermal growth factor receptor signaling play integral roles in estrogen-stimulated proliferation of estrogen receptor-positive breast cancer cells. Mol Endocrinol 22:1781–1796
7. Herynk MH, Fuqua SA (2004) Estrogen receptor mutations in human disease. Endocr Rev 25:869–898
8. Biscardi JS, Ishizawar RC, Silva CM, Parsons SJ (2000) Tyrosine kinase signalling in breast cancer: epidermal growth factor receptor and c-Src interactions in breast cancer. Breast Cancer Res 2:203–210
9. Silva CM, Shupnik MA (2007) Integration of steroid and growth factor pathways in breast cancer: focus on signal transducers and activators of transcription and their potential role in resistance. Mol Endocrinol 21:1499–1512
10. Nilsson S, Makela S, Treuter E et al (2001) Mechanisms of estrogen action. Physiol Rev 81:1535–1565
11. Shupnik MA (2004) Crosstalk between steroid receptors and the c-Src-receptor tyrosine kinase pathways: implications for cell proliferation. Oncogene 23:7979–7989
12. Levin ER (2003) Bidirectional signaling between the estrogen receptor and the epidermal growth factor receptor. Mol Endocrinol 17:309–317
13. Hammes SR, Levin ER (2007) Extranuclear steroid receptors: nature and actions. Endocr Rev 28:726–741
14. Prossnitz ER, Oprea TI, Sklar LA, Arterburn JB (2008) The ins and outs of GPR30: a transmembrane estrogen receptor. J Steroid Biochem Mol Biol 109:350–353
15. Song RX, McPherson RA, Adam L et al (2002) Linkage of rapid estrogen action to MAPK activation by ERalpha-Shc association and Shc pathway activation. Mol Endocrinol 16:116–127
16. Song RX, Barnes CJ, Zhang Z, Bao Y, Kumar R, Santen RJ (2004) The role of Shc and insulin-like growth factor 1 receptor in mediating the translocation of estrogen receptor alpha to the plasma membrane. Proc Natl Acad Sci U S A 101:2076–2081
17. Pedram A, Razandi M, Levin ER (2006) Nature of functional estrogen receptor at the plasma membrane. Mol Endocrinol 20:1996–2009
18. Ahola TM, Alkio N, Manninen T, Ylikomi T (2002) Progestin and G protein-coupled receptor 30 inhibit mitogen-activated protein kinase activity in MCF-7 breast cancer cells. Endocrinology 143:4620–4626
19. Bjornstrom L, Sjoberg M (2005) Mechanisms of estrogen receptor signaling: convergence of genomic and nongenomic actions on target genes. Mol Endocrinol 19:833–842
20. Fox EM, Andrade J, Shupnik MA (2009) Novel actions of estrogen to promote proliferation: integration of cytoplasmic and nuclear pathways. Steroids 74:622–627
21. Cabodi S, Moro L, Baj G et al (2004) p130Cas interacts with estrogen receptor alpha and modulates non-genomic estrogen signaling in breast cancer cells. J Cell Sci 117:1603–1611
22. Barletta F, Wong CW, McNally C, Komm BS, Katzenellenbogen B, Cheskis BJ (2004) Characterization of the interactions of estrogen receptor and MNAR in the activation of cSrc. Mol Endocrinol 18:1096–1108
23. Edwards DP, Boonyaratanakornkit V (2003) Rapid extranuclear signaling by the estrogen receptor (ER): MNAR couples ER and Src to the MAP kinase signaling pathway. Mol Interv 3:12–315
24. Summy JM, Gallick GE (2003) Src family kinases in tumor progression and metastasis. Cancer Metastasis Rev 22:337–358
25. Thomas SM, Brugge JS (1997) Cellular functions regulated by Src family kinases. Annu Rev Cell Dev Biol 13:513–609
26. Brown MT, Cooper JA (1996) Regulation, substrates and functions of src. Biochim Biophys Acta 1287:121–149

27. Arnold SF, Obourn JD, Jaffe H, Notides AC (1995) Phosphorylation of the human estrogen receptor on tyrosine 537 in vivo and by src family tyrosine kinases in vitro. Mol Endocrinol 9:24–33
28. Castoria G, Migliaccio A, Bilancio A et al (2001) PI3-kinase in concert with Src promotes the S-phase entry of oestradiol-stimulated MCF-7 cells. EMBO J 20:6050–6059
29. Kraus S, Gioeli D, Vomastek T, Gordon V, Weber MJ (2006) Receptor for activated C kinase 1 (RACK1) and Src regulate the tyrosine phosphorylation and function of the androgen receptor. Cancer Res 66:11047–11054
30. Cheng CY, Kuo CT, Lin CC, Hsieh HL, Yang CM (2010) IL-1beta induces expression of matrix metalloproteinase-9 and cell migration via a c-Src-dependent, growth factor receptor transactivation in A549 cells. Br J Pharmacol 160:1595–1610
31. Lee CW, Lin CC, Lin WN et al (2007) TNF-alpha induces MMP-9 expression via activation of Src/EGFR, PDGFR/PI3K/Akt cascade and promotion of NF-kappaB/p300 binding in human tracheal smooth muscle cells. Am J Physiol Lung Cell Mol Physiol 292:L799–812
32. Wu CY, Hsieh HL, Sun CC, Tseng CP, Yang CM (2008) IL-1 beta induces proMMP-9 expression via c-Src-dependent PDGFR/PI3K/Akt/p300 cascade in rat brain astrocytes. J Neurochem 105:1499–1512
33. Migliaccio A, Di Domenico M, Castoria G et al (1996) Tyrosine kinase/p21ras/MAP-kinase pathway activation by estradiol-receptor complex in MCF-7 cells. EMBO J 15:1292–1300
34. Kumar P, Wu Q, Chambliss KL et al (2007) Direct Interactions with G alpha i and G betagamma mediate nongenomic signaling by estrogen receptor alpha. Mol Endocrinol 21:1370–1380
35. Migliaccio A, Piccolo D, Castoria G et al (1998) Activation of the Src/p21ras/Erk pathway by progesterone receptor via cross-talk with estrogen receptor. EMBO J 17:2008–2018
36. Arnold SF, Vorojeikina DP, Notides AC (1995) Phosphorylation of tyrosine 537 on the human estrogen receptor is required for binding to an estrogen response element. J Biol Chem 270:30205–30212
37. Yudt MR, Vorojeikina D, Zhong L et al (1999) Function of estrogen receptor tyrosine 537 in hormone binding, DNA binding, and transactivation. Biochemistry 38:14146–14156
38. Wong CW, McNally C, Nickbarg E, Komm BS, Cheskis BJ (2002) Estrogen receptor-interacting protein that modulates its nongenomic activity-crosstalk with Src/Erk phosphorylation cascade. Proc Natl Acad Sci U S A 99:14783–14788
39. Cheskis BJ, Greger J, Cooch N et al (2008) MNAR plays an important role in ERa activation of Src/MAPK and PI3K/Akt signaling pathways. Steroids 73:901–905
40. Vadlamudi RK, Wang RA, Mazumdar A et al (2001) Molecular cloning and characterization of PELP1, a novel human coregulator of estrogen receptor alpha. J Biol Chem 276:38272–38279
41. Riggins RB, Thomas KS, Ta HQ et al (2006) Physical and functional interactions between Cas and c-Src induce tamoxifen resistance of breast cancer cells through pathways involving epidermal growth factor receptor and signal transducer and activator of transcription 5b. Cancer Res 66:7007–7015
42. Chen Y, Alvarez EA, Azzam D et al (2010) Combined Src and ER blockade impairs human breast cancer proliferation in vitro and in vivo. Breast Cancer Res Treat
43. Manavathi B, Acconcia F, Rayala SK, Kumar R (2006) An inherent role of microtubule network in the action of nuclear receptor. Proc Natl Acad Sci U S A 103:15981–15986
44. Wang X, Yang Z, Zhang H et al (2008) The estrogen receptor-interacting protein HPIP increases estrogen-responsive gene expression through activation of MAPK and AKT. Biochim Biophys Acta 1783:1220–1228
45. Alam SM, Rajendran M, Ouyang S, Veeramani S, Zhang L, Lin MF (2009) A novel role of Shc adaptor proteins in steroid hormone-regulated cancers. Endocr Relat Cancer 16:1–16
46. Kousteni S, Bellido T, Plotkin LI et al (2001) Nongenotropic, sex-nonspecific signaling through the estrogen or androgen receptors: dissociation from transcriptional activity. Cell 104:719–730

47. Migliaccio A, Di Domenico M, Castoria G et al (2005) Steroid receptor regulation of epidermal growth factor signaling through Src in breast and prostate cancer cells: steroid antagonist action. Cancer Res 65:10585–10593
48. Wells A (1999) EGF receptor. Int J Biochem Cell Biol 31:637–643
49. Normanno N, De Luca A, Bianco C et al (2006) Epidermal growth factor receptor (EGFR) signaling in cancer. Gene 366:2–16
50. Zhang H, Berezov A, Wang Q et al (2007) ErbB receptors: from oncogenes to targeted cancer therapies. J Clin Invest 117:2051–2058
51. Bogdan S, Klambt C (2001) Epidermal growth factor receptor signaling. Curr Biol 11:R292–295
52. Mendelsohn J (2002) Targeting the epidermal growth factor receptor for cancer therapy. J Clin Oncol 20:1S–13S
53. Nicholson RI, Gee JM, Harper ME (2001) EGFR and cancer prognosis. Eur J Cancer 37 Suppl 4:S9-15
54. Velu TJ, Beguinot L, Vass WC et al (1987) Epidermal-growth-factor-dependent transformation by a human EGF receptor proto-oncogene. Science 238:1408–1410
55. Jorissen RN, Walker F, Pouliot N, Garrett TP, Ward CW, Burgess AW (2003) Epidermal growth factor receptor: mechanisms of activation and signalling. Exp Cell Res 284:31–53
56. Ren W, Korchin B, Zhu QS et al (2008) Epidermal growth factor receptor blockade in combination with conventional chemotherapy inhibits soft tissue sarcoma cell growth in vitro and in vivo. Clin Cancer Res 14:2785–2795
57. Lopez JP, Wang-Rodriguez J, Chang C et al (2007) Gefitinib inhibition of drug resistance to doxorubicin by inactivating ABCG2 in thyroid cancer cell lines. Arch Otolaryngol Head Neck Surg 133:1022–1027
58. Harari D, Yarden Y (2000) Molecular mechanisms underlying ErbB2/HER2 action in breast cancer. Oncogene 19:6102–6114
59. Schiffer IB, Gebhard S, Heimerdinger CK et al (2003) Switching off HER-2/neu in a tetracycline-controlled mouse tumor model leads to apoptosis and tumor-size-dependent remission. Cancer Res 63:7221–7231
60. Piccart-Gebhart MJ, Procter M, Leyland-Jones B et al (2005) Trastuzumab after adjuvant chemotherapy in HER2-positive breast cancer. N Engl J Med 353:1659–1672
61. Vogel CL, Cobleigh MA, Tripathy D et al (2002) Efficacy and safety of trastuzumab as a single agent in first-line treatment of HER2-overexpressing metastatic breast cancer. J Clin Oncol 20:719–726
62. Tiezzi DG, Andrade JM, Ribeiro-Silva A, Zola FE, Marana HR, Tiezzi MG (2007) HER-2, p53, p21 and hormonal receptors proteins expression as predictive factors of response and prognosis in locally advanced breast cancer treated with neoadjuvant docetaxel plus epirubicin combination. BMC Cancer 7:36
63. Pritchard KI, Shepherd LE, O'Malley FP et al (2006) HER2 and responsiveness of breast cancer to adjuvant chemotherapy. N Engl J Med 354:2103–2111
64. Tubbs R, Barlow WE, Budd GT et al (2009) Outcome of patients with early-stage breast cancer treated with doxorubicin-based adjuvant chemotherapy as a function of HER2 and TOP2A status. J Clin Oncol 27:3881–3886
65. Del Mastro L, Bruzzi P, Nicolo G et al (2005) HER2 expression and efficacy of dose-dense anthracycline-containing adjuvant chemotherapy in breast cancer patients. Br J Cancer 93:7–14
66. Gilcrease MZ, Woodward WA, Nicolas MM et al (2009) Even low-level HER2 expression may be associated with worse outcome in node-positive breast cancer. Am J Surg Pathol 33:759–767
67. Witton CJ, Reeves JR, Going JJ, Cooke TG, Bartlett JM (2003) Expression of the HER1–4 family of receptor tyrosine kinases in breast cancer. J Pathol 200:290–297
68. Frogne T, Laenkholm AV, Lyng MB, Henriksen KL, Lykkesfeldt AE (2009) Determination of HER2 phosphorylation at tyrosine 1221/1222 improves prediction of poor survival for breast cancer patients with hormone receptor-positive tumors. Breast Cancer Res 11:R11

69. Petit T, Wilt M, Velten M et al (2010) Semi-quantitative evaluation of estrogen receptor expression is a strong predictive factor of pathological complete response after anthracycline-based neo-adjuvant chemotherapy in hormonal-sensitive breast cancer. Breast Cancer Res Treat 124:387–391
70. Huober J, von Minckwitz G, Denkert C et al (2010) Effect of neoadjuvant anthracycline-taxane-based chemotherapy in different biological breast cancer phenotypes: overall results from the GeparTrio study. Breast Cancer Res Treat 124:133–140
71. Darb-Esfahani S, Loibl S, Muller BM et al (2009) Identification of biology-based breast cancer types with distinct predictive and prognostic features: role of steroid hormone and HER2 receptor expression in patients treated with neoadjuvant anthracycline/taxane-based chemotherapy. Breast Cancer Res 11:R69
72. Andre F, Mazouni C, Liedtke C et al (2008) HER2 expression and efficacy of preoperative paclitaxel/FAC chemotherapy in breast cancer. Breast Cancer Res Treat 108:183–190
73. Stoica GE, Franke TF, Moroni M et al (2003) Effect of estradiol on estrogen receptor-alpha gene expression and activity can be modulated by the ErbB2/PI 3-K/Akt pathway. Oncogene 22:7998–8011
74. Oh AS, Lorant LA, Holloway JN, Miller DL, Kern FG, El-Ashry D (2001) Hyperactivation of MAPK induces loss of ERalpha expression in breast cancer cells. Mol Endocrinol 15:1344–1359
75. Zhu Y, Sullivan LL, Nair SS et al (2006) Coregulation of estrogen receptor by ERBB4/HER4 establishes a growth-promoting autocrine signal in breast tumor cells. Cancer Res 66:7991–7998
76. Mendez P, Azcoitia I, Garcia-Segura LM (2003) Estrogen receptor alpha forms estrogen-dependent multimolecular complexes with insulin-like growth factor receptor and phosphatidylinositol 3-kinase in the adult rat brain. Brain Res Mol Brain Res 112:170–176
77. Santen RJ, Fan P, Zhang Z, Bao Y, Song RX, Yue W (2009) Estrogen signals via an extra-nuclear pathway involving IGF-1R and EGFR in tamoxifen-sensitive and -resistant breast cancer cells. Steroids 74:586–594
78. Song RX, Zhang Z, Chen Y, Bao Y, Santen RJ (2007) Estrogen signaling via a linear pathway involving insulin-like growth factor I receptor, matrix metalloproteinases, and epidermal growth factor receptor to activate mitogen-activated protein kinase in MCF-7 breast cancer cells. Endocrinology 148:4091–4101
79. Song RX, Chen Y, Zhang Z et al (2010) Estrogen utilization of IGF-1-R and EGF-R to signal in breast cancer cells. J Steroid Biochem Mol Biol 118:219–230
80. Hewitt SC, Li Y, Li L, Korach KS (2010) Estrogen-mediated regulation of Igf1 transcription and uterine growth involves direct binding of estrogen receptor alpha to estrogen-responsive elements. J Biol Chem 285:2676–2685
81. Madeo A, Maggiolini M (2010) Nuclear alternate estrogen receptor GPR30 mediates 17beta-estradiol-induced gene expression and migration in breast cancer-associated fibroblasts. Cancer Res 70:6036–6046
82. Filardo EJ (2002) Epidermal growth factor receptor (EGFR) transactivation by estrogen via the G-protein-coupled receptor, GPR30: a novel signaling pathway with potential significance for breast cancer. J Steroid Biochem Mol Biol 80:231–238
83. Filardo EJ, Quinn JA, Bland KI, Frackelton AR Jr (2000) Estrogen-induced activation of Erk-1 and Erk-2 requires the G protein-coupled receptor homolog, GPR30, and occurs via trans-activation of the epidermal growth factor receptor through release of HB-EGF. Mol Endocrinol 14:1649–1660
84. Vivacqua A, Lappano R, De Marco P et al (2009) G protein-coupled receptor 30 expression is up-regulated by EGF and TGF alpha in estrogen receptor alpha-positive cancer cells. Mol Endocrinol 23:1815–1826
85. Naresh A, Thor AD, Edgerton SM, Torkko KC, Kumar R, Jones FE (2008) The HER4/4ICD estrogen receptor coactivator and BH3-only protein is an effector of tamoxifen-induced apoptosis. Cancer Res 68:6387–6395

86. Chen JQ, Delannoy M, Cooke C, Yager JD (2004) Mitochondrial localization of ERalpha and ERbeta in human MCF7 cells. Am J Physiol Endocrinol Metab 286:E1011–1022
87. Vidal GA, Naresh A, Marrero L, Jones FE (2005) Presenilin-dependent gamma-secretase processing regulates multiple ERBB4/HER4 activities. J Biol Chem 280:19777–19783
88. Naresh A, Long W, Vidal GA et al (2006) The ERBB4/HER4 intracellular domain 4ICD is a BH3-only protein promoting apoptosis of breast cancer cells. Cancer Res 66:6412–6420
89. Kato S, Endoh H, Masuhiro Y et al (1995) Activation of the estrogen receptor through phosphorylation by mitogen-activated protein kinase. Science 270:1491–1494
90. Bunone G, Briand PA, Miksicek RJ, Picard D (1996) Activation of the unliganded estrogen receptor by EGF involves the MAP kinase pathway and direct phosphorylation. Embo J 15:2174–2183
91. Marquez DC, Lee J, Lin T, Pietras RJ (2001) Epidermal growth factor receptor and tyrosine phosphorylation of estrogen receptor. Endocrine 16:73–81
92. Curtis SW, Washburn T, Sewall C et al (1996) Physiological coupling of growth factor and steroid receptor signaling pathways: estrogen receptor knockout mice lack estrogen-like response to epidermal growth factor. Proc Natl Acad Sci U S A 93:12626–12630
93. Vignon F, Bouton MM, Rochefort H (1987) Antiestrogens inhibit the mitogenic effect of growth factors on breast cancer cells in the total absence of estrogens. Biochem Biophys Res Commun 146:1502–1508
94. Montero JC, Rodriguez-Barrueco R, Ocana A, Diaz-Rodriguez E, Esparis-Ogando A, Pandiella A (2008) Neuregulins and cancer. Clin Cancer Res 14:3237–3241
95. Loi S, Sotiriou C, Haibe-Kains B et al (2009) Gene expression profiling identifies activated growth factor signaling in poor prognosis (Luminal-B) estrogen receptor positive breast cancer. BMC Med Genomics 2:37
96. St-Laurent V, Sanchez M, Charbonneau C, Tremblay A (2005) Selective hormone-dependent repression of estrogen receptor beta by a p38-activated ErbB2/ErbB3 pathway. J Steroid Biochem Mol Biol 94:23–37
97. Lindberg K, Helguero LA, Omoto Y, Gustafsson JA, Haldosen LA (2011) EstrogenEstrogen receptor beta represses Akt signaling in breast cancer cells via downregulation of HER2/HER3 and upregulation of PTEN - implications for tamoxifen sensitivity. Breast Cancer Res 13:R43
98. Ballare C, Uhrig M, Bechtold T et al (2003) Two domains of the progesterone receptor interact with the estrogen receptor and are required for progesterone activation of the c-Src/Erk pathway in mammalian cells. Mol Cell Biol 23:1994–2008
99. Novaro V, Roskelley CD, Bissell MJ (2003) Collagen-IV and laminin-1 regulate estrogen receptor alpha expression and function in mouse mammary epithelial cells. J Cell Sci 116: 2975–2986
100. Sisci D, Aquila S, Middea E et al (2004) Fibronectin and type IV collagen activate ERalpha AF-1 by c-Src pathway: effect on breast cancer cell motility. Oncogene 23:8920–8930
101. Biscardi JS, Tice DA, Parsons SJ (1999) c-Src, receptor tyrosine kinases, and human cancer. Adv Cancer Res 76:61–119
102. Ishizawar R, Parsons SJ (2004) c-Src and cooperating partners in human cancer. Cancer Cell 6:209–214
103. Boerner JL, Biscardi JS, Silva CM, Parsons SJ (2005) Transactivating agonists of the EGF receptor require Tyr 845 phosphorylation for induction of DNA synthesis. Mol Carcinog 44:262–273
104. Weaver AM, Silva CM (2007) Signal transducer and activator of transcription 5b: a new target of breast tumor kinase/protein tyrosine kinase 6. Breast Cancer Res 9:R79
105. Boerner JL, Demory ML, Silva C, Parsons SJ (2004) Phosphorylation of Y845 on the epidermal growth factor receptor mediates binding to the mitochondrial protein cytochrome c oxidase subunit II. Mol Cell Biol 24:7059–7071
106. Demory ML, Boerner JL, Davidson R et al (2009) Epidermal growth factor receptor translocation to the mitochondria: regulation and effect. J Biol Chem 284:36592–6604

107. Cao X, Zhu H, Ali-Osman F, Lo HW (2011) EGFR and EGFRvIII undergo stress- and EGFR kinase inhibitor-induced mitochondrial translocalization: a potential mechanism of EGFR-driven antagonism of apoptosis. Mol Cancer 10:26
108. Garcia R, Bowman TL, Niu G et al (2001) Constitutive activation of Stat3 by the Src and JAK tyrosine kinases participates in growth regulation of human breast carcinoma cells. Oncogene 20:2499–2513
109. Bernaciak TM, Zareno J, Parsons JT, Silva CM (2009) A novel role for signal transducer and activator of transcription 5b (STAT5b) in beta1-integrin-mediated human breast cancer cell migration. Breast Cancer Res 11:R52
110. Miyake T, Parsons SJ (2011) Functional interactions link choline kinase to EGFR and c-Src in breast cancer cell proliferation. Oncogene (Epub ahead of print)
111. Al-Saffar NM, Jackson LE, Raynaud FI et al (2010) The phosphoinositide 3-kinase inhibitor PI-103 downregulates choline kinase alpha leading to phosphocholine and total choline decrease detected by magnetic resonance spectroscopy. Cancer Res 70:5507–5517
112. Cuadrado A, Carnero A, Dolfi F, Jimenez B, Lacal JC (1993) Phosphorycholine: a novel second messenger essential for mitogenic activity of growth factors. Oncogene 8:2959–2968
113. Parsons SJ, Parsons JT (2004) Src family kinases, key regulators of signal transduction. Oncogene 23:7906–7909
114. Bromann PA, Korkaya H, Courtneidge SA (2004) The interplay between Src family kinases and receptor tyrosine kinases. Oncogene 23:7957–7968
115. Reynolds AB, Roczniak-Ferguson A (2004) Emerging roles for p120-catenin in cell adhesion and cancer. Oncogene 23:7947–7956
116. Ischenko I, Camaj P, Seeliger H et al (2008) Inhibition of Src tyrosine kinase reverts chemoresistance toward 5-fluorouracil in human pancreatic carcinoma cells: an involvement of epidermal growth factor receptor signaling. Oncogene 27:7212–7222
117. Lurje G, Lenz HJ (2009) EGFR signaling and drug discovery. Oncology 77:400–410
118. Belsches-Jablonski AP, Biscardi JS, Peavy DR, Tice DA, Romney DA, Parsons SJ (2001) Src family kinases and HER2 interactions in human breast cancer cell growth and survival. Oncogene 20:1465–1475
119. Ishizawar RC, Miyake T, Parsons SJ (2007) c-Src modulates ErbB2 and ErbB3 heterocomplex formation and function. Oncogene 26:3503–3510
120. Cabioglu N, Summy J, Miller C et al (2005) CXCL-12/stromal cell-derived factor-1alpha transactivates HER2-neu in breast cancer cells by a novel pathway involving Src kinase activation. Cancer Res 65:6493–6497
121. Wang SE, Xiang B, Zent R, Quaranta V, Pozzi A, Arteaga CL (2009) Transforming growth factor beta induces clustering of HER2 and integrins by activating Src-focal adhesion kinase and receptor association to the cytoskeleton. Cancer Res 69:475–482
122. Peters AA, Buchanan G, Ricciardelli C et al (2009) Androgen receptor inhibits estrogen receptor-alpha activity and is prognostic in breast cancer. Cancer Res 69:6131–6140
123. Castellano I, Allia E, Accortanzo V et al (2010) Androgen receptor expression is a significant prognostic factor in estrogen receptor positive breast cancers. Breast Cancer Res Treat 124:607–617
124. Hu R, Dawood S, Holmes MD et al (2011) Androgen receptor expression and breast cancer survival in postmenopausal women. Clin Cancer Res
125. Migliaccio A, Castoria G, Di Domenico M et al (2000) Steroid-induced androgen receptor-oestradiol receptor beta-Src complex triggers prostate cancer cell proliferation. Embo J 19:5406–5417
126. Hamzeh M, Robaire B (2011) Androgens activate mitogen-activated protein kinase via epidermal growth factor receptor/insulin-like growth factor 1 receptor in the mouse PC-1 cell line. J Endocrinol 209:55–64
127. Migliaccio A, Varricchio L, De Falco A et al (2007) Inhibition of the SH3 domain-mediated binding of Src to the androgen receptor and its effect on tumor growth. Oncogene 26: 6619–6629

128. Zhou J, Hernandez G, Tu SW et al (2005) Synergistic induction of DOC-2/DAB2 gene expression in transitional cell carcinoma in the presence of GATA6 and histone deacetylase inhibitor. Cancer Res 65:6089–6096
129. Cops EJ, Bianco-Miotto T, Moore NL et al (2008) Antiproliferative actions of the synthetic androgen, mibolerone, in breast cancer cells are mediated by both androgen and progesterone receptors. J Steroid Biochem Mol Biol 110:236–243
130. Birrell SN, Butler LM, Harris JM, Buchanan G, Tilley WD (2007) Disruption of androgen receptor signaling by synthetic progestins may increase risk of developing breast cancer. Faseb J 21:2285–2293
131. Sanga S, Broom BM, Cristini V, Edgerton ME (2009) Gene expression meta-analysis supports existence of molecular apocrine breast cancer with a role for androgen receptor and implies interactions with ErbB family. BMC Med Genomics 2:59
132. Naderi A, Chia KM, Liu J (2011) Synergy between inhibitors of androgen receptor and MEK has therapeutic implications in estrogen receptor-negative breast cancer. Breast Cancer Res 13:R36
133. Lange CA (2004) Making sense of cross-talk between steroid hormone receptors and intracellular signaling pathways: who will have the last word? Mol Endocrinol 18:269–278
134. Richer JK, Jacobsen BM, Manning NG, Abel MG, Wolf DM, Horwitz KB (2002) Differential gene regulation by the two progesterone receptor isoforms in human breast cancer cells. J Biol Chem 277:5209–5218
135. Ward RD, Weigel NL (2009) Steroid receptor phosphorylation: Assigning function to site-specific phosphorylation. Biofactors 35:528–536
136. Faivre EJ, Daniel AR, Hillard CJ, Lange CA (2008) Progesterone receptor rapid signaling mediates serine 345 phosphorylation and tethering to specificity protein 1 transcription factors. Mol Endocrinol 22:823–837
137. Daniel AR, Qiu M, Faivre EJ, Ostrander JH, Skildum A, Lange CA (2007) Linkage of progestin and epidermal growth factor signaling: phosphorylation of progesterone receptors mediates transcriptional hypersensitivity and increased ligand-independent breast cancer cell growth. Steroids 72:188–201
138. Abdel-Hafiz H, Dudevoir ML, Horwitz KB (2009) Mechanisms underlying the control of progesterone receptor transcriptional activity by SUMOylation. J Biol Chem 284: 9099–9108
139. Daniel AR, Lange CA (2009) Protein kinases mediate ligand-independent derepression of sumoylated progesterone receptors in breast cancer cells. Proc Natl Acad Sci U S A 106:14287–14292
140. Boonyaratanakornkit V, McGowan E, Sherman L, Mancini MA, Cheskis BJ, Edwards DP (2007) The role of extranuclear signaling actions of progesterone receptor in mediating progesterone regulation of gene expression and the cell cycle. Mol Endocrinol 21:359–375
141. Boonyaratanakornkit V, Scott MP, Ribon V et al (2001) Progesterone receptor contains a proline-rich motif that directly interacts with SH3 domains and activates c-Src family tyrosine kinases. Mol Cell 8:269–280
142. Skildum A, Faivre E, Lange CA (2005) Progesterone receptors induce cell cycle progression via activation of mitogen-activated protein kinases. Mol Endocrinol 19: 327–339
143. Hagan CR, Faivre EJ, Lange CA (2009) Scaffolding actions of membrane-associated progesterone receptors. Steroids 74:568–572
144. Kabat GC, Etgen AM, Rohan TE (2010) Do steroid hormones play a role in the etiology of glioma? Cancer Epidemiol Biomarkers Prev 19:2421–2427
145. Rashid F, Khan RN, Iftikhar SY (2010) Probing the link between oestrogen receptors and oesophageal cancer. World J Surg Oncol 8:9
146. Issa JP, Ottaviano YL, Celano P, Hamilton SR, Davidson NE, Baylin SB (1994) Methylation of the oestrogen receptor CpG island links ageing and neoplasia in human colon. Nat Genet 7:536–540

147. Grodstein F, Newcomb PA, Stampfer MJ (1999) Postmenopausal hormone therapy and the risk of colorectal cancer: a review and meta-analysis. Am J Med 106:574–582
148. Li LC, Chui R, Nakajima K, Oh BR, Au HC, Dahiya R (2000) Frequent methylation of estrogen receptor in prostate cancer: correlation with tumor progression. Cancer Res 60:702–706
149. Tanaka Y, Sasaki M, Kaneuchi M, Shiina H, Igawa M, Dahiya R (2003) Polymorphisms of estrogen receptor alpha in prostate cancer. Mol Carcinog 37:202–208
150. Kavanagh DO, McIlroy M, Myers E et al (2010) The role of oestrogen receptor alpha in human thyroid cancer: contributions from coregulatory proteins and the tyrosine kinase receptor HER2. Endocr Relat Cancer 17:255–264
151. Konduri S, Schwarz RE (2007) Estrogen receptor beta/alpha ratio predicts response of pancreatic cancer cells to estrogens and phytoestrogens. J Surg Res 140:55–66
152. Kawai H, Ishii A, Washiya K et al (2005) Estrogen receptor alpha and beta are prognostic factors in non-small cell lung cancer. Clin Cancer Res 11:5084–5089
153. Jacobs C, Rubsamen H (1983) Expression of pp60c-src protein kinase in adult and fetal human tissue: high activities in some sarcomas and mammary carcinomas. Cancer Res 43:1696–1702
154. Ottenhoff-Kalff AE, Rijksen G, van Beurden EA, Hennipman A, Michels AA, Staal GE (1992) Characterization of protein tyrosine kinases from human breast cancer: involvement of the c-src oncogene product. Cancer Res 52:4773–4778
155. Vallabhaneni S, Nair BC, Cortez V et al (2010) Significance of ER-Src axis in hormonal therapy resistance. Breast Cancer Res Treat
156. Duxbury MS, Ito H, Zinner MJ, Ashley SW, Whang EE (2004) Inhibition of SRC tyrosine kinase impairs inherent and acquired gemcitabine resistance in human pancreatic adenocarcinoma cells. Clin Cancer Res 10:2307–2318
157. George JA, Chen T, Taylor CC (2005) SRC tyrosine kinase and multidrug resistance protein-1 inhibitions act independently but cooperatively to restore paclitaxel sensitivity to paclitaxel-resistant ovarian cancer cells. Cancer Res 65:10381–10388
158. Kopetz S, Lesslie DP, Dallas NA et al (2009) Synergistic activity of the SRC family kinase inhibitor dasatinib and oxaliplatin in colon carcinoma cells is mediated by oxidative stress. Cancer Res 69:3842–3849
159. Ta HQ, Thomas KS, Schrecengost RS, Bouton AH (2008) A novel association between p130Cas and resistance to the chemotherapeutic drug adriamycin in human breast cancer cells. Cancer Res 68:8796–8804
160. Pritchard JE, Conaway MR, Silva CM, Parsons SJ (2011) A mechanistic study of the effect of doxorubicin/adriamycin on the estrogen response in a breast cancer model. Submitted
161. Rhee J, Han SW, Cha Y et al (2010) High serum TGF-alpha predicts poor response to lapatinib and capecitabine in HER2-positive breast cancer. Breast Cancer Res Treat 125:107–114
162. Li X, Lewis MT, Huang J et al (2008) Intrinsic resistance of tumorigenic breast cancer cells to chemotherapy. J Natl Cancer Inst 100:672–679
163. Mueller KL, Yang ZQ, Haddad R, Ethier SP, Boerner JL (2010) EGFR/Met association regulates EGFR TKI resistance in breast cancer. J Mol Signal 5:8
164. Balzer EM, Whipple RA, Thompson K et al (2010) c-Src differentially regulates the functions of microtentacles and invadopodia. Oncogene 29:6402–6408
165. Zhang S, Huang WC, Li P et al (2011) Combating trastuzumab resistance by targeting SRC, a common node downstream of multiple resistance pathways. Nat Med 17:461–469
166. Rexer BN, Ham AJ, Rinehart C et al (2011) Phosphoproteomic mass spectrometry profiling links Src family kinases to escape from HER2 tyrosine kinase inhibition. Oncogene
167. Mayer EL, Krop IE (2010) Advances in targeting SRC in the treatment of breast cancer and other solid malignancies. Clin Cancer Res 16:3526–3532
168. Puls LN, Eadens M, Messersmith W (2011) Current status of SRC inhibitors in solid tumor malignancies. Oncologist 16:566–578

169. Hudis CA (2007) Trastuzumab–mechanism of action and use in clinical practice. N Engl J Med 357:39–51
170. Boschelli F, Arndt K, Gambacorti-Passerini C (2010) Bosutinib: a review of preclinical studies in chronic myelogenous leukaemia. Eur J Cancer 46:1781–1789
171. Araujo J, Logothetis C (2010) Dasatinib: a potent SRC inhibitor in clinical development for the treatment of solid tumors. Cancer Treat Rev 36:492–500
172. Somlo G, Atzori F, Strauss L et al (2009) Dasatinib plus capecitabine (Cap) for progressive advanced breast cancer(ABC): Phase I study CA180004. J Clin Oncol 27:43s
173. Mayer E, Baurain J, Sparano J et al (2009) Dasatinib in advanced HER2/neu amplified and ER/PR-positive breast cancer: Phase II study CA180088. J Clin Oncol 27:43s
174. NCI (2011) Clinical Trials Database. National Cancer Institute
175. Green TP, Fennell M, Whittaker R et al (2009) Preclinical anticancer activity of the potent, oral Src inhibitor AZD0530. Mol Oncol
176. Moon C, Chae YK, Lee J (2010) Targeting epidermal growth factor receptor in head and neck cancer: lessons learned from cetuximab. Exp Biol Med (Maywood) 235:907–920
177. NCI (2011) Cancer Drug Information. National Cancer Institute
178. Buzdar AU (2009) Role of biologic therapy and chemotherapy in hormone receptor- and HER2-positive breast cancer. Ann Oncol 20:993–999
179. Cleator SJ, Ahamed E, Coombes RC, Palmieri C (2009) A 2009 update on the treatment of patients with hormone receptor-positive breast cancer. Clin Breast Cancer 9 Suppl 1:S6-S17
180. Lin SX, Chen J, Mazumdar M et al (2010) Molecular therapy of breast cancer: progress and future directions. Nat Rev Endocrinol 6:485–493

Cross Talk Between ERα and Src Signaling and Its Relevance to ER Status and Hormone Responsiveness

Jun Sun, Wen Zhou, Zafar Nawaz and Joyce M. Slingerland

Abstract While two thirds of breast cancers are ER positive and a majority of these are responsive to endocrine therapies, up to one third of newly diagnosed breast cancers lack detectable ER protein. ER negative breast cancers are thought to be resistance to endocrine therapy. Here we review several potential mechanisms underlying the ER negative status of these breast cancers. The role of cross-talk between ER and Src-activated signal transduction as a mediator of both ER proteolysis and ER transactivation is discussed. Src kinase is often activated in breast cancer. Liganded ER rapidly and transiently activates Src which phosphorylates ER. For a subset of ER-responsive promoters, ER phosphorylation by Src leads to enhanced ER binding to the promoter, increased interactions with E3 ubiquitin ligases, and rapid ER degradation, in a process in which ER activation is coupled to its degradation. Thus, the function of ER may not be solely dependent

J. Sun · W. Zhou · Z. Nawaz · J. M. Slingerland
Braman Family Breast Cancer Institute, University of Miami Sylvester
Comprehensive Cancer Center, Miami, FL 33136, USA
e-mail: jsun@med.miami.edu

W. Zhou
e-mail: wzhou@med.miami.edu

Z. Nawaz
e-mail: znawaz@med.miami.edu

J. M. Slingerland
Departments of Medicine, University of Miami Miller School of Medicine,
Miami, FL 33136, USA

W. Zhou · Z. Nawaz · J. M. Slingerland (✉)
Biochemistry & Molecular Biology, University of Miami Miller School of Medicine,
Miami, FL 33136, USA
e-mail: jslingerland@med.miami.edu

G. Castoria and A. Migliaccio (eds.), *Advances in Rapid Sex-Steroid Action*,
DOI: 10.1007/978-1-4614-1764-4_4, © Springer Science+Business Media, LLC 2012

on the steady state levels of ER protein. A subset of ER negative breast cancers that have ER mRNA but lack detectable ER protein levels may ultimately prove to be responsive to estrogen. These observations may have broader implications for estrogen driven gene expression. Cells of estrogen responsive tissues (ovary, bone, brain and intestine) could have low ER protein levels, but retain responses to estrogen through estrogen driven ER proteolysis-coupled transcriptional activity.

Keywords Estrogen receptor · Src kinase · Breast cancer · Signal transduction · Ubiquitin · Proteolysis

Abbreviations

EGF	Epidermal growth factor
EGFR	Epidermal growth factor receptor
ER	Estrogen receptor
ERK	Extracellular signal-regulated kinase
Her 2	Human epidermal growth factor receptor 2
IGF	Insulin growth factor
IGF-IR	IGF-I receptor
MAPK	Mitogen activated protein kinase
MEK	Mitogen-activated protein (MAP) kinase kinase
PI3K	Phosphatidylinositol 3-kinase
Ras	Rat sarcoma

Contents

1 Estrogen Receptor in Breast Cancer

Estrogen regulates proliferation of many cell types expressing its cognate receptors and is a risk factor for breast cancer development. Estrogen exerts its biological functions through binding to its intracellular receptors, the estrogen receptors, ERα and ERβ, which are members of the nuclear hormone receptor superfamily [1]. The two different types of ER identified in humans, ERα and ERβ are encoded by different genes [2–4]. ERα is expressed in the epithelium of the breast, endometrium, ovary, bone and brain in the adult human [2]. ERβ is widely expressed throughout the body. ERα co-exists with ERβ in the mammary epithelium, uterus, adipose tissue, skeletal muscle, liver, pancreas and the central nervous system. ERβ is also expressed in ERα-negative tissues including the prostatic and pulmonary epithelium [5]. While ERβ is expressed in some breast cancers, the prognostic implications of this have not been fully defined [6]. The vast majority of studies of ER in breast cancer pertain to ERα [7]. Since this review addresses ERα, exclusively, hereafter ER refers to only ERα.

When activated by estrogen binding, ER dissociates from heat shock protein, dimerizes, translocates into the nucleus, and recruits coregulators to the regulatory regions in the target genes to modulate gene transcription. ER coregulators have been shown with diverse functions which include acetylation, methylation, ubiquitination and phosphorylation [8].

ER protein is assayed in breast cancer because it is a clinically useful prognostic factor and is predictive of response to endocrine therapy. A majority of newly diagnosed breast cancers express levels of ER protein that are clinically detectable either by immunohistochemistry or by cytosolic ligand-binding assay. In the past, ligand-binding assay was used to examine the level of ER in breast tumors. Tumors with an ER content of $\geq$10 fmol/mg protein were considered to be ER-positive [9]. Immunohistochemistry is less costly and is now more widely used to assess ER status in breast tumors which can predict response to endocrine therapy, although the ER status determined by immunohistochemistry is not always in agreement with the ligand-binding assay method [10]. Tumors that show detectable ER protein is at least 10% of tumor nuclei are designated ER positive. About two thirds of newly diagnosed breast cancers are ER positive and one third are ER negative. Endocrine therapies utilized in breast cancer care oppose estrogen action and are comprised of either ER-blocking agents (tamoxifen, raloxifene) or aromatase inhibitors (letrozole, anastrozole or exemestane). These are used to prevent breast cancer development or recurrence, or to treat metastatic disease [7, 11].

2 Mechanisms Underlying ER Loss in Breast Cancer

ER negative breast cancers have a worse prognosis and are resistant to antiestrogen therapy [7]. While estrogen is a mitogen for cultured ER positive breast cancer cell lines and primary ER positive cancers, the proliferation of ER negative breast cancer has been thought to be estrogen independent. This conclusion has been based on the observations that ER negative cancers do not respond to therapeutic ER blockade [12, 13] and that, when grown in tissue culture, ER-negative breast cancer lines do not require the presence of estrogens to sustain proliferation and are thus, estrogen independent for growth. The mechanisms underlying the lack of ER protein expression in these breast cancers is not entirely clear and appears to be multifactorial.

2.1 *ER Gene Changes*

Homozygous deletion of the ER locus on chromosome 6q has not been reported in breast cancers and loss of homozygosity (hemizygous loss) at 6q affects ER positive and negative cancers equally [14, 15]. ER gene mutations are relatively uncommon. A study of 200 primary breast cancers revealed few polymorphisms and only one ER mutation in an ER negative cancer [16]. Thus, ER gene changes are too uncommon to account for ER negative breast cancer [15, 16].

2.2 *ER Promoter Hypermethylation*

ER promoter hypermethylation was observed in six ER negative lines and demethylating agents restored ER mRNA expression [17, 18]. However, ER promoter methylation was detected in only a small portion of primary ER negative breast cancers examined (in nine of thirty nine cases or 23%) [19]. Indeed a comprehensive analysis of large number of primary breast cancers has yet to be done and the true frequency of ER hypermethylation in breast cancers is not established. Histone deacetylase inhibitors (trichostatin A) and 5-aza-2′-deoxycytidine have been shown to restore ER mRNA expression and ER protein levels in ER negative breast cancer lines [20, 21], raising the provocative possibility that histone deacetylase inhibitor drugs may have value in converting some ER-negative cancers to ER-positive, opening the possibility of this therapy to restore ER expression and anti-estrogen responsiveness [22]. This has led to the development of clinical trials for HDAC inhibitors in ER negative breast cancer, but these are still in clinical development.

2.3 ER mRNA Expression in Breast Cancers

Three early studies, using relatively insensitive non-quantitative dot blot, Northern and PCR showed a majority (43/64 assayed) of ER negative cancers express ER mRNA [23–25]. With the development of more sensitive and quantitative techniques, quantitative real-time PCR detected ER mRNA in all of 56 ER negative cancers [26, 27]. ER positive tumors tended to have higher ER mRNA levels, with significant overlap in ER mRNA values between ER positive and negative [26, 27]. ER promoter methylation may account for the lowest ER mRNA levels observed [27]. Our highly sensitive real-time PCR quantitation showed ER mRNA expression in all of 250 primary breast cancers assayed, with high variability and overlap in concentrations of ER mRNA between ER positive and negative [28]. We also observed a trend to higher ER mRNA in the ER positive cancers.

Although microarray studies have shown reduced ER gene expression in ER negative breast cancer [29–31], in these studies, individual breast cancer ER mRNA was compared to a reference of pooled cRNAs from ER positive and negative tumors [29] or to the average signal from all tumors [30, 31]. These findings are thus consistent with RT-PCR data showing ER mRNA in all breast cancers. Other array studies show variable ER [32]. QPCR from fixed paraffin embedded tissues using the Oncotype Dx analysis also indicate lower ER mRNA in ER- cancers [33–35]. However, the expression array types of analysis exhibit only about five fold variability in ER mRNA levels while QPCR from fresh frozen tissue yields up to seven logs variability in ER mRNA levels and higher sensitivity. It is noteworthy that other QPCR analysis using paraffin embedded breast cancer samples also revealed ER mRNA detection in ER negative tumors. Ma et al. [36] also showed ER mRNA values overlap between ER positive and negative tumors in over 800 primary breast cancers with lower values in the ER negative. Since highly sensitive real-time PCR shows uniform expression with variable and overlapping ER mRNA levels in ER positive and ER negative primary breast cancers, post-transcriptional and/or post-translational control of ER may also play a role in regulating ER protein levels in breast tumors [26–28].

2.4 MAPK Activated Loss of ER Expression

Recent work has implicated activation of several oncogenes upstream of MAPK in the loss of ER expression in breast cancers. El-Ashry's group developed MCF-7-derived models with inducible EGFR [37], and constitutively active (ca) c-erbB-2 [38], c-Raf1 [39], and MEK1 [40] and showed that activation of these EGFR and erbB-2 effectors decreased levels of ER and caused estrogen-independent growth [40]. SiRNA to MAPK restored ER levels in these lines, indicating that MAPK activation is causally linked to ER loss and MAPK may mediate ER negativity in at least a subset of tumors with EGFR or erbB-2 overexpression [41]. In three other established ER- breast cancer cell lines, SUM 229 (high EGFR), SUM 190 (high EGFR and erbB-2), and SUM 149 (high RhoC and EGFR), MAPK inhibition by MEK inhibitor U0126 also increased ER [42]. This mechanism appears relevant to cells that may have initially expressed high ER protein and RNA levels, but in which oncogenic activation of MAPK arises during malignant progression. This mechanism involved both ER protein and later RNA loss and arises during long term estrogen deprivation in vitro. Recent work has identified that the ER can be targeted by miRNA 222 and this was shown to be overexpressed more frequently in ER negative than ER positive breast cancers in a limited retrospective analysis [43]. The extent to which this underlies ER negative breast cancers is yet to be defined. MAPK has been shown to upregulate miRNA 222 and may underlie the MEK/MAPK mediated ER loss (El-Ashry et al., unpublished).

3 EGFR Family and Src Kinase Activation in Breast Cancer

EGFR family activation is strongly linked to ER negative breast cancer. Different studies showed the ErbB2/Her2 gene is amplified [44] and EGFR overexpressed [45] in up to 30% of primary invasive breast cancers. Both are associated with poor prognosis [45] and ER negativity in primary breast cancers [46, 47]. EGFR activation is frequent in triple negative breast cancers [48]. EGFR and erbB2 activate the Raf/MEK/MAPK pathway. The MAPK pathway is often hyperactivated in breast cancers compared to benign tissue [49], due to activation of upstream regulators, Raf-1 and MEK. MAPK hyperactivation is more frequent in ER negative compared to ER positive breast cancer. EGFR and ErbB2/Her2 each bind Src to catalyze mutual kinase activation and stimulate cell proliferation [50].

The first non-receptor tyrosine kinase identified was the v-Src oncogenic protein which plays a role in oncogenesis [51]. The vertebrate counterpart of v-Src, c-Src was identified shortly after [52]. It belongs to a family of closely related non-receptor tyrosine kinases called Src family kinases that include Src, Yes, Fyn, Fgr, Lck, Lyn, Hck, and Blk. They are closely related with a wide variety of functionality depending on cell type and cell growth. They can be involved in signal transduction, cellular proliferation, migration, differentiation and transformation [53, 54]. Src, Yes and Fyn are ubiquitously expressed in many human tissues [55]. Others are mainly expressed in hemopoietic tissues. Of these, Src is the best studied and is known to be deregulated in multiple tumor types, including breast, prostate, lung and pancreatic cancers [56].

Src is a 60 kDa tyrosine kinase and is the best-studied member of Src family kinases. Src-deficient mammary epithelial cells have been shown to have impairment of signaling pathways in response to estrogen, suggesting Src plays a role in ER signaling in vivo [57]. Src expression and or activity is elevated in many different epithelial cancers, including breast and ovarian cancers [58–66]. Our recent immunohistochemical analysis of activated Src used a phospho-specific antibody (pY416-Src) in 482 tumors. Of these approximately 39% showed strong Src activation. ER negative status was strongly correlated with Src activation ($p = 0.002$) (unpublished data and [67]. The increased levels and activation of Src in human breast cancer provide a rationale for targeting Src in breast cancer [68]. Src specific inhibitor as a single agent to treat the breast cancer showed modest activity. The trials of combination with other agents are ongoing [69].

4 ER Cross-Talk with Signaling Transduction Pathways

In addition to genomic function, which modulates ER target gene transcription, ER also plays a role in the rapid transient actions of estrogen that do not require gene expression and have been termed non-genomic action. While the highest steady state levels are detected in the cell nucleus, there is evidence that some of the regulatory actions of ER may be extranuclear. Liganded ER rapidly and transiently activates Src and Shc, leading to Ras/MAPK as well as PI3K/AKT activation (see Fig. 1) [70–72]. Indeed recent elegant work has indicated that liganded ER is recruited to the cell surface via interaction with the cytoplasmic portion of the IGF-1R [73, 74]. ER interaction with Src is modulated by Src interacting proteins, MNAR/PELP1 and p130CAS [75–77].

The activation of signal transduction pathways by the cross-talk with liganded ER leads to ER phosphorylation at multiple sites by various kinases. ER is predominantly phosphorylated on S118 by MAPK [78], and to a lesser extent on S104 and S106 by CyclinA-CDK2 [79]. S167 may be phosphorylated by RSK1 or AKT [80, 81]. These phosphorylation events all affect the N-terminal region of ER which contains ligand independent activation function 1. PKA has been shown to phosphorylate S236, which is in the DNA-binding domain [82], and S305, which is at the start of ligand binding domain (LBD) [83]. These phosphorylation events appear to modulate ER function by altering binding to ligand, promoter DNA binding, and ER coactivators [84].

Even in the absence of estrogen, ER can be activated by several growth factors through activated receptor tyrosine kinases like EGFR and IGF-1R, which also activate Src, MAPK, PI3K/AKT pathways and lead to ER phosphorylation [85–88].

5 ER Phosphorylation by Src

Tyrosine phosphorylation of the ER has been implied the earliest in ER signaling [89, 90] and is stimulated by estrogen [91]. Early work indicated that ER-Tyrosine 537 (Y537) can be phosphorylated by Src [92]. However this was for years

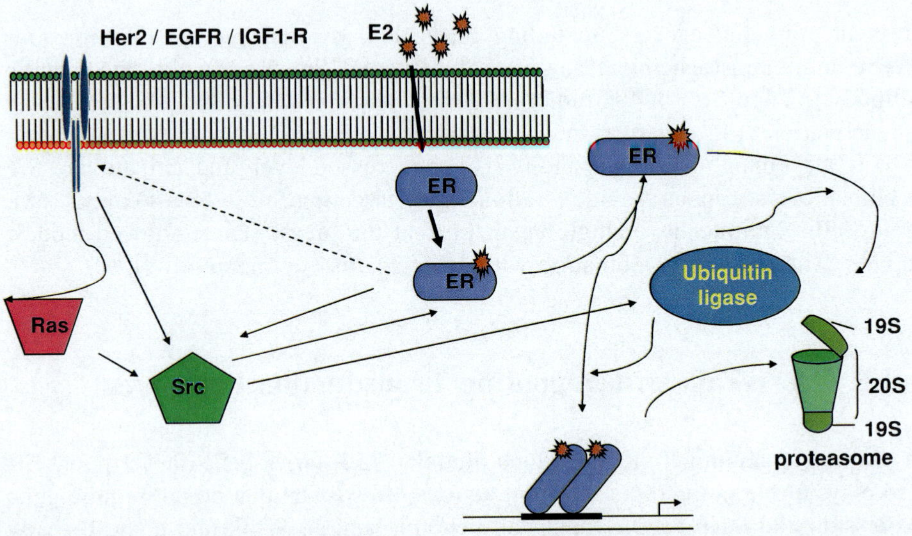

Fig. 1 Liganded ER and Src recruit proteins that serve dual roles as coactivator/ubiquitin ligases to couple ER target gene activation with ER proteolysis. This would serve to facilitate ER removal and recharging of the promoter once fired and fine tune receptor transcriptional activity. In addition, in the context of high levels of EGF and IGF-1R activation, high constitutive Src family action may permit rapid turnover of the ER in a context in which estrogen and Src are constitutively driving ER transcriptional activation. In tissues in which hormone stimulates rapid cell growth such as the uterus, ovary and breast epithelium this scenario may occur in the context of low steady state ER levels

considered controversial and a role for this phosphorylation event in ER action was not known. There are twenty-three tyrosine residues in the full length human ER. While multiple tyrosine sites in ER could be potential Src targets, in vitro Src kinase reaction generate phosphorylation of on average about two tyrosine sites per ER molecule and Y537 is one of these major sites [93]. Using a phosphorylation site prediction program [84], our analysis showed Y537 to be the single site mostly likely to be phosphorylated by Src among five tyrosine residues in the ER LBD, based on estradiol/ER LBD structure [94], consistent with early experimental results [95]. Tyrosine phosphorylation of the ER increases its affinity for estradiol [93]. A peptide containing the sequences around the phosphotyrosine residue Y537 in ER can block the ER/Src interaction and cell growth stimulated by estrogen [96]. Src also affects activation function 1 of ER [97]. Recent data indicated two additional tyrosine residues in the amino-terminal half of ER, Y52 and Y219 can be phosphorylated by Abl non-receptor tyrosine kinase in vitro. Those two may also be Src targets in ER at its amino- terminus [98]. Phosphorylation of Y537 could potentially affect ER coactivator binding, ER degradation as well as ER transactivation. This notion is supported by recent work from our lab [99].

6 The Link Between Steroid Hormone Receptor Activation and Receptor Degradation

The ubiquitin-proteasome pathway regulates eukaryotic gene transcription in a number of important ways. For many transcription factors the very phosphorylation events and protein–protein interactions that stimulate their transcriptional activity also trigger factor proteolysis [100–102]. Signaling pathways that activate many transcription factors, including NFκB, c-Jun, c-Myc, Gcn4, and E2F-1 also trigger their ubiquitin dependent degradation [100]. Components of the basal transcription apparatus can phosphorylate and activate transcription factor proteolysis [100]. Ubiquitin-mediated degradation can efficiently limit transactivator availability and action [103, 104]. In addition, ubiquitylation is required for the activity of certain transcription factors [100, 105] and may influence co-activator binding [100]. Co-activators can also enhance transcription factor ubiquitylation [100–102, 106].

Ligand mediated proteolysis regulates the turnover of most nuclear hormone receptors (NHR) including progesterone [107], thyroid hormone [108], retinoic X [109] and estrogen receptors [110–112]. The magnitude and duration of NHR transcriptional activity is also regulated by the ubiquitin proteasome pathway. Many ubiquitin proteasome components are co-activators of steroid hormone receptors [113], including the ubiquitin ligases E6AP [114], receptor potentiation factor 1/reverse Spt phenotype 5 (RPF1/RSP5) [115], MDM2 [116, 117], and BRCA1 [118, 119]; the sumo-conjugating enzyme ubc9 [120, 121]; and the 19S proteasomal subunit, yeast suppressor of gal1/thyroid receptor interacting protein 1(SUG1/TRIP1/rpt6) [122]. Overexpression of the ubiquitin ligase component NEDD8 can impair ER transcriptional activity [123, 124]. Several E2-Ubcs also regulate the levels and activities of NHR co-activators [125] and ubiquitin conjugating enzyme UbcH7 can itself act as a steroid receptor coactivator [125, 126]. Thus, the proteasome pathway can facilitate co-repressor/coactivator exchange and transcription complex remodeling [113, 125, 127].

7 Src Promotes Ligand Activated ER Degradation and ER Target Gene Transcription

Cellular ER protein levels are delicately regulated [128]. Estrogen binding to ER not only activates ER transactivation, but also leads to ubiquitin-dependent ER proteolysis [112, 129, 130]. Certain ubiquitin ligases have been identified as ER coactivators, including E6AP [114], MDM2 [116], and BRCA1 [118, 119]. The binding of these E3 ligase/coactivators may regulate both ER transcriptional activation and its proteolysis. Paradoxically, proteasome inhibition decreases ER transcriptional activity at some ER target promoters, despite an increase in ER protein levels [130].

As noted above, the phosphorylation-dependent activation of many transcription factors is linked to their proteolysis. Many ubiquitin ligases recognize and bind only appropriately phosphorylated substrates to facilitate their ubiquitylation and proteolysis [131]. Substrate phosphorylation is usually tightly regulated to ensure the proper timing and extent of its recognition by the ubiquitin ligase that mediates its proteolysis. Specific phosphorylation event that trigger proteasomal degradation has been identified for progesterone receptor which is a member of nuclear receptor superfamily [132].

We have found that Src regulates ER transcriptional activity and also its proteolysis. Tyrosine phosphorylation of ER by Src in vitro increases ER ubiquitylation and 26S proteasome mediated ER degradation. In vivo, Src inhibitor PP1 impairs estrogen stimulated ER ubiquitylation. We have constructed MCF-7 human breast cancer cell line with induced expression of constitutive active Src. Estrogen stimulated ER proteolysis was accelerated when Src expression was induced. At the same time, estrogen stimulated ER target gene expression, like GREB1 and pS2, was elevated. Among 101 primary breast tumors tested, Src and ER levels were inversely correlated. In ER negative BT-20 cell line, ER protein was detected although at a very low levels in proliferating cells, but increased when cells were deprived of estrogen, and Src knockdown increased ER levels [29].

The mammary tissue of E6AP null mouse shows increased ER protein compared to wild-type littermates. The transgenic mouse which over expresses E6AP in mammary tissue has reduced ER protein level [133]. We recently also show that E6AP can act as ubiquitin ligase for ER in vitro and E6AP-mediated ER ubiquitylation was increased by pre-treatment of ER with Src. ER-phosphorylation by Src at Y537 enhances ER recognition by E6AP and promotes both ER proteolysis and ER target gene transcription [99].

8 Implications for the Definition of an "Estrogen Responsive" Tissue

The data above and increasing data in the field support a model in which liganded and/or appropriately phosphorylated ER recruits co-activators that include ubiquitin conjugating enzymes and ubiquitin ligase components to promote not only transcriptional activation of certain target genes, but also ER degradation. Our findings indicate that Src plays an active role in ER signaling and that ER activity may not be solely dependent on the steady state level of ER protein. This mechanism of coupled ER activation and proteolysis may be at play in a number of hormonally regulated cancers, including ER "negative" breast, ovarian and endometrial cancers, certain forms of colon cancer and malignancies of bone and brain. Thus one could conceive of tumor tissues, and indeed of scenarios during rapid growth factor receptor and steroid stimulated proliferation of normal hormone responsive tissues in which low steady state levels of receptor are present, but the receptor itself is disproportionately activated, such as would be the case with rapid turnover of ER when Src is highly active. These data permit the possibility that a subset of ER "negative" breast tumors and indeed certain states of hormonally regulated normal tissue growth may prove to be estrogen regulated: they express ER mRNA, but ER protein levels are low or undetectable due to accelerated ligand and Src mediated ER proteolysis.

Liganded receptor cross talk with different signaling kinases, including Src, may predicate promoter selection and occupancy in the presence of estrogen in different tissue contexts. As we explore the relationship between steroid receptor turnover and transcriptional activation, we may find ways in which different cross talk-mediated receptor phosphorylation events drive differences in broad patterns of target gene expression, coactivator or repressor binding and chromatin conformational changes in the presence of various activated signal transduction pathways that are germane to receptor action at low to undetectable receptor levels. There may indeed be situations in hormone driven normal and malignant tissues where receptor levels are present at vanishingly low levels, but receptor driven transcriptional activation brisk. These concepts open a new way of viewing hormone sensitive physiology in tissue with low to undetectable hormone receptor levels.

References

1. Mangelsdorf DJ, Thummel C, Beato M, Herrlich P, Schutz G, Umesono K et al (1995) The nuclear receptor superfamily: the second decade. Cell 83:835–839
2. Green S, Walter P, Kumar V, Krust A, Bornert JM, Argos P et al (1986) Human oestrogen receptor cDNA: sequence, expression and homology to v-erb-A. Nature 320:134–139
3. Greene GL, Gilna P, Waterfield M, Baker A, Hort Y, Shine J (1986) Sequence and expression of human estrogen receptor complementary DNA. Science 231:1150–1154
4. Mosselman S, Polman J, Dijkema R (1996) ER beta: identification and characterization of a novel human estrogen receptor. FEBS Lett 392:49–53
5. Morani A, Warner M, Gustafsson JA (2008) Biological functions and clinical implications of oestrogen receptors alfa and beta in epithelial tissues. J Intern Med 264:128–142
6. Skliris GP, Leygue E, Curtis-Snell L, Watson PH, Murphy LC (2006) Expression of oestrogen receptor-beta in oestrogen receptor-alpha negative human breast tumours 1. Br J Cancer 95:616–626
7. Jordan VC (1995) Studies on the estrogen receptor in breast cancer - 20 years as a target for the treatment and prevention of cancer. Breast Cancer Res Treat 36:267–285
8. Lonard DM, O'Malley BW (2007) Nuclear receptor coregulators: judges, juries, and executioners of cellular regulation. Mol Cell 27:691–700
9. McGuire WL, De La Garza M, Chamness GC (1977) Evaluation of estrogen receptor assays in human breast cancer tissue. Cancer Res 37:637–639

10. Harvey JM, Clark GM, Osborne CK, Allred DC (1999) Estrogen receptor status by immunohistochemistry is superior to the ligand-binding assay for predicting response to adjuvant endocrine therapy in breast cancer. J Clin Oncol 17:1474
11. Wong ZW, Ellis MJ (2004) First-line endocrine treatment of breast cancer: aromatase inhibitor or antioestrogen? Br J Cancer 90:20–25
12. Clarke M, Collins R, Davies C, Godwin J, Gray R, Peto R (1998) Tamoxifen for early breast cancer: an overview of the randomised trials. Lancet 351:1451–1467
13. Abe O, Abe R, Enomoto K, Kikuchi K, Koyama H, Masuda H et al (2005) Effects of chemotherapy and hormonal therapy for early breast cancer on recurrence and 15-year survival: an overview of the randomised trials. Lancet 365:1687–1717
14. Ferguson AT, Vertino PM, Spitzner JR, Baylin SB, Muller MT, Davidson NE (1997) Role of estrogen receptor gene demethylation and DNA methyltransferase DNA adduct formation in 5-Aza-2′-deoxycytidine-induced cytotoxicity in human breast cancer cells. J Cell Biochem 272:32260–32266
15. Ferguson AT, Davidson NE (1997) Regulation of estrogen receptor alpha function in breast cancer. Crit Rev Oncog 8:29–46
16. Roodi N, Bailey LR, Kao WY, Verrier CS, Yee CJ, Dupong WD et al (1995) Estrogen receptor gene analysis in estrogen receptor-positive and receptor-negative primary breast cancer. J Natl Cancer Inst 87:446–451
17. Ottaviano YL, Issa JP, Parl FF, Smith HS, Baylin SB, Davidson NE (1994) Methylation of the estrogen receptor gene CpG island marks loss of estrogen receptor expression in human breast cancer cells. Cancer Res 54:2552–2555
18. Ferguson AT, Lapidus RG, Baylin SB, Davidson NE (1995) Demethylation of the estrogen receptor gene in estrogen receptor-negative breast cancer cells can reactivate estrogen receptor gene expression. Cancer Res 55:2279–2283
19. Lapidus RG, Ferguson AT, Ottaviano YL, Parl FF, Smith HS, Wetizman SA et al (1996) Methylation of estrogen and progesterone receptor gene 5′ CpG islands correlates with lack of estrogen and progesterone receptor gene expression in breast tumors. Clin Cancer Res 2:805–810
20. Sharma D, Blum J, Yang X, Beaulieu N, Macleod AR, Davidson NE (2005) Release of methyl CpG binding proteins and histone deacetylase 1 from the estrogen receptor alpha (ER) promoter upon reactivation in ER-negative human breast cancer cells. Mol Endocrinol 19:1740–1751
21. Zhou Q, Atadja P, Davidson NE (2007) Histone deacetylase inhibitor LBH589 reactivates silenced estrogen receptor alpha (ER) gene expression without loss of DNA hypermethylation. Cancer Biol Ther 6:64–69
22. Yang X, Ferguson AT, Nass SJ, Phillips DL, Butash KA, Wang SM et al (2000) Transcriptional activation of estrogen receptor alpha in human breast cancer cells by histone deacetylase inhibition. Cancer Res 60:6890–6894
23. Carmeci C, DeConinck EC, Lawton T, Bloch DA, Weigel RJ (1997) Analysis of estrogen receptor messenger RNA in breast carcinomas from archival specimens is predictive of tumor biology. Am J Pathol 150:1563–1570
24. Henry JA, Nicholson S, Farndon JR, Westley BR, May FEB (1988) Measurement of oestrogen receptor mRNA levels in human breast tumours. Br J Cancer 58:600–605
25. Garcia T, Lehrer S, Bloomer WD, Schachter B (1988) A variant estrogen receptor messenger ribonucleic acid is associated wity reduced levels of estrogen binding in human mammary tumors. Mol Endocrinol 2:785–791
26. Iwao K, Miyoshi Y, Egawa C, Ikeda N, Tsukamoto F, Noguchi S (2000) Quantitative analysis of estrogen receptor-alpha and -beta messenger RNA expression in breast carcinoma by real-time polymerase chain reaction. Cancer 89:1732–1738
27. Iwao K, Miyoshi Y, Egawa C, Ikeda N, Noguchi S (2000) Quantitative analysis of estrogen receptor-beta mRNA and its variants in human breast cancer. Int J Cancer 88:733–736
28. Chu I, Arnaout A, Loiseau S, Sun J, Seth A, McMahon C et al (2007) Src promotes estrogen-dependent estrogen receptor alpha proteolysis in human breast cancer. J Clin Invest 117:2205–2215

29. Van't Veer LJ, Dai H, van de Vijver MJ, He YD, Hart AA, Mao M et al (2002) Gene expression profiling predicts clinical outcome of breast cancer. Nature 415:530–536
30. Gruvberger S, Ringner M, Chen Y, Panavally S, Saal LH, Borg A et al (2001) Estrogen receptor status in breast cancer is associated with remarkably distinct gene expression patterns. Cancer Res 61:5979–5984
31. West M, Blanchette C, Dressman H, Huang E, Ishida S, Spang R et al (2001) Predicting the clinical status of human breast cancer by using gene expression profiles. Proc Natl Acad Sci U S A 98:11462–11467
32. Perou CM, Sorlie T, Eisen MB, Van De RM, Jeffrey SS, Rees CA et al (2000) Molecular portraits of human breast tumours. Nature 406:747–752
33. Paik S, Shak S, Tang G, Kim C, Baker J, Cronin M et al (2004) A multigene assay to predict recurrence of tamoxifen-treated, node-negative breast cancer. N Engl J Med 351:2817–2826
34. Drury S, Salter J, Baehner FL, Shak S, Dowsett M (2010) Feasibility of using tissue microarray cores of paraffin-embedded breast cancer tissue for measurement of gene expression: a proof-of-concept study. J Clin Pathol 63:513–517
35. Badve SS, Baehner FL, Gray RP, Childs BH, Maddala T, Liu ML et al (2008) Estrogen- and progesterone-receptor status in ECOG 2197: comparison of immunohistochemistry by local and central laboratories and quantitative reverse transcription polymerase chain reaction by central laboratory. J Clin Oncol 26:2473–2481
36. Ma XJ, Hilsenbeck SG, Wang W, Ding L, Sgroi DC, Bender RA et al (2006) The HOXB13:IL17BR expression index is a prognostic factor in early-stage breast cancer. J Clin Oncol 24:4611–4619
37. Miller DL, El-Ashry D, Cheville AL, Liu Y, McLeskey SW, Kern FG (1994) Emergence of MCF-7 cells overexpressing a transfected epidermal growth factor receptor (EGFR) under estrogen-depleted conditions: evidence for a role of EGFR in breast cancer growth and progression. Cell Growth Differ 5:1263–1274
38. Liu Y, El Ashry D, Chen D, Ding IY, Kern FG (1995) MCF-7 breast cancer cells overexpressing transfected c-erbB-2 have an in vitro growth advantage in estrogen-depleted conditions and reduced estrogen-dependence and tamoxifen-sensitivity in vivo. Breast Cancer Res Treat 34:97–117
39. El-Ashry D, Miller D, Kharbanda S, Lippman ME, Kern FG (1997) Constitutive Raf-1 kinase activity in breast cancer cells induces both estrogen-independent growth and apoptosis. Oncogene 15:435
40. Oh AS, Lorant LA, Holloway JN, Miller DL, Kern FG, El-Ashry D (2001) Hyperactivation of MAPK induces loss of ERalpha expression in breast cancer cells. Mol Endocrinol 15:1344–1359
41. Holloway JN, Murthy S, El Ashry D (2004) A cytoplasmic substrate of mitogen-activated protein kinase is responsible for estrogen receptor-alpha down-regulation in breast cancer cells: the role of nuclear factor-kappaB. Mol Endocrinol 18:1396–1410
42. Bayliss J, Hilger A, Vishnu P, Diehl K, El-Ashry D (2007) Reversal of the estrogen receptor negative phenotype in breast cancer and restoration of antiestrogen response. Clin Cancer Res 13:7029–7036
43. Di LG, Gasparini P, Piovan C, Ngankeu A, Garofalo M, Taccioli C et al (2010) MicroRNA cluster 221–222 and estrogen receptor alpha interactions in breast cancer. J Natl Cancer Inst 102:706–721
44. Slamon DJ, Clark GM, Wong SG, Levin WJ, Ullrich A, McGuire WL (1987) Human breast cancer: correlation of relapse and survival with amplification of the HER-2/neu oncogene. Science 235:177–182
45. Tsutsui S, Ohno S, Murakami S, Hachitanda Y, Oda S (2002) Prognostic value of epidermal growth factor receptor (EGFR) and its relationship to the estrogen receptor status in 1029 patients with breast cancer. Breast Cancer Res Treat 71:67–75
46. Pegram MD, Pauletti G, Slamon DJ (1998) HER-2/neu as a predictive marker of response to breast cancer therapy. Breast Cancer Res Treat 52:65–77

47. Klijn JG, Berns PM, Schmitz PI, Foekens JA (1992) The clinical significance of epidermal growth factor receptor (EGF-R) in human breast cancer: a review on 5232 patients. Endocr Rev 13:3–17
48. Cleator S, Heller W, Coombes RC (2007) Triple-negative breast cancer: therapeutic options. Lancet Oncol 8:235–244
49. Sivaraman VS, Wang HY, Nuovo GJ, Malbon CC (1997) Hyperexpression of mitogen-activated protein kinase in human breast cancer. J Clin Invest 99:1478–1483
50. Ishizawar R, Parsons SJ (2004) c-Srcc-Src and cooperating partners in human cancer. Cancer Cell 6:209–214
51. Stehelin D, Fujita DJ, Padgett T, Varmus HE, Bishop JM (1977) Detection and enumeration of transformation-defective strains of avian sarcoma virus with molecular hybridization. Virology 76:675–684
52. Oppermann H, Levinson AD, Varmus HE, Levintow L, Bishop JM (1979) Uninfected vertebrate cells contain a protein that is closely related to the product of the avian sarcoma virus transforming gene (src). Proc Natl Acad Sci U S A 76:1804–1808
53. Parsons JT, Parsons SJ (1997) Src family protein tyrosine kinases: cooperating with growth factor and adhesion signaling pathways. Curr Opin Cell Biol 9:187–192
54. Parsons SJ, Parsons JT (2004) Src family kinases, key regulators of signal transduction. Oncogene 23:7906–7909
55. Benati D, Baldari CT (2008) SRC family kinases as potential therapeutic targets for malignancies and immunological disorders. Curr Med Chem 15:1154–1165
56. Johnson FM, Gallick GE (2007) SRC family nonreceptor tyrosine kinases as molecular targets for cancer therapy. Anticancer Agents Med Chem 7:651–659
57. Kim H, Laing M, Muller W (2005) c-Srcc-Src-null mice exhibit defects in normal mammary gland development and ERalpha signaling. Oncogene 24:5629–5636
58. Rosen N, Bolen JB, Schwartz AM, Cohen P, DeSeau V, Israel MA (1986) Analysis of pp60c-src protein kinase activity in human tumor cell lines and tissues. J Biol Chem 261:13754–13759
59. Hennipman A, van Oirschot BA, Smits J, Rijksen G, Staal GEJ (1989) Tyrosine kinase activity in breast cancer, benign breast disease and normal breast tissue. Cancer Res 49: 519–521
60. Lehrer S, O'Shaughnessy J, Song HK, Levine E, Savoretti P, Dalton J et al (1989) Activity of pp60c-src protein kinase in human breast cancer. Mt Sinai J Med 56:83–85
61. Ottenhoff-Kalff AE, Rijksen G, van Beurden EA, Hennipman A, Michels AA, Staal GE (1992) Characterization of protein tyrosine kinases from human breast cancer: involvement of the c-src oncogene product. Cancer Res 52:4773–4778
62. Lower EE, Franco RS, Miller MA, Martelo OJ (1993) Enzymatic and immunohistochemical evaluation of tyrosine phosphorylation in breast cancer specimens. Breast Cancer Res Treat 26:217–224
63. Verbeek BS, Vroom TM, Adriaansen-Slot SS, Ottenhoff-Kalff AE, Geertzema JG, Hennipman A et al (1996) c-Srcc-Src protein expression is increased in human breast cancer. An immunohistochemical and biochemical analysis. J Pathol 180:383–388
64. Reissig D, Clement J, Sanger J, Berndt A, Kosmehl H, Bohmer FD (2001) Elevated activity and expression of Src-family kinases in human breast carcinoma tissue versus matched non-tumor tissue. J Cancer Res Clin Oncol 127:226–230
65. Frame MC (2002) Src in cancer: deregulation and consequences for cell behaviour. Biochim Biophys Acta 1602:114–130
66. Summy JM, Gallick GE (2003) Src family kinases in tumor progression and metastasis. Cancer Metastasis Rev 22:337–358
67. Chu I, Sun J, Arnaout A, Kahn H, Hanna W, Narod S et al (2007) p27 phosphorylation by Src regulates inhibition of cyclin E-Cdk2. Cell 128:281–294
68. Finn RS (2008) Targeting Src in breast cancer. Ann Oncol 19:1379–1386
69. Mayer EL, Krop IE (2010) Advances in targeting SRC in the treatment of breast cancer and other solid malignancies. Clin Cancer Res 16:3526–3532

70. Improta-Bears T, Whorton AR, Codazzi F, York JD, Meyer T, McDonnell DP (1990) Estrogen-induced activation of mitogen-activated protein kinase requires mobilization of intracellular calcium. Proc Natl Acad Sci U S A 96:4686–4691
71. Aronica SM, Kraus WL, Katzenellenbogen BS (1994) Estrogen action via the cAMP signaling pathway: Stimulation of adenylate cyclase and cAMP-regulated gene transcription. Proc Natl Acad Sci U S A 91:8517–8521
72. Migliaccio A, Castoria G, Di Domenico M, de Falco A, Bilancio A, Lombardi M et al (2000) Steroid-induced androgen receptor-oestradiol receptor beta-Src complex triggers prostate cancer cell proliferation. EMBO J 19:5406–5417
73. Song RX, Barnes CJ, Zhang ZG, Bao YD, Kumar R, Santen RJ (2004) The role of Shc and insulin-like qrowth factor 1 receptor in mediating the translocation of estrogen receptor a to the plasma membrane. Proc Natl Acad Sci U S A 101:2076–2081
74. Song RXD, McPherson RA, Adam L, Bao YD, Shupnik M, Kumar R et al (2002) Linkage of rapid estrogen action to MAPK activation by ER alpha-Shc association and Shc pathway activation. Mol Endocrinol 16:116–127
75. Vadlamudi RK, Wang RA, Mazumdar A, Kim Y, Shin J, Sahin A et al (2001) Molecular cloning and characterization of PELP1, a novel human coregulator of estrogen receptor alpha. J Biol Chem 276:38272–38279
76. Wong CW, McNally C, Nickbarg E, Komm BS, Cheskis BJ (2002) Estrogen receptor-interacting protein that modulates its nongenomic activity-crosstalk with Src/Erk phosphorylation cascade. Proc Natl Acad Sci U S A 99:14783–14788
77. Cabodi S, Moro L, Baj G, Smeriglio M, Di Stefano P, Gippone S et al (2004) p130Cas interacts with estrogen receptor alpha and modulates non-genomic estrogen signaling in breast cancer cells. J Cell Sci 117:1603–1611
78. Joel PB, Traish AM, Lannigan DA (1995) Estradiol and phorbol ester cause phosphorylation of serine 118 in the human estrogen receptor. Mol Endocrinol 9:1041–1052
79. Rogatsky I, Trowbridge JM, Garabedian MJ (1999) Potentiation of human estrogen receptor alpha transcriptional activation through phosphorylation of serines 104 and 106 by the cyclin A-CDK2 complex. J Biol Chem 274:22296–22302
80. Joel PB, Smith J, Sturgill TW, Fisher TL, Blenis J, Lannigan DA (1998) pp90rsk1 regulates estrogen receptor-mediated transcription through phosphorylation of Ser-167. Mol Cell Biol 18:1978–1984
81. Arnold SF, Obourn JD, Jaffe H, Notides AC (1994) Serine 167 is the major estradiol-induced phosphorylation site on the human estrogen receptor. Mol Endocrinol 8:1208–1214
82. Lannigan DA (2003) Estrogen receptor phosphorylation. Steroids 68:1–9
83. Michalides R, Griekspoor A, Balkenende A, Verwoerd D, Janssen L, Jalink K et al (2004) Tamoxifen resistance by a conformational arrest of the estrogen receptor alpha after PKA activation in breast cancer. Cancer Cell 5:597–605
84. Durek P, Schudoma C, Weckwerth W, Selbig J, Walther D (2009) Detection and characterization of 3D-signature phosphorylation site motifs and their contribution towards improved phosphorylation site prediction in proteins. BMC Bioinf 10:117
85. Ignar-Trowbridge DM, Nelson KG, Bidwell MC, Curtis SW, Washburn TF, McLachlan JA et al (1992) Coupling of dual signaling pathways: epidermal growth factor action involves the estrogen receptor. Proc Natl Acad Sci U S A 89:4658–4662
86. Ignar-Trowbridge DM, Teng CT, Ross KA, Parker MG, Korach KS, McLachlan JA (1993) Peptide growth factors elicit estrogen receptor-dependent transcriptional activation of an estrogen-responsive element. Mol Endocrinol 7:992–998
87. Bunone G, Briand PA, Miksicek RJ, Picard D (1996) Activation of the unliganded estrogen receptor by EGF involves the MAP kinase pathway and direct phosphorylation. EMBO J 15:2174–2183
88. Aronica SM, Katzenellenbogen BS (1993) Stimulation of estrogen receptor-mediated transcription and alteration in the phosphorylation state of the rat uterine estrogen receptor by estrogen, cyclic adenosine monophosphate, and insulin-like growth factor-I. Mol Endocrinol 7:743–752

89. Migliaccio A, Rotondi A, Auricchio F (1984) Calmodulin-stimulated phosphorylation of 17 beta-estradiol receptor on tyrosine. Proc Natl Acad Sci U S A 81:5921–5925
90. Migliaccio A, Rotondi A, Auricchio F (1986) Estradiol receptor: phosphorylation on tyrosine in uterus and interaction with anti-phosphotyrosine antibody. EMBO J 5: 2867–2872
91. Auricchio F, Migliaccio A, Di DM, Nola E (1987) Oestradiol stimulates tyrosine phosphorylation and hormone binding activity of its own receptor in a cell-free system. EMBO J 6:2923–2929
92. Arnold SF, Obourn JD, Jaffe H, Notides AC (1995) Phosphorylation of the human estrogen receptor on tyrosine 537 in vivo and by Src family tyrosine kinases in vitro. Mol Endocrinol 9:24–33
93. Likhite VS, Stossi F, Kim K, Katzenellenbogen BS, Katzenellenbogen JA (2006) Kinase-specific phosphorylation of the estrogen receptor changes receptor interactions with ligand, DNA, and coregulators associated with alterations in estrogen and tamoxifen activity. Mol Endocrinol 20:3120–3132
94. Brzozowski AM, Pike AC, Dauter Z, Hubbard RE, Bonn T, Engstrom O et al (1997) Molecular basis of agonism and antagonism in the oestrogen receptor. Nature 389:753–758
95. Castoria G, Migliaccio A, Green S, DiDomenico M, Chambon P, Auricchio F (1993) Properties of a purified estradiol-dependent calf uterus tyrosine kinase. Biochemistry 32:1740–1750
96. Varricchio L, Migliaccio A, Castoria G, Yamaguchi H, De FA, Di DM et al (2007) Inhibition of estradiol receptor/Src association and cell growth by an estradiol receptor alpha tyrosine-phosphorylated peptide. Mol Cancer Res 5:1213–1221
97. Feng W, Webb P, Nguyen P, Liu X, Li J, Karin M et al (2001) Potentiation of estrogen receptorestrogen receptor activation function 1 (AF-1) by Src/JNK through a serine 118-independent pathway. Mol Endocrinol 15:32–45
98. He X, Zheng Z, Song T, Wei C, Ma H, Ma Q et al (2010) c-Abl regulates estrogen receptor alpha transcription activity through its stabilization by phosphorylation. Oncogene 29:2238–2251
99. Sun J, Zhou W, Kaliappan K, Nawaz Z, Slingerland JM (2011) ERα phosphorylation at Y537 by Src couples ligand-activated transcription and ERα proteolysisproteolysis. Submitted
100. Tansey WP (2001) Transcriptional activation: risky business. Genes Dev 15:1045–1050
101. Collins GA, Tansey WP (2006) The proteasome: a utility tool for transcription? Curr Opin Genet Dev 16:197–202
102. Muratani M, Tansey WP (2003) How the ubiquitin-proteasome system controls transcription. Nat Rev Mol Cell Biol 4:192–201
103. Kim TK, Maniatis T (1996) Regulation of interferon-g-activated STAT1 by the ubiquitin-proteasome pathway. Science 273:1717–1719
104. Li S, Li Y, Carthew RW, Lai ZC (1997) Photoreceptor cell differentiation requires regulated proteolysis of the transcriptional repressor tramtrack. Cell 90:469–476
105. Salghetti SE, Caudy AA, Chenoweth JG, Tansey WP (2001) Regulation of transcriptional activation domain function by ubiquitin. Science 293:1651–1653
106. Fukuchi M, Imamura T, Chiba T, Ebisawa T, Kawabata M, Tanaka K et al (2001) Ligand-dependent degradation of Smad3 by a ubiquitin ligase complex of ROC1 and associated proteins. Mol Biol Cell 12:1431–1443
107. Syvala H, Vienonen A, Zhuang YH, Kivineva M, Ylikomi T, Tuohimaa P (1998) Evidence for enhanced ubiquitin-mediated proteolysis of the chicken progesterone receptor by progesterone. Life Sci 63:1505–1512
108. Syvala H, Vienonen A, Zhuang YH, Kivineva M, Ylikomi T, Tuohimaa P (1998) Evidence for enhanced ubiquitin-mediated proteolysis of the chicken progesterone receptor by progesterone. Life Sci 63:1505–1512
109. Dace A, Zhao L, Park KS, Furuno T, Takamura N, Nakanishi M et al (2000) Hormone binding induces rapid proteasome-mediated degradation of thyroid hormone receptors. Proc Natl Acad Sci U S A 97:8985–8990

110. Nomura Y, Nagaya T, Hayashi Y, Kambe F, Seo H (1999) 9-cis-retinoic acid decreases the level of its cognate receptor, retinoid X receptor, through acceleration of the turnover. Biochem Biophys Res Commun 260:729–733
111. Nirmala PB, Thampan RV (1995) Ubiquitination of the rat uterine estrogen receptor: Dependence on estradiol. Biochem Biophys Res Commun 213:24–31
112. Alarid ET, Bakopoulos N, Solodin N (1999) Proteasome-mediated proteolysis of estrogen receptor: A novel component in autologous Down-regulation. Mol Endocrinol 13: 1522–1534
113. Nawaz Z, Lonard DM, Dennis AP, Smith CL, O'Malley BW (1999) Proteasome-dependent degradation of the human estrogen receptor. Proc Natl Acad Sci U S A 96:1858–1862
114. Nawaz Z, O'Malley BW (2004) Urban renewal in the nucleus: is protein turnover by proteasomes absolutely required for nuclear receptor-regulated transcription? Mol Endocrinol 18:493–499
115. Nawaz Z, Lonard DM, Smith CL, Lev-Lehman E, Tsai SY, Tsai MJ et al (1999) The Angelman syndrome-associated protein, E6-AP, is a coactivator for the nuclear hormone receptor superfamily. Mol Cell Biol 19:1182–1189
116. Imhof MO, McDonnell DP (1996) Yeast RSP5 and its human homolog hRPF1 potentiate hormone-dependent activation of transcription by human progesterone and glucocorticoid receptor. Mol Cell Biol 16:2594–2605
117. Saji S, Okumura N, Eguchi H, Nakashima S, Suzuki A, Toi M et al (2001) MDM2 enhances the function of estrogen receptor alpha in human breast cancer cells. Biochem Biophys Res Commun 281:259–265
118. Reid G, Hubner MR, Metivier R, Brand H, Denger S, Manu D et al (2003) Cyclic, proteasome-mediated turnover of unliganded and liganded ERalpha on responsive promoters is an integral feature of estrogen signaling. Mol Cell 11:695–707
119. Ruffner H, Joazeiro CA, Hemmati D, Hunter T, Verma IM (2001) Cancer-predisposing mutations within the RING domain of BRCA1: loss of ubiquitin protein ligase activity and protection from radiation hypersensitivity. Proc Natl Acad Sci U S A 98:5134–5139
120. Fan S, Wang J, Yuan R, Ma Y, Meng Q, Erdos MR et al (1999) BRCA1 inhibition of estrogen receptor signaling in transfected cells. Science 284:1354–1356
121. Poukka H, Aarnisalo P, Karvonen U, Palvimo JJ, Janne OA (1999) Ubc9 interacts with the androgen receptor and activates receptor-dependent transcription. J Biol Chem 274: 19441–19446
122. Gottlicher M, Heck S, Doucas V, Wade E, Kullmann M, Cato ACB et al (1996) Interaction of the Ubc9 human homologue with c-Jun and with the glucocorticoid receptor. Steroids 61:257–262
123. von Baur E, Zechel C, Heery D, Heine MJS, Garnier JM, Vivat V et al (1996) Differential ligand-dependent interactions between the AF-2 activating domain of nuclear receptors and the putative transcriptional intermediary factors mSUG1 and TIF1. EMBO J 15:110–124
124. Fan M, Bigsby RM, Nephew KP (2003) The NEDD8 pathway is required for proteasome-mediated degradation of human estrogen receptor (ER)-alpha and essential for the antiproliferative activity of ICI 182, 780 in ERalpha-positive breast cancer cells. Mol Endocrinol 17:356–365
125. Huibregtse JM, Scheffner M, Beaudenon S, Howley PM (1995) A family of proteins structurally and functionally related to the E6-AP ubiquitin-protein ligase. Proc Natl Acad Sci U S A 92:2563–2567
126. Yan F, Gao X, Lonard DM, Nawaz Z (2003) Specific ubiquitin-conjugating enzymes promote degradation of specific nuclear receptor coactivators. Mol Endocrinol 17: 1315–1331
127. Verma S, Ismail A, Gao X, Fu G, Li X, O'Malley BW et al (2004) The ubiquitin-conjugating enzyme UBCH7 acts as a coactivator for steroid hormone receptors. Mol Cell Biol 24:8716–8726
128. Reid G, Denger S, Kos M, Gannon F (2002) Human estrogen receptor-alpha: regulation by synthesis, modification and degradation. Cell Mol Life Sci 59:821–831

129. Horigome T, Ogata F, Golding TS, Korach KS (1988) Estradiol-stimulated proteolytic cleavage of the estrogen receptor in mouse uterus. Endocrinology 123:2540–2548
130. Lonard DM, Nawaz Z, Smith CL, O'Malley BW (2000) The 26S proteasome is required for estrogen receptor-alpha and coactivator turnover and for efficient estrogen reeptor-alpha transactivation. Mol Cell 5:939–948
131. Joazeiro CA, Weissman AM (2000) RING finger proteins: mediators of ubiquitin ligase activity. Cell 102:549–552
132. Lange CA, Shen T, Horwitz KB (2000) Phosphorylation of human progesterone receptor at serine-294 by mitogen-activated protein kinase signals their degradation by the 26S proteasome. Proc Natl Acad Sci U S A 97:1032–1037
133. Ramamoorthy S, Dhananjayan SC, Demayo FJ, Nawaz Z (2010) Isoform-specific degradation of PR-B by E6-AP is critical for normal mammary gland development. Mol Endocrinol 24:2099–2113

Post-translational Modifications of ER Alpha in Rapid Estrogen's Action

Muriel Le Romancer, Coralie Poulard, Stéphanie Sentis and Laura Corbo

Abstract Estrogen receptor α (ERα) is a member of a large conserved superfamily of steroid hormone nuclear receptors that regulate many physiological processes, notably the growth and survival of breast tumor cells. In addition to their well-described effect on transcription, estrogens also induce rapid signaling outside of the nucleus through activation of kinase cascades. Although these effects have been extensively described, the mechanisms underlying this non-genomic function remain unclear. To fully understand how ERα functions are regulated, we must consider the role of post-translational modifications (PTMs) that modulate its activity. This review will focus particularly on PTMs regulating extranuclear signaling and on their deregulation in breast cancer. A thorough understanding of the role of these modifications in carcinogenesis might open new

---

M. Le Romancer · C. Poulard · S. Sentis · L. Corbo (✉)
Université de Lyon, F-69000 Lyon, France
e-mail: laura.corbo@lyon.unicancer.fr

M. Le Romancer
e-mail: muriel.leromancer@lyon.unicancer.fr

C. Poulard
e-mail: coralie.poulard@lyon.unicancer.fr

S. Sentis
e-mail: stephanie.sentis@lyon.unicancer.fr

M. Le Romancer · C. Poulard · S. Sentis · L. Corbo
Université Lyon 1, F-69000 Lyon, France

S. Sentis
Université de Lyon 1, ISPB, 69003 Lyon, France

M. Le Romancer · C. Poulard · S. Sentis · L. Corbo
Equipe Labellisée "La Ligue", UMR INSERM 1052 - CNRS 5286
Cancer Research Center of Lyon, Centre Léon Bérard,
28 rue Laennec, 69008 Lyon, France

G. Castoria and A. Migliaccio (eds.), *Advances in Rapid Sex-Steroid Action*,
DOI: 10.1007/978-1-4614-1764-4_5, © Springer Science+Business Media, LLC 2012

avenues not only for identifying new predictors of response to endocrine therapy, but also for promoting the development of novel therapeutic strategies.

Keywords Estrogen receptors α • Breast cancer • Estrogen signaling • Post-translational modifications • Arginine methylation • Palmitoylation

Abbreviations

AF-1	Activation function-1
AF-2	Activation function-2
AI	aromatase inhibitor
E_2	Estrogens
ER	estrogen receptor
FAK	Focal Adhesion Kinase
JMJD6	Jumonji domain-containing 6 protein
LBD	ligand-binding domain
PAT	palmitoyl acyltransferase
PAD	peptidylarginine deiminase
PI3K	phosphatidylinositol 3-kinase
PKA	protein kinase A
PLA	Proximity ligation assay
PRMT1	protein arginine N methyltransferase 1
PTM	post-translational modification
SERD	selective ER down-regulator
SERM	selective ER modulator

Contents

1 Introduction

Estrogens (E_2) mediate a broad spectrum of physiological processes, including reproduction, cardiovascular health, bone integrity, cognition and behaviour [1] through two receptors, ERα and ERβ [2], which "communicate" most of estrogen's mitogenic and survival stimuli via direct modulation of gene expression (genomic action) [3] or via activation of signal transduction cascades (non-genomic action) [4].

ERα is responsible for many of the effects of estrogens on normal breast development. Indeed, ERα-null mice develop a rudimentary mammary gland, indicating that ERα expression is essential to mammary development [1]. The involvement of E_2 and ERα in breast cancer development and progression is based on data from both clinical and animal studies. Compelling clinical and experimental evidence has demonstrated that lifetime exposure to E_2 and to estrogenic components constitutes a major risk factor for breast cancer and promotes cancer progression by stimulating malignant cell proliferation [5].

Although in the normal breast ERα is expressed at low levels [6], 70% of breast cancers are ERα-positive [7], supporting the use of agents that suppress receptor function (anti-estrogens) or estrogen synthesis (aromatase inhibitors) for breast cancer treatment [8]. ERα is a well-established predictive marker for hormone sensitivity and a good prognostic marker in breast cancer; it helps identify tumors that are likely to respond to endocrine treatment. However, de novo or acquired resistance to these treatments develops and is associated with aggressive, hormone-independent tumor growth [9]. The metastatic potential and poorer prognosis of these resistant tumors raise the need for novel therapeutic strategies to overcome drug resistance. A focus on estrogen signaling could help understand its deregulations in patients prone to develop resistance to endocrine therapy.

The biological function of ERα is based on its ability to regulate a range of cellular functions through genomic and non-genomic mechanisms. Moreover, there is growing knowledge and understanding of rapid extra-nuclear actions of ERα. First, some reports have indicated that a subpopulation of ERα localized at or near the plasma membrane mediates ERα extra-nuclear signaling [10]. However, the identity of the receptor and its exact localization, to or close to the plasma membrane, are the subject of intense effort and debate [11–13]. Biochemical and cellular evidences indicate that membrane and nuclear forms of ERα derive from the same gene [14]. In addition, various truncated ERs have been identified as the mediators of E_2 non genomic-signaling [15, 16]. ERα receptors have no intrinsic ability to signal because they lack structural domains such as those of tyrosine kinase receptors, but they can activate multiple signal transduction cascades through direct interactions with various proteins, including the tyrosine kinase Src, phosphatidylinositol 3-kinase (PI3K) and adaptor proteins [17–21]. ERα localization to the membrane can also be mediated by interactions with the membrane adaptor protein Shc [22] and with a variety of proximal signaling molecules such as G proteins [23]. ERα interactions with Src and PI3K can also be activated by other accessory proteins such as the adaptor protein p130Cas which regulates the activation of Src kinase in T47D human breast carcinoma cells [24]. Other partners may be involved, like the caveolin-binding protein striatin which targets ERα to the plasma membrane [25]. The estradiol-dependent formation of complexes between ERα and Src or the PI3K subunit p85 activates two major pathways: the Src/ras/MAPK and the PI3K/Akt pathways. Finally, PTMs of ERα have been described as a crucial component of non-genomic signaling, which not only triggers ERα interactions with membrane or cytoplamic proteins but also promotes the signaling cascades.

In this review, we focus on ERα PTMs involved in non-genomic signaling, and we discuss whether deregulation of these processes can contribute to the neoplastic transformation of breast cells.

2 PTMs Involved in ER Non-genomic Signaling

Protein PTMs are highly versatile tools that regulate the activity of key proteins. PTMs include the addition of simple chemical groups, such as a phosphate, acetyl, methyl or hydroxyl groups; larger protein complexes, such as AMP, ADP-ribose, sugars or lipids; or small polypeptides, such as ubiquitin or ubiquitin-like proteins. They also include modifications of specific amino acid side chains (e.g., deamidation of glutamine residues) and the cleavage of peptide bonds (i.e., proteolysis). ERα and its coregulators are subject to a variety of covalent PTMs [26] most of which have been linked to estrogen genomic signaling. Nevertheless, a number of recent studies have also described PTMs regulating ERα non-genomic signaling, which gives new insight into this pathway. Figure 1 illustrates the PTMs involved in ERα non-genomic signaling.

2.1 Palmitoylation

To explain the rapid non-genomic effect of E_2, it has been postulated that a small population of ERα localizes to the plasma membrane, allowing its association to signal transduction molecules [10, 27, 28]. Consistently, the presence of a fraction of ERα has been reported in caveolae or caveolar-like membrane microdomains [29, 30], and more recent reports have described the involvement of post-translational lipid modifications such as palmitoylation in facilitating ERα membrane localization [31]. Palmitoylation consists of the attachment of a long fatty acyl chain, generally a C16-carbon saturated fatty acyl chain, either to cytoplasmic cysteine residues via a thioester linkage (S-palmitoylation) or to glycine/cysteine residues via an amide linkage (N-palmitoylation). S-palmitoylation, the only reversible fatty reaction, affects the lipophilicity of target proteins by changing their subcellular distribution, from the endoplasmic reticulum to the plasma membrane for instance, or increasing their affinity for lipid rafts in membranes [32]. ERα has been identified as the target of *S*-palmitoylation mediated by an unknown palmitoyl acyltransferase (PAT) at cysteine 447, located in the human ERα ligand-binding region [31]. This site seems to be required for both the localization of ERα to the membrane and for E_2 rapid signaling. Indeed, mutation of ERα at the Cys447 residue impairs receptor membrane localization and interaction with caveolin-1 and

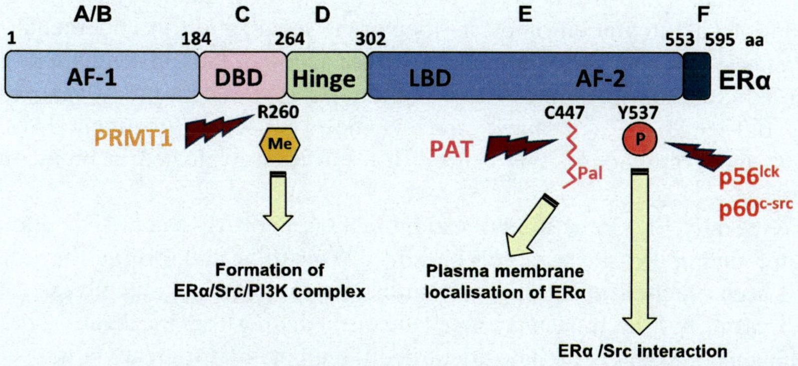

Fig. 1 Post-translational modifications of ERα involved in non-nuclear ERα signaling Functional domains of ERα. The structure of ERα is shown in linear fashion, with the N- to C-terminal domains designated A–F. The amino acid spans of the domains are indicated. A/B domain contains the activation function 1 domain (AF-1). C domain is composed of the DNA binding domain (DBD). D domain is the Hinge region that includes nuclear localisation signals. E domain is composed of Ligand Binding Domain (LBD) and Activation function 2 (AF-2). F domain is important for the ligand specificity. Localisation of Post-translational modifications of ERα. Specific residues are modified as shown, with phosphorylation (P) in red, arginine methylation (Me) in orange and palmitoylation (Pal) in pink. Proteins responsible for these modifications are shown in matching colours

limits the E_2-induced rapid activation of the ERK/MAPK signaling pathway [22, 33]. Furthermore, inhibition of PAT activity by 2-bromopalmitate prevents ERK/MAPK and PI3K/Akt activation, thus supporting the central role of palmitoylation in rapid E_2 signaling. The group of M. Marino has shown that the plant-derived flavanone naringenin inhibits estrogen non-genomic signaling through rapid depalmitoylation of membrane-ERα [34]. The functional impact of this regulation is not currently understood. As S-palmitoylation is a reversible PTM, ERα palmitoylation can be modulated in response to cell stimulation, notably through E_2 induction. The accepted model proposes that palmitoylation triggers ERα to the plasma membrane through interaction with caveolin. Upon E_2 binding, ERα undergoes de-palmitoylation and dissociates from caveolin-1, thereby facilitating its association with signaling molecules.

Subsequent studies have identified a palmitoylation motif of nine amino acids (445–453 in ERα) including the cysteine palmitoylation site, which is highly conserved in the E domains of ERα, ERβ, the progesterone receptor (PR) and the androgen receptor (AR) [35]. Recently, using a proteomic approach and conjugation to a palmitoylation motif peptide, Levin's group has shown that the heat shock protein Hsp27 interacts with the palmitoylation motif of ERα and that this protein is required for ERα palmitoylation, membrane translocation and rapid signaling [36].

In addition to the full-length classic transcript of ERα, mRNA splice variants generated through alternative splicing or alternative promoters also have membrane localization. The ERα46 variant lacking the AF-1 domain has been identified in MCF-7 breast cancer cells [37], osteoblasts [38], human macrophages [39] and endothelial cells [15]. It has been shown that ERα46 is palmitoylated and that inhibitors of palmitoylation block its membrane localization in endothelial cells [15]. In breast cell lines, this variant inhibits the action of the full-length ERα [40]. Interestingly, the transfection of ERα46 in tamoxifen–resistant breast cancer cells inhibits full-length ERα response and enhances endocrine treatment [41, 42]. However, the expression of this isoform has not been evaluated in breast tumor samples.

More recently ERα36, a 36 kDa variant lacking both AF-1 and AF-2 domains, has been found in breast cancer cell lines [43]. This truncated form of the receptor has also been reported to localize predominantly to the plasma membrane and to the cytoplasm, but the molecular mechanism mediating this localization has not been elucidated. Wang et al. have identified three potential myristoylation sites in ERα36 and propose that also this ERα isoform may be localized to the plasma membrane by posttranslational modification [16, 43]. This truncated ERα is also characterized by the presence of a unique 27–amino-acid region at the C-terminus, which most likely changes its ligand-binding specificity. ERα36 inhibits the transactivation activities of wild-type ERα. Notably, it mediates membrane-initiated signaling of both estrogens and antiestrogens [16], leading to activation of the MAPK signaling pathway and cell proliferation in breast cancer cells, suggesting the involvement of ERα36 in the development of tamoxifen-resistant breast cancer [44, 45]. Indeed patients who express high levels of ERα36 are less likely to respond to tamoxifen treatment.

The enzymes catalyzing palmitoylation have not yet been clearly identified and very little is known about the enzymes responsible for reversing these modifications. Discovering the molecular identity of PATs has increased the interest in palmitoylation, partly because many of the genes encoding PATs have been shown to be associated with human disease, particularly with cancer [46, 47]. Notably, numerous PAT genes have been implicated in tumorigenesis and metastasis [48, 49], suggesting that the substrates of these PATs can be associated with regulatory signaling networks. The identification of these networks will potentially provide new therapeutic targets for the prevention or the reversal of cancer progression. Given that ERα is one of the few known targets of palmitoylation, particular attention will be paid to the identification of the PAT responsible for ERα modification. While some progress has been made in identifying pharmacological modulators of palmitoylation [50–52], the strategy for specifically targeting individual PATs is not known yet. From a practical standpoint, inhibiting specific PATs may be a simpler process than developing specific PAT agonists.

2.2 *Phosphorylation on Tyrosine (Y)*

The phosphorylation of Y537 located within the ligand-binding domain of ERα was first reported in rat uterus [53] and then confirmed in MCF-7 cells where the residue is basally phosphorylated. In vitro data indicate that Src tyrosine kinases

($p56^{lck}$ and $p60^{c\text{-}src}$) could be responsible for this phosphorylation which is necessary for ERα dimerization. Cheskis's group has confirmed that ERα interacts with the SH2 domain of Src through this phosphorylated site [54]. Research by the group of Aurrichio has recently shown interesting results demonstrating that this phosphorylation is involved in estrogen non-genomic action. A six-amino-acid peptide that mimics the sequence around the phosphoY537 residue disrupts ERα/Src interaction in MCF-7 cells, and inhibits cyclin D1 expression and cell proliferation [55]. The phospho-peptide also reduces E_2 protective effect against apoptosis. Interestingly, injection of the phospho-peptide inhibits the growth of MCF-7 cell xenografts in nude mice, supporting the relevance of this strategy in vivo and confirming a potential therapeutic interest in ERα-positive tumors.

Src is a protooncogene involved in signaling that culminates in the control of multiple biological functions such as cell proliferation, cell differentiation, migration, angiogenesis and survival. Src is thought to play a key role in tumor formation and progression.

The non-receptor tyrosine kinase Src is overexpressed and activated in a large number of human malignancies and has long been associated with the development of cancer and progression to distant metastases. In recent years, in vitro observations have led to the hypothesis that, in addition to increasing cellular proliferation, one of the primary roles of Src in cancer is to regulate cell adhesion, invasion and motility [56].

Unfortunately, because of the lack of a specific antibody, the expression of phosphorylated ERα in breast tumors cannot be detected. Given the deregulation of Src activity, one could expect that ERα is hyperphosphorylated in these tumors. This could be circumvent by the use of the Proximity ligation assay (PLA) developed by Olink Bioscience to detect in situ protein interaction in fixed tissues. The study of ERα/Src interactions in breast tumors would help determine whether this pathway is deregulated in breast cancer and can be targeted by disruption of the complex. If ERα is found to be hyperphosphorylated on Y537, a possible treatment strategy could be to inhibit Src activity. The Src inhibitor dasatinib is available for clinical trials [57].

However, results from Katzenellenbogen's group strongly indicate that Src phosphorylates ERα on different other tyrosine residues, as confirmed by the fact that a truncated ERα isoform, ERα36, triggers non-genomic signaling through Src/MAPK activation and this isoform lacks tyrosine 537, suggesting that other mechanisms are involved in ERα/Src interaction [58].

2.3 *Arginine Methylation*

The methylation of arginine residues is catalyzed by the protein arginine N-methyltransferase (PRMT) family of enzymes. The PRMT family comprises 10 members classified as type I or type II, depending on whether they catalyze symmetric or asymmetric dimethylation, respectively. These enzymes are involved in different cellular processes including transcriptional regulation, DNA repair, RNA metabolism and signal transduction [59, 60]. Arginine methylation regulates these processes mainly through modifications of protein–protein interactions. Our team has reported a novel paradigm for ERα regulation through PRMT1-mediated methylation of arginine 260 within the ERα DNA-binding domain [61, 62]. Mutation of arginine 260 to alanine specifically abolishes the modification induced by PRMT1. An antibody specific to the methylated form of ERα (R260met) has been generated and used to confirm ERα methylation in living cells. A variety of consequences of ERα methylation has been described, as well as the possible underlying mechanisms. Indeed estrogen treatment induces rapid and transient methylation of ERα and this methylation event is required for mediating the extra-nuclear function of the receptor. Biochemical and cellular approaches have provided evidence that PRMT1 activation initiates the rapid estrogen action responsible for methylating ERα, which thereby interacts with Src and PI3K, and propagates the signal to downstream transduction cascades that orchestrate cell proliferation and survival. Additionally, ERα methylation seems to depend on the activation of the Src family of tyrosine kinases, as E_2 -induced methylation of ERα has been shown to be reversed by the Src family tyrosine kinase inhibitors PP1 and SU6656. In line with this, we have found that the Src substrate FAK (Focal Adhesion kinase), participates in this signaling complex and that Src activity is required both for FAK interaction with Src and for the stability of the complex. Given the key role of the dual kinases Src/FAK in cell migration, we can speculate that the complex containing methylated ERα/Src/PI3K/FAK is involved in cell adhesion and migration. Rapid down-regulation of ERα methylation and/or Src activity may serve to control rapid physiological responses of estrogen, inducing the dissociation of the complex and ultimately the extinction of downstream kinase activation [61, 62].

As mentioned before, the methylation of ERα is transient after estrogen treatment, suggesting that an enzyme could remove the methyl mark. Indeed, the disappearance of the methylated receptor is not due to ERα degradation by the proteasome. So far the only enzyme reported to be able to reverse the methylation of arginine residues is JMJD6 [26], although it remains unclear whether JMJD6 is able to demethylate nonhistone proteins. Another class of enzymes capable of removing methyl marks is the peptidylarginine deiminases (PADIs), previously characterized as capable of catalyzing the conversion of arginines to citrullines by deimination which, as a consequence, prevents methylation by PRMTs [63, 64]. To date, five human PADI homologs with a relatively broad substrate specificity have been identified, PADI1-4 and PADI1-6 [65].

Immunohistochemical studies in a cohort of breast cancer patients have demonstrated that ERα is methylated in normal epithelial breast cells and is hypermethylated in a subset of breast cancer cells. Importantly, the presence or absence of methylated ERα does not correlate with the clinical classification as ERα negative or positive tumors. Actually, tumors with high levels of methylated ERα belong equally to ERα positive and negative cases. This apparent paradox is easily resolved since only tumors showing ERα nuclear staining are included in the

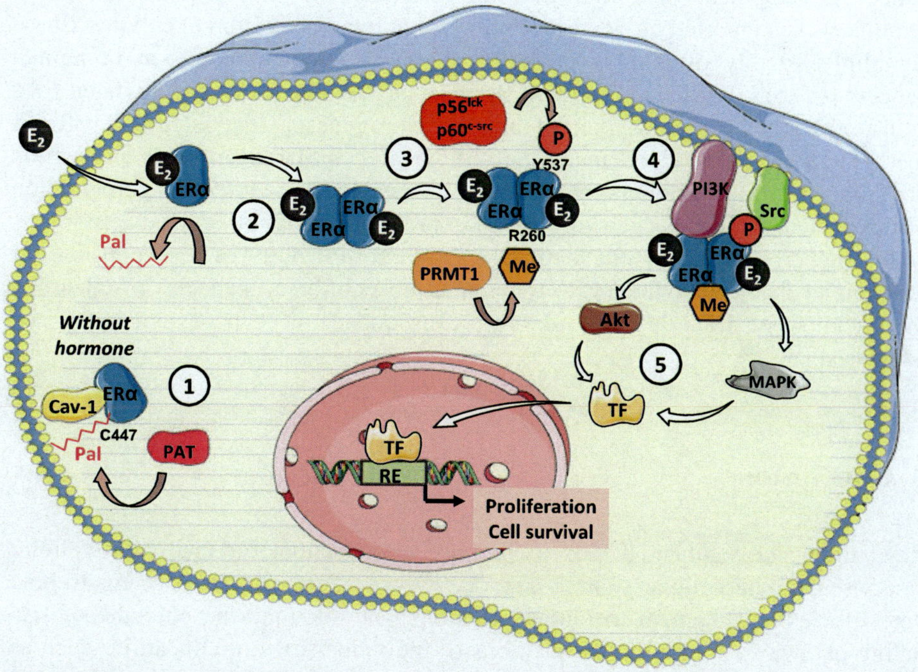

Fig. 2 Model integrating ERα post-transcriptional modifications in rapid estrogen's signaling (**1**) without hormone, a small population of ERα is palmitoylated on Cys447 by an unknown palmitoyltransferase (PAT) localized at the plasma membrane through caveolin-1 association (**2**) E2 binding, promotes ERα depalmitoylation, dissociation from caveolin-1 and consecutive receptor dimerization; leading to (**3**) its methylation on the arginine 260 by PRMT1 and phosphorylation on the tyrosine 537 by $p56^{lck}$, $p60^{c\text{-}src}$. Both modifications promote (**4**) the formation of a signaling complex propagating the signal to downstream transduction cascades that orchestrate cell proliferation and survival (**5**) Indeed, methylation on R260 promotes the formation of the ERα/PI3K/Src complex and phosphorylation on Y537 is a prerequisite for the interaction between Src and ERα. It has not been established whether phosphorylation and methylation act sequentially or in concert

population of ERα-positive cases and tumors with negative or extra-nuclear expression of the receptor belong to the population of ERα-negative patients [66]. One cannot rule out that the cytoplasmic methylated form of ERα revealed by this immunohystochemical study corresponds, at least in part, to the methylated truncated forms of the receptors (ERα46 or ERα36) described above. Studies in progress in our laboratory, using different approaches such as PLA and real-time RT-PCR, should answer this question. Our analysis should also determine whether subgroups of breast tumors overexpressing different isoforms of methylated ERα exist. Several questions remain about the physiological role of ERα methylation, how it is regulated in breast tumors, and if a relationship exists between ERα hypermethylation and breast cancer development and/or progression. One can hypothesize that the deregulation of ERα methylation may be involved in breast cancer development and contribute to resistance to hormone therapy. This hypothesis is supported by previous findings that hyperactivation of cellular kinase signaling, notably of Akt, is probably the most frequent alteration in human cancers [67, 68]. Further studies will be necessary to determine if methylated ERα could constitute a new marker of breast tumorigenesis. In conclusion, ERα is methylated in breast cells under physiological conditions and this process is deregulated in breast tumors by an unknown mechanism. Moreover, deregulation of the demethylation mechanism (loss of expression or loss of enzyme activity) as well as hyper-activation of the methylase activity of PRMT1 can be responsible for the high levels of methylated ERα found in a subset of breast cancers. Whether this modification of ERα is a cause or a consequence of cancer remains to be addressed.

3 Conclusions

Reversible and regulated PTMs of proteins are essential for mediating cellular responses to extracellular signals. The occurrence of several PTMs seems to be a very efficient mechanism to initiate, terminate or fine-tune the outcome of signaling pathways. While the implications of individual ERα modifications such as phosphorylation, acetylation and methylation have been relatively well-documented, interactions between the PTMs involved in ERα non-genomic signaling remain to be elucidated. We can reasonably postulate that one modification is coupled to the enhancement or suppression of another. In this context, we will discuss the potential interplays between these ERα PTMs involved in estrogen rapid action (Fig. 2). Without hormones, a small population of ERα, palmitoylated on Cys447 by an unidentified PAT, localizes at the plasma membrane through caveolin-1 association. Estrogen treatment promotes ERα depalmitoylation although an unknown mechanism, and induces its dissociation from caveolin-1 and consecutive receptor dimerization thereby leading to its methylation on the arginine 260 by PRMT1 and phosphorylation on the tyrosine 537 by $p56^{lck}$, $p60^{c\text{-}src}$. Both modifications will promote the assembly of the signaling complex which propagates the signal to downstream transduction cascades that orchestrate cell proliferation and survival. Although, as discussed before, both PRMT1 and Src activities are required for ERα methylation on R260 and for the stability of the ERα/Src/PI3K complex and that also phosphorylation on Y537 is a prerequisite for the interaction between Src and ERα, to date we don't know whether these PTMs act sequentially or in concert. It will be interesting to test if the peptide derived from the sequence around the phosphoY537 residue, which prevents ERα/Src interaction, may inhibit ERα methylation.

At present, ERα status is the only factor used routinely for prediction of response to endocrine therapy and patient selection in breast cancer. Current breast cancer therapies can target the interaction of estrogen to its receptor by blocking the activity of ERα with drugs like tamoxifen [69] or other selective estrogen receptor modulators (SERMs); by inducing the destabilization and degradation of ERα by treatment with selective estrogen receptor down-regulators (SERDs) such as fulvestrant (Faslodex, formerly known as ICI 182,780) [70, 71] and by reducing the production of estrogens in peripheral tissues and within the tumor using aromatase inhibitors [72, 73]. Understanding how PTMs regulate ERα actions remains a crucial goal to dissect the mechanisms by which breast cancers evade anti estrogen-mediated growth arrest and to design new anticancer strategies based on this pathway. Certainly, our knowledge of these dynamic modifications is still at an early stage due to the lack of appropriate tools to monitor modifications of endogenous proteins. It is important to note that most the effect of the described PTMs come from in vitro or transfection studies and, because of the unavailability of specific antibodies, their in vivo significance is poorly understood. It will be crucial to verify their relevance in vivo, or at least by targeted mutations in breast cell lines. This is essential, as transfection studies present intrinsic difficulties in accurately reproducing stoichiometric relationships between members of the ERα network. Future studies should investigate how the different modifications act, sequentially and/or in concert, under physiological and pathological conditions. Using proteomic approaches, including developing site- and modification-specific antibodies and employing mass spectrometry techniques, would allow a better understanding of the regulation of these dynamic modifications in vivo. Furthermore, genetic approaches, such as the creation of mice with specific mutations in individual amino acid residues that are target sites of PTMs would provide useful in testing the role of these modifications in ERα physiological functions. In addition, crosses of these modification-deficient ERα knock-in animals would help to dissect the interplay of these various PTM. While these types of approaches are often labour-intensive and relatively expensive, these models can serve as in vivo targets to test new cancer treatments and permit the generation of genetically defined cells for in vitro experiments. Important efforts should also be made to better define the actors involved in PTM regulation, notably the enzymes responsible for reversing ERα PTMs.

New treatments targeting the molecules responsible for modifying or reversing PTMs could advantageously be used in combination with endocrine therapies or after treatment failure or acquired resistance. However, specifically targeting the PTMs present in breast cancer cells is a prerequisite to reduce therapy-related risks, as most of the enzymes involved in such modifications are present in both the tumor and healthy tissues and treatment may cause a wide range of unwanted side effects.

Acknowledgments We thank M. D. Reynaud for reading the manuscript. This work was supported by the Ligue Nationale Contre le Cancer (Equipe labellisée 2009), and the Association pour la Recherche sur le Cancer. C.P. is supported by a fellowship from the French Ministry of Research. Figures were produced using Servier Medical Art.

The authors have nothing to disclose.

References

1. Couse JF, Korach KS (1999) Estrogen receptor null mice: what have we learned and where will they lead us? Endocr Rev 20:358–417
2. Enmark E, Gustafsson JA (1999) Oestrogen receptors—an overview. J Intern Med 246: 133–138
3. McDonnell DP, Norris JD (2002) Connections and regulation of the human estrogen receptor. Science 296:1642–1644
4. Levin ER (2009) Membrane oestrogen receptor alpha signalling to cell functions. J Physiol 587:5019–5023
5. Santen RJ, Allred DC (2007) The estrogen paradox. Nat Clin Pract Endocrinol Metab 3: 496–497
6. Crandall DL, Busler DE, Novak TJ, Weber RV, Kral JG (1998) Identification of estrogen receptor beta RNA in human breast and abdominal subcutaneous adipose tissue. Biochem Biophys Res Commun 248:523–526
7. Colditz GA (1998) Relationship between estrogen levels, use of hormone replacement therapy, and breast cancer. J Natl Cancer Inst 90:814–823
8. Harvey JM, Clark GM, Osborne CK, Allred DC (1999) Estrogen receptor status by immunohistochemistry is superior to the ligand-binding assay for predicting response to adjuvant endocrine therapy in breast cancer. J Clin Oncol 17:1474–1481
9. Ali S, Coombes RC (2002) Endocrine-responsive breast cancer and strategies for combating resistance. Nat Rev Cancer 2:101–112
10. Pietras RJ, Szego CM (1977) Specific binding sites for oestrogen at the outer surfaces of isolated endometrial cells. Nature 265:69–72
11. Hammes SR, Levin ER (2007) Extranuclear steroid receptors: nature and actions. Endocr Rev 28:726–741
12. Olde B, Leeb-Lundberg LM (2009) GPR30/GPER1: searching for a role in estrogen physiology. Trends Endocrinol Metab 20:409–416
13. Pappas TC, Gametchu B, Watson CS (1995) Membrane estrogen receptor-enriched GH(3)/ B6 cells have an enhanced non-genomic response to estrogen. Endocrine 3:743–749
14. Levin ER (2009) Plasma membrane estrogen receptors. Trends Endocrinol Metab 20: 477–482
15. Li L, Haynes MP, Bender JR (2003) Plasma membrane localization and function of the estrogen receptor alpha variant (ER46) in human endothelial cells. Proc Natl Acad Sci U S A 100:4807–4812
16. Wang Z, Zhang X, Shen P, Loggie BW, Chang Y, Deuel TF (2006) A variant of estrogen receptor-{alpha}, hER-{alpha}36: transduction of estrogen- and antiestrogen-dependent membrane-initiated mitogenic signaling. Proc Natl Acad Sci U S A 103:9063–9068
17. Acconcia F, Manavathi B, Mascarenhas J, Talukder AH, Mills G, Kumar R (2006) An inherent role of integrin-linked kinase-estrogen receptor alpha interaction in cell migration. Cancer Res 66:11030–11038
18. Bjornstrom L, Sjoberg M (2005) Mechanisms of estrogen receptor signaling: convergence of genomic and nongenomic actions on target genes. Mol Endocrinol 19:833–842
19. Castoria G, Migliaccio A, Bilancio A, Di Domenico M, de Falco A, Lombardi M, Fiorentino R, Varricchio L, Barone MV, Auricchio F (2001) PI3-kinase in concert with Src promotes the S-phase entry of oestradiol-stimulated MCF-7 cells. EMBO J 20:6050–6059
20. Simoncini T, Hafezi-Moghadam A, Brazil DP, Ley K, Chin WW, Liao JK (2000) Interaction of oestrogen receptor with the regulatory subunit of phosphatidylinositol-3-OH kinase. Nature 407:538–541
21. Song RX, Zhang Z, Santen RJ (2005) Estrogen rapid action via protein complex formation involving ERalpha and Src. Trends Endocrinol Metab 16:347–353

22. Song RX, Barnes CJ, Zhang Z, Bao Y, Kumar R, Santen RJ (2004) The role of Shc and insulin-like growth factor 1 receptor in mediating the translocation of estrogen receptor alpha to the plasma membrane. Proc Natl Acad Sci USA 101:2076–2081
23. Kumar P, Wu Q, Chambliss KL, Yuhanna IS, Mumby SM, Mineo C, Tall GG, Shaul PW (2007) Direct Interactions with G alpha i and G betagamma mediate nongenomic signaling by estrogen receptor alpha. Mol Endocrinol 21:1370–1380
24. Cabodi S, Moro L, Baj G, Smeriglio M, Di Stefano P, Gippone S, Surico N, Silengo L, Turco E, Tarone G, Defilippi P (2004) p130Cas interacts with estrogen receptor alpha and modulates non-genomic estrogen signaling in breast cancer cells. J Cell Sci 117:1603–1611
25. Lu Q, Pallas DC, Surks HK, Baur WE, Mendelsohn ME, Karas RH (2004) Striatin assembles a membrane signaling complex necessary for rapid, nongenomic activation of endothelial NO synthase by estrogen receptor alpha. Proc Natl Acad Sci USA 101:17126–17131
26. O'Malley BW, Qin J, Lanz RB (2008) Cracking the coregulator codes. Curr Opin Cell Biol 20:310–315
27. Levin ER (1999) Cellular functions of the plasma membrane estrogen receptor. Trends Endocrinol Metab 10:374–377
28. Pedram A, Razandi M, Levin ER (2006) Nature of functional estrogen receptors at the plasma membrane. Mol Endocrinol 20:1996–2009
29. Razandi M, Oh P, Pedram A, Schnitzer J, Levin ER (2002) ERs associate with and regulate the production of caveolin: implications for signaling and cellular actions. Mol Endocrinol 16:100–115
30. Kim HP, Lee JY, Jeong JK, Bae SW, Lee HK, Jo I (1999) Nongenomic stimulation of nitric oxide release by estrogen is mediated by estrogen receptor alpha localized in caveolae. Biochem Biophys Res Commun 263:257–262
31. Acconcia F, Ascenzi P, Fabozzi G, Visca P, Marino M (2004) S-palmitoylation modulates human estrogen receptor-alpha functions. Biochem Biophys Res Commun 316:878–883
32. Salaun C, Greaves J, Chamberlain LH (2010) The intracellular dynamic of protein palmitoylation. J Cell Biol 191:1229–1238
33. Acconcia F, Ascenzi P, Bocedi A, Spisni E, Tomasi V, Trentalance A, Visca P, Marino M (2005) Palmitoylation-dependent estrogen receptor alpha membrane localization: regulation by 17beta-estradiol. Mol Biol Cell 16:231–237
34. Galluzzo P, Ascenzi P, Bulzomi P, Marino M (2008) The nutritional flavanone naringenin triggers antiestrogenic effects by regulating estrogen receptor alpha-palmitoylation. Endocrinology 149:2567–2575
35. Pedram A, Razandi M, Sainson RC, Kim JK, Hughes CC, Levin ER (2007) A conserved mechanism for steroid receptor translocation to the plasma membrane. J Biol Chem 282:22278–22288
36. Razandi M, Pedram A, Levin ER (2010) Heat shock protein 27 is required for sex steroid receptor trafficking to and functioning at the plasma membrane. Mol Cell Biol 30:3249–3261
37. Trivedi S, Piccart M, Muquardt C, Gilot N, Hadiy S, Patel D, Leclercq G (1996) Tamoxifen aziridine labeling of the estrogen receptor-potential utility in detecting biologically aggressive breast tumors. Breast Cancer Res Treat 40:231–241
38. Denger S, Reid G, Kos M, Flouriot G, Parsch D, Brand H, Korach KS, Sonntag-Buck V, Gannon F (2001) ERalpha gene expression in human primary osteoblasts: evidence for the expression of two receptor proteins. Mol Endocrinol 15:2064–2077
39. Murphy AJ, Guyre PM, Wira CR, Pioli PA (2009) Estradiol regulates expression of estrogen receptor ERalpha46 in human macrophages. PLoS One 4:e5539
40. Fuqua SA, Fitzgerald SD, Allred DC, Elledge RM, Nawaz Z, McDonnell DP, O'Malley BW, Greene GL, McGuire WL (1992) Inhibition of estrogen receptor action by a naturally occurring variant in human breast tumors. Cancer Res 52:483–486
41. Penot G, Le Peron C, Merot Y, Grimaud-Fanouillere E, Ferriere F, Boujrad N, Kah O, Saligaut C, Ducouret B, Metivier R, Flouriot G (2005) The human estrogen receptor-alpha isoform hERalpha46 antagonizes the proliferative influence of hERalpha66 in MCF7 breast cancer cells. Endocrinology 146:5474–5484

42. Klinge CM, Riggs KA, Wickramasinghe NS, Emberts CG, McConda DB, Barry PN, Magnusen JE (2010) Estrogen receptor alpha 46 is reduced in tamoxifen resistant breast cancer cells and re-expression inhibits cell proliferation and estrogen receptor alpha 66-regulated target gene transcription. Mol Cell Endocrinol 323:268–276
43. Wang Z, Zhang X, Shen P, Loggie BW, Chang Y, Deuel TF (2005) Identification, cloning, and expression of human estrogen receptor-alpha36, a novel variant of human estrogen receptor-alpha66. Biochem Biophys Res Commun 336:1023–1027
44. Zhang XT, Kang LG, Ding L, Vranic S, Gatalica Z, Wang ZY (2011) A positive feedback loop of ER-alpha36/EGFR promotes malignant growth of ER-negative breast cancer cells. Oncogene 30:770–780
45. Lin SL, Yan LY, Zhang XT, Yuan J, Li M, Qiao J, Wang ZY, Sun QY (2010) ER-alpha36, a variant of ER-alpha, promotes tamoxifen agonist action in endometrial cancer cells via the MAPK/ERK and PI3K/Akt pathways. PLoS One 5:e9013
46. Planey SL, Zacharias DA (2009) Palmitoyl acyltransferases, their substrates, and novel assays to connect them (Review). Mol Membr Biol 26:14–31
47. Saleem AN, Chen YH, Baek HJ, Hsiao YW, Huang HW, Kao HJ, Liu KM, Shen LF, Song IW, Tu CP, Wu JY, Kikuchi T, Justice MJ, Yen JJ, Chen YT (2010) Mice with alopecia, osteoporosis, and systemic amyloidosis due to mutation in Zdhhc13, a gene coding for palmitoyl acyltransferase. PLoS Genet 6:e1000985
48. Draper JM, Smith CD (2010) DHHC20: a human palmitoyl acyltransferase that causes cellular transformation. Mol Membr Biol 27:123–136
49. Planey SL, Keay SK, Zhang CO, Zacharias DA (2009) Palmitoylation of cytoskeleton associated protein 4 by DHHC2 regulates antiproliferative factor-mediated signaling. Mol Biol Cell 20:1454–1463
50. Jennings BC, Nadolski MJ, Ling Y, Baker MB, Harrison ML, Deschenes RJ, Linder ME (2009) 2-Bromopalmitate and 2-(2-hydroxy-5-nitro-benzylidene)-benzo[b]thiophen-3-one inhibit DHHC-mediated palmitoylation in vitro. J Lipid Res 50:233–242
51. Ducker CE, Griffel LK, Smith RA, Keller SN, Zhuang Y, Xia Z, Diller JD, Smith CD (2006) Discovery and characterization of inhibitors of human palmitoyl acyltransferases. Mol Cancer Ther 5:1647–1659
52. Resh MD (2006) Use of analogs and inhibitors to study the functional significance of protein palmitoylation. Methods 40:191–197
53. Migliaccio A, Rotondi A, Auricchio F (1986) Estradiol receptor: phosphorylation on tyrosine in uterus and interaction with anti-phosphotyrosine antibody. EMBO J 5:2867–2872
54. Barletta F, Wong CW, McNally C, Komm BS, Katzenellenbogen B, Cheskis BJ (2004) Characterization of the interactions of estrogen receptor and MNAR in the activation of cSrc. Mol Endocrinol 18:1096–1108
55. Varricchio L, Migliaccio A, Castoria G, Yamaguchi H, De FA, Di DM, Giovannelli P, Farrar W, Appella E, Auricchio F (2007) Inhibition of estradiol receptor/Src association and cell growth by an estradiol receptor alpha tyrosine-phosphorylated peptide. Mol Cancer Res 5:1213–1221
56. Biscardi JS, Ishizawar RC, Silva CM, Parsons SJ (2000) Tyrosine kinase signalling in breast cancer: epidermal growth factor receptor and c-Srcc-Src interactions in breast cancer. Breast Cancer Res 2:203–210
57. Burstein HJ (2011) Novel agents and future directions for refractory breast cancer. Semin Oncol 38(2):S17–S24
58. Likhite VS, Stossi F, Kim K, Katzenellenbogen BS, Katzenellenbogen JA (2006) Kinase-specific phosphorylation of the estrogen receptor changes receptor interactions with ligand, deoxyribonucleic acid, and coregulators associated with alterations in estrogen and tamoxifen activity. Mol Endocrinol 20:3120–3132
59. Bedford MT, Clarke SG (2009) Protein arginine methylation in mammals: who, what, and why. Mol Cell 33:1–13

60. Teyssier C, Le Romancer M, Sentis S, Jalaguier S, Corbo L, Cavailles V (2010) Protein arginine methylation in estrogen signaling and estrogen-related cancers. Trends Endocrinol Metab 21:181–189
61. Le Romancer M, Treilleux I, Leconte N, Robin-Lespinasse Y, Sentis S, Bouchekioua-Bouzaghou K, Goddard S, Gobert-Gosse S, Corbo L (2008) Regulation of estrogen rapid signaling through arginine methylation by PRMT1. Mol Cell 31:212–221
62. Le Romancer M, Treilleux I, Bouchekioua-Bouzaghou K, Sentis S, Corbo L (2010) Methylation, a key step for nongenomic estrogen signaling in breast tumors. Steroids 75: 560–564
63. Wang Y, Wysocka J, Sayegh J, Lee YH, Perlin JR, Leonelli L, Sonbuchner LS, McDonald CH, Cook RG, Dou Y, Roeder RG, Clarke S, Stallcup MR, Allis CD, Coonrod SA (2004) Human PAD4 regulates histone arginine methylation levels via demethylimination. Science 306:279–283
64. Cuthbert GL, Daujat S, Snowden AW, Erdjument-Bromage H, Hagiwara T, Yamada M, Schneider R, Gregory PD, Tempst P, Bannister AJ, Kouzarides T (2004) Histone deimination antagonizes arginine methylation. Cell 118:545–553
65. Klose RJ, Zhang Y (2007) Regulation of histone methylation by demethylimination and demethylation. Nat Rev Mol Cell Biol 8:307–318
66. Kim R, Kaneko M, Arihiro K, Emi M, Tanabe K, Murakami S, Osaki A, Inai K (2006) Extranuclear expression of hormone receptors in primary breast cancer. Ann Oncol 17: 1213–1220
67. Altomare DA, Testa JR (2005) Perturbations of the AKT signaling pathway in human cancer. Oncogene 24:7455–7464
68. Hennessy BT, Smith DL, Ram PT, Lu Y, Mills GB (2005) Exploiting the PI3K/AKT pathway for cancer drug discovery. Nat Rev Drug Discov 4:988–1004
69. MacGregor JI, Jordan VC (1998) Basic guide to the mechanisms of antiestrogen action. Pharmacol Rev 50:151–196
70. Lonard DM, Nawaz Z, Smith CL, O'Malley BW (2000) The 26S proteasome is required for estrogen receptor-alpha and coactivator turnover and for efficient estrogen receptor-alpha transactivation. Mol Cell 5:939–948
71. Wijayaratne AL, McDonnell DP (2001) The human estrogen receptor-alpha is a ubiquitinated protein whose stability is affected differentially by agonists, antagonists, and selective estrogen receptor modulators. J Biol Chem 276:35684–35692
72. Johnston SR, Dowsett M (2003) Aromatase inhibitors for breast cancer: lessons from the laboratory. Nat Rev Cancer 3:821–831
73. Jordan VC (2004) Aromatase inhibitors that regulate estrogen target tissues selectively? Bone 34:372–375

Sex-Steroid Rapid Action and Its Role in Invasiveness and Metastasis of Breast Cancer

Marina Ines Flamini, Angel Matias Sanchez, Xiao-Dong Fu and Tommaso Simoncini

Abstract Through a variety of rapidly recruited intracellular mediators steroid receptors enact quick changes in the function of cells in different settings. Emerging evidence indicates that the interaction with the extracellular environment and cell movement are regulated by sex steroids through such rapid mechanisms. Exposure of different cell types to estrogen, progesterone or other steroids results in swift changes in the morphology of the cells, primarily because of changes in the position and organization of actin fibers. These changes are coupled with the formation of a variety of specialized cell membrane structures that are necessary for the cell interaction with high-molecular weight extracellular proteins or nearby cells, and thus to move around or to cross-talk with neighbor cells. Prominent actions on horizontal cell movement or on the ability to invade matrices have also been observed during exposure to estrogen or other steroids, which indicate that these steroids are powerful regulators of cell movement. Many of these actions are enacted via the rapid activation on extra-nuclear signaling cascades of sex steroid receptors that lead to the recruitment of small GTPases such as

M. I. Flamini · A. M. Sanchez · T. Simoncini (✉)
Molecular and Cellular Gynecological Endocrinology Laboratory (MCGEL),
Department of Reproductive Medicine and Child Development,
Division of Obstetrics and Gynecology, University of Pisa,
Via Roma 57, 56100 PI, Italy
e-mail: tommaso.simoncini@med.unipi.it; t.simoncini@obgyn.med.unipi.it

M. I. Flamini
e-mail: flaminimarinaines@hotmail.com

A. M. Sanchez
e-mail: angelsanchez2001@hotmail.com

X.-D. Fu
Department of Physiology, Zhongshan School of Medicine, Sun Yat-Sen University,
510080, Guangzhou, People's Republic of China
e-mail: mcgel@obgyn.med.unipi.it

G. Castoria and A. Migliaccio (eds.), *Advances in Rapid Sex-Steroid Action*,
DOI: 10.1007/978-1-4614-1764-4_6,

RhoA or Rac, which therefore drive the changes in actin positioning. These actions of sex steroids appear to be fundamental for migration and invasion in endocrine-sensitive breast cancer cells, and may therefore have relevance for local progression and metastasis. The characterization of these rapid actions of estrogens and other steroids will help to understand the effects of these hormones in the setting of breast cancer metastasis, and may eventually lead to new therapeutic strategies.

Keywords Breast cancer · Metastasis · Estrogen · Estrogen receptor · Extra-nuclear signaling

Contents

1 Introduction

Breast cancer is the most frequently diagnosed cancer and it is the main cause of mortality in women. About one woman in ten will develop breast cancer at some stage in her life. Extensive research has clearly demonstrated that the abnormal changes in the levels, frequencies, and types of steroid hormones are important contributors to the development of major cancer types such as the cancers of the prostate, testes, breast, ovary, uterine endometrium, and thyroid [1]. Thus, many studies have been focused on the involvement of steroids in the regulation of tumor development, cancer cell proliferation, progression, and metastatic processes [2].

The sex steroid hormones, estrogen and progesterone play an important role in normal mammary gland development, and breast cancer progression is influenced by estrogen, progesterone and their receptors. At the onset of puberty, female sex steroids are the fundamental regulators of ductal morphogenesis. On the other side, prolonged exposure to estrogen (i.e. early menarche, late menopause or postmenopausal hormone replacement therapy) is associated with a greater risk of developing breast cancer [3, 4]. All these factors stimulate epithelial cell proliferation and induce genotoxic effects and aneuplody, resulting in breast cancer initiation [5].

Local breast cancer spread and its later diffusion to the lymph nodes or to distant sites are the main cause of morbidity and death [6]. The generation of cancer cell movement in the surrounding environment is the first step in these processes and involves a complex set of cellular actions. A critical step is represented by the remodeling of the actin cytoskeleton toward the cell membrane, which allows the formation of bridges between the backbone of the cell and the extracellular matrix mediated by anchorage proteins [7].

Currently, the exact roles of sex steroids on breast cancer metastasis are controversial and may possibly be dual. There are clinical data showing that the adjuvant therapy with aromatase inhibitors reduces early distant metastasis and improves disease-free survival in breast cancer patients [8], suggesting that sex steroids promotes breast cancer progression. However, the opposite clinical observations have been reported that among the women using hormone replacement therapy, breast tumors are less invasive to distant sites [9, 10]. Moreover, expression of sex steroids receptors, including estrogen receptors (ERs) and progesterone receptors (PRs), is associated with more differentiated and less invasive breast cancers [11].

Furthermore endocrine therapy using the progesterone receptor (PR) antagonist RU486 prevents the development of mammary tumors and induces the regression of lymph node and lung metastases in mouse breast cancer models [12, 13], supporting a role for PR in these processes. In addition, PR agonists enhance the invasiveness of breast cancer cells by increasing tissue factor or vascular endothelial growth factor expression [14, 15]. However, definitive mechanistic explanations of the effects of ER or PR on breast cancer cell movement or invasion are not available. Therefore, further explorations on the relevance between sex steroids and breast cancer metastasis are needed to ascertain this discrepancy.

In common with other tumors, to undergo metastasis breast cancer cells acquire a migratory phenotype and these cells degrade underlying basement membrane and detach from the primary tumor site. Following entrance of circulation, breast cancer cells are arrested and homed to specific secondary sites such as bone and lung [16]. Recently, a large body of evidence has indicated that sex steroids and their receptors impact on these steps through non-genomic and genomic actions. In this chapter we will describe the rapid action of sex steroids and its role in invasiveness and metastasis of breast cancer.

2 Non-genomic Actions by Steroid Hormones

A number of studies demonstrated the involvement of non-genomic actions of steroid hormones, including androgens and estrogens, in cellular processes such as cell proliferation and motility [17–19]. Non-genomic, or extra-nuclear effects of steroids are enacted quickly, and do not rely on signaling of nuclear receptors to gene expression. Non-genomic effects of steroids are mediated by multiple pathways; those relevant for breast cancer metastasis are discussed below.

2.1 *Rapid Action of Steroids Involving Classical Intracellular Steroid Receptors*

Steroids may bind to the classical intracellular steroid receptors and activate second messenger pathways such as c-Src kinase that rapidly stimulate MAPK/ERK and PI3K/AKT kinase pathways [20]. Interestingly, an androgen receptor (AR)/Src/modulator of non-genomic action of estrogen receptor (MNAR) complex and the cooperative association of c-Src, estrogen receptors (ERs), and AR activates MAPK and c-Src kinase pathways respectively [21, 22]. Estrogens on binding to ERα may also serve as a transcriptional co-activators regulating several transcriptional factors, such as activator protein 1 (AP-1), nuclear factor kappa B (NF-κB), and SP-1 in a non-genomic manner [23–25]. Steroids can also activate cAMP dependent protein kinase A (PKA) in cooperation with transmembrane G-protein-coupled receptors (GPCR) [26, 27]. The activation of PKA via the induction of cAMP is observed in both prostate and breast cancer cells [28, 29].

2.2 *Rapid Action of Steroids Involving Non-classical Membrane-Bound Steroid Receptors*

Steroids may enact non-genomic actions by binding to distinct non-classical membrane bound steroid receptors. Several reports have presumed the presence of androgen- and estrogen-binding sites in a number of cells [30, 31]. Interestingly, both the membrane androgen receptor (mAR) and the membrane ER (mER) are found to be associated with an integral membrane protein caveolin that facilitates the assembling of several signaling complexes, including phosphatidylinositol 3-kinase (PI3K), Ras, and Src kinase in their scaffold domain [32, 33]. Furthermore, mER perhaps exists as in a cytoplasmic pool and the rapid action requires its interaction with caveolin in association with MNAR, Shc and growth factor receptors, along with the scaffolding protein striatin that translocates ER to the plasma membrane [34, 35].

2.3 Rapid Action of Membrane Steroid Receptors Involving G Protein-Coupled Receptors (GPCR)

The most preserved non-genomic action of steroid hormones is the rapid increase in intracellular calcium concentration [Ca^{2+}] mediated via GPCR [36, 37], which ultimately results in the rapid activation of MAPK/ERK and PI3K/AKT pathways, leading to the activation of PKC and PKA [38, 39]. The interaction of mAR with GPCR results in the dissociation of Gα-subunit and the signal is transmitted from G$\beta\gamma$ through the activation of effector molecules including c-Src, Raf, and phospholipase C (PLC) [40]. GPCR itself may also serve as the membrane receptor, i.e., binding of E2 to an orphan GPCR, termed GPR30, plays a critical role in the rapid signaling of E2 [41, 42] and stimulates the Ras-dependent MAPK activation through phosphorylation of Shc [43].

2.4 Rapid Action of Membrane Steroid Receptors via Trans-Activation of Growth Factor Receptors

Rapid non-genomic actions of membrane steroid receptors may function via trans-activation of growth factor receptors [44]. The phenomenon is further confirmed by the co-existence of endogenous membrane receptors, including AR and ER, G proteins, GPCR, growth factor receptors (EGFR, IGFR), non-receptor tyrosine kinases (Src, Ras), and linker proteins such as MNAR and striatin in the plasma membrane termed as 'signalosomes' [45]. Alternatively, steroids may activate growth factor receptor kinase activity by inhibiting the regulatory phosphatases [46].

2.5 Rapid Non-transcriptional Action of Membrane Steroid Receptors

Steroids also elicit non-transcriptional effects via membrane receptors that provoke post-translational amendments of signaling proteins, including phosphorylation. By regulating kinases and phosphatases, steroids influence cell functions such as cell motility via modifying the architecture of the actin cytoskeleton [44, 47].

3 Sex Steroids and Actin Cytoskeleton Remodeling

The cytoskeleton forms the backbone of human cells and provides the basic infrastructure for cell motility. Actin is one of the most important cytoskeletal proteins and it exists as two forms: globular, non-polymerized G-actin and polymerized double-helical actin filaments (F-actin). When cells are polarized by extracellular stimuli, G-actin readily polymerizes to form F-actin through the "tread milling" mechanism and de novo actin polymerization occurs at the leading edge, resulting in the formation of membrane protrusions such as filopodia (thin projections), lamellipodia (broad, sheet-like membrane protrusions) as well as invadopodia (moderate-width extensions). The above process is known as actin cytoskeleton remodeling, the primary mechanism for most types of cell migration [48]. These protrusions interact with the extracellular matrix (ECM) via anchorage proteins and focal adhesions, which provide the platform to generate the locomotive force that enables cells to move via the activation of the actomyosin contractile machinery [49].

Growing evidence shows that sex steroids are powerful modulators on these steps through activation of actin-binding proteins and signalling molecules [50]. We and others have demonstrated that sex steroids promote breast cancer metastasis in vitro [7, 51, 52]. Estrogen and progesterone alone or in combination enhance T47-D or MCF-7 breast cancer cell horizontal migration distance and promote three-dimensional invasion into matrigel matrices [7, 51, 52]. These effects are attributed to sex steroids abilities to provoke actin cytoskeleton remodelling. At baseline, actin predominantly exists as monomers (G-actin) and actin fibers are arranged longitudinally in the cytoplasm and the cell membrane is regular. When stimulated with estrogen or progesterone, G-actin rapidly shifts to F-actin and actin fibers concentrate toward the edge of the membrane, in association with a significant increase of the thickness of the cell membrane and increased membrane ruffles, filopodia and lamellipodia that supports horizontal cell movement and invasion [7, 51, 52].

3.1 Sex Steroids and Ezrin/Radixin/Moesin

The actions of sex steroids on actin cytoskeleton remodelling are mediated by the activation of moesin, an actin-binding protein that belongs to the ezrin/radixin/moesin (ERM) family [7, 51, 52]. In quiescent conditions moesin exists in an autoinhibited conformation and phosphorylation of Thr^{558} within the C-terminal actin-binding domain leads to its activation that links the actin cytoskeleton to a variety of membrane-anchoring proteins [53, 54]. Both estrogen and progesterone induce the non-genomic activation of moesin in breast cancer cells. Silencing of moesin abolishes sex steroids actions on cytoskeleton remodelling and cell movement, indicating that moesin is an important intermediate for the sex steroids-induced breast cancer metastasis [7, 51, 52]. Moreover, activation of moesin is rapidly triggered by a complex of non-genomic intracellular events that requires the interaction of membrane sex steroids receptors (including membrane ER and PR) with the G protein $G\alpha13$ with the following involvement of the ubiquitous cytoskeletal modulator RhoA and of the Rho-associated kinase, ROCK, which is

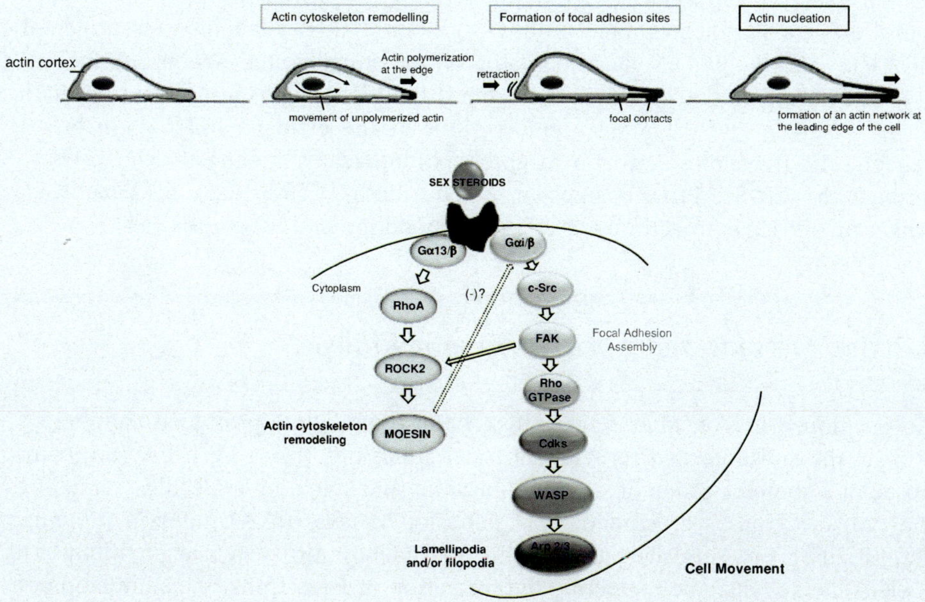

Fig. 1 Depicts the mechanism by which rapid activation of signaling pathways by sex steroids lead to cytoskeleton changes and cell movement in breast cancer cells

responsible for the phosphorylation of moesin [7, 51, 52]. Figure 1 depicts the model of regulation of cell motility by sex steroids.

Estrogen and progesterone enhance horizontal migration and invasion of three-dimensional matrices of ER+/PR+ breast cancer cells by recruiting the actin-binding protein, moesin. This pathway leads to the formation of membrane ruffles and pseudopodia which interact with the extracellular matrix and with nearby cells, thus promoting cell migration. Non-genomic signaling of ER/PR to ERM proteins and actin may thus serve as a mechanism of general relevance for the determination of cell movement [7, 51, 52].

Ezrin is another important member of ERM family. Abnormal ezrin localization is associated with clinical pathological features in invasive breast carcinomas [55]. Sex steroids can modulate Ezrin protein expression or activity. For instance, in the presence of progesterone, PRA induces redistribution of ezrin and actin cytoskeleton remodeling in breast cancer cells [56]. Fu XD et al. recently indicated that estrogen increases ezrin phosphorylation and protein expression, leading to cytoskeleton remodeling and breast cancer cell metastasis (Fu XD, unpublished data).

The GTP-binding proteins Rho, Rac and Cdc42 are known to regulate actin organization [57, 58]. Generally it is believed that Rho induces the assembly of contractile actin-based filaments such as stress fibres, Rac regulates the formation of lamellipodia and membrane ruffles, while Cdc42 is required for filopodium extension [59]. There has been evidence that estrogen increases the activities of Rac and Cdc42, leading to the formation of filopodia and lamellipodia that facilitate breast cancer cell movement. However, the signaling pathways responsible for Rho GTPase activation remain unrevealed [60]. In this aspect, latest evidence indicates that proline-, glutamic acid-, leucine-rich protein-1 (PELP1), also known as the modulator of the nongenomic actions of the ER (MNAR), is the pivotal signaling molecule [61]. PELP1 plays important roles both in the genomic and the nongenomic actions of the estrogen [62–64]. In breast cancer cells it couples estrogen receptor extranuclear signaling to Rho GTPase through the ER-Src-PELP1- integrin-linked kinase 1(ILK)-Rac/Cdc42 pathway, which finally leads to actin cytoskeleton remodeling and metastasis [61].

3.2 Sex Steroids and Focal Adhesion Kinase

As mentioned before, after actin cytoskeleton remodeling, protruded membranes contact the substrate and form novel focal adhesions (FAs) [49]. FAs are composed of a complex group of structural proteins and signaling molecules, including the tyrosine kinases c-Src and focal adhesion kinase (FAK), integrin proteins, actin-binding proteins such as vinculin and adaptor proteins like paxillin [65]. FAK is the key enzyme regulating the formation of FAs. Under the stimulation of multiple factors, FAK is activated via the phosphorylation at Tyr^{397} and begins to partner with cell-membrane integrins with the assistance of other proteins such as p130CAS, paxillin and vinculin, resulting in FAs formation and endowing cells with higher motility [66].

FAK influences the dynamic regulation of integrin-associated adhesions, and the actin cytoskeleton through diverse molecular interactions, controlling cell migration through assembly/disassembly cycle at the leading edge of migrating cells, while also controlling adhesion disassembly at the trailing edge.

Clinical data have indicated that high FAK expression is associated with an aggressive phenotype in breast carcinomas [67, 68]. Over-expression of FAK is related to the metastatic behavior of various tumors, such as lung cancer [69], ovarian cancer [70] and melanoma [71]. In animal models, inhibition of FAK activity in a rat breast cancer metastasis model abrogates cancer diffusion to the lung [72], and targeted deletion of FAK in mouse mammary epithelium reduces the pool of cancer stem/progenitor cells in primary tumors and their self-renewal and migration [73]. On the opposite, silencing of FAK in human and mouse mammary tumor cells results in cell senescence and in loss of invasive ability [74]. Overall, these findings highlight the relevance of the activity of focal adhesion kinase for cancer progression.

Sex steroids are capable to modulate the activity and expression of FAK in breast cancer cells. In a PR-positive but ER-negative breast cancer cell model, progesterone increases tyrosine phosphorylation of FAK, in association with increased FAs formation [75, 76]. Recently the molecular mechanism of FAK activation induced by progesterone in T47-D breast cancer cells has been described. In the presence of progesterone, PR recruits c-Src and PI3K/Akt, leading to RhoA/ROCK-2 activation, which eventually phosphorylates FAK at

Tyr^{397} and results in novel FAs formation. Silencing of FAK with specific siRNAs prevents the invasive behavior, suggesting that FAK plays important role in progesterone's effect on breast cancer metastasis [77].

Estrogen is also known to regulate FAs formation. In MDA-MB-231 human breast cancer cells, estrogen increases lamellipodia and FAs that are integral for cell migration [78]. Although there is evidence that FAK expression or activity is enhanced by estrogen in other type of cells [79, 80], the exact effect of estrogen on FAK in breast cancer cells is less understood. For example, in MCF-7 cells, treatment with estrogen for 7 days results in decreased tyrosine phosphorylation of FAK [81], while Sanchez et al. have shown that estrogen induces a rapid phosphorylation of FAK [82]. This apparent discrepancy may be explained by the dual functions of FAK on cell motility: an initial increase in FAK phosphotyrosine content, cell spread, and focal contact formation is followed by the gradual loss of FAK phosphorylation which coincides with disruption of focal contacts and conversion to a motile phenotype [83, 84].

Sanchez et al. have recently shown that estrogen rapidly activates FAK via phosphorylation on Tyr^{397} in human breast carcinoma cell line T47-D, leading to the formation of focal adhesion complexes. They identify the recruitment of PI3K after activation of c-Src by estrogen, and they show that this step is required for FAK phosphorylation on Tyr^{397}. This is consistent with previous reports showing that the c-Src/PI3K pathway is implicated in Tyr^{397} FAK phosphorylation [85, 86]. ERα-dependent PI3K activation results in the recruitment of the Gαi/Gβ/c-Src pathway and through this means it increases FAK activity in breast cancer cells [82].

The identification of FAK regulation by estrogen may thus offer important mechanistic insights to better understand the role of this hormone on breast cancer metastasis. This work shows that estrogen controls FAK and cell movement by regulating Cdc42 and its effector N-WASP [82]. N-WASP is a scaffold that links upstream signals to the activation of the Arp2/3 complex, leading to a burst of actin polymerization. Actin nucleation by the Arp2/3-complex appears to be critical for the rapid formation of an actin network at the leading edge of the cell [87–89] that provides the protrusive force required for the extension of filopodia and lamellipodia during cell movement [90]. Interestingly, in the presence of estrogen, FAK only associates with Cdc42-activated N-WASP and does not activate N-WASP itself. Although FAK phosphorylation of N-WASP does not affect N-WASP activity toward Arp-2/3, it seems important for maintaining the cytoplasmic distribution of N-WASP and for promoting cell motility [91]. As Cdc42 regulates actin dynamics in cell membrane projections, interaction of FAK with Cdc42-activated N-WASP might couple actin polymerization with membrane protrusion during cell movement [92].

In conclusion, within the broader range of actions of estrogen receptors, rapid extra-nuclear signaling to the actin cytoskeleton through the Gαi/Gβ/c-Src/PI3K/FAK/Cdc42/N-WASP/Arp-2/3 cascade is relevant for the generation of estrogen-dependent breast cancer cell movement and invasion. Through this cascade, estradiol leads to rapid changes of cell membrane morphology with a rearrangement of the actin cytoskeleton and the formation of focal adhesion complexes at sites where structures related with cell movement are formed.

4 Sex Steroids and Tyrosine Kinase Receptor

The epidermal growth factor receptor (EGFR) is a member of the EGFR/ErbB/HER family of type I transmembrane tyrosine kinase receptors which play essential roles in organ development and growth by regulating both the differentiation and morphology of cells and tissues [93]. EGFR is frequently overexpressed in a wide array of human cancers and signaling initiated from EGFR evokes invasive activities in breast cancer cells [94]. By using in vivo mouse models of breast cancer, the EGFR inhibitor gefitinib inhibits tumor cell motility and invasion [95]. A recent small randomized study shows that endocrine therapy with gefitinib is associated with a better advantage in progression-free survival in patients with hormone receptor-positive metastatic breast cancer [96]. Currently anti-EGFR therapy is regarded as a promising treatment for breast cancer patients with improved specificity, activity, and safety [93].

Sex steroids signal in breast cancer cells and promote cancer metastasis by the interaction of sex steroids receptors with EGFR. Recently, a new model of crosstalk between extranuclear steroid receptors and EGFR has been proposed. In this model, estrogen triggers the release of the membrane-tethered proHB-EGF, which, in turn, binds to unoccupied EGFR resulting in their activation [97]. This action is believed to be mediated by the membrane estrogen receptor GPR30, an orphan member of the seven transmembrane receptor [97] that has been attracted much attention in breast cancer progression. Clinical analysis has indicated that GPR30 expression associated positively with tumor size and extra mammary metastases [98]. In ER-negative human breast cancer cells the activation of GPR30 induces a transcription factor network that promotes metastasis-related proteins gene expression, leading to stimulation of breast cancer cell migration [99]. Therefore, GPR30 may support alternative pathways through which estrogen impacts on metastasis in ER-negative or tamoxifen resistant breast cancers [100].

Likewise, estrogen causes an association of membrane ERα with Shc, Src, leading to Insulin-like Growth Factor Receptor (IGFR) activation [101, 102]. Activated EGFR and IGFR recruit downstream signaling avenues such as MAPK and Akt that promote breast cancer metastasis [103]. Interestingly, sex steroids receptors are also directly implicated in epidermal growth factor (EGF) actions. EGF stimulates ER phosphorylation on tyrosine and promotes the association of a complex between EGFR, ER, androgen receptor and the non-receptor tyrosine kinase Src. The complex assembly triggers Src activity, EGFR phosphorylation and the activation of EGFR downstream signaling in breast cancer cells [104].

In the crosstalk between sex steroid receptors and growth receptors, the non-receptor tyrosine kinase c-Src is identified to be the critical intermediate. Indeed, c-Src mediates signal transduction pathways that regulate breast cancer cell proliferation, survival, invasion, and metastasis [105]. Fu et al. have demostrated that medroxyprogesterone acetate (MPA) promotes breast cancer metastasis by the interaction of progesterone receptor with c-Src [7]. Furthermore, in the presence of E2, ERα recruits a $G\alpha_i/G\beta$-dependent signaling that triggers the formation of a multiprotein complex where ERα, c- Src, PI3K, and FAK interact promoting the branching of actin filaments and cell membrane remodeling [82]. Recently it has been shown that estrogen activates c-Src through the release of nitric oxide (NO), leading to breast cancer cell invasion and metastasis [106].

5 Sex Steroids and Other Metastasis-Associated Molecules

5.1 Chemokines and Their Receptors

Chemokines are small cytokine-like proteins that elicit directional cell migration. Expression of some of the chemokines and their receptors in breast tumors has been correlated with a poor prognosis, increased metastasis, resistance to conventional therapeutic agents and a poor outcome in the pathogenesis of breast cancer [107, 108].

Several reports demonstrate that the levels of chemokines or chemokine receptors are dependent on sex steroids. For example, in experimental breast cancer, estrogen increases IL-8 whereas the anti-estrogen tamoxifen inhibits the secretion of IL-8 both in vitro and extracellularly in vivo in tumors of nude mice [109, 110]. In MCF-7 cells estrogen has synergetic effects with tumor necrosis factor to increase IL-8 and monocyte chemoattractant protein 1 (MCP-1) production [111]. In addition, estrogen increases CXCR4 protein expression via PI3K/AKT, MAPK and mTOR pathways in breast cancer cells [112]. However, current understanding in this area is poor and the next step will be definitely to analyze the effects of sex steroids on the expression patterns of chemokines and their receptors in breast cancer cells.

5.2 Integrins

Integrins play a vital role in cancer progression because of their ability to regulate various intracellular signaling molecules that are essential for cell motility, cell survival, and proliferation [113, 114]. Integrins are heterodimers composed of non-covalently associated α and β subunits and they directly bind components of the extracellular matrix and provide the traction that regulate cell motility and invasion [115]. While several integrins, such as $\beta1$, $\alpha2$, and $\alpha6$ are known to be decreased in invasive breast carcinoma, others, such as $\alpha3$, $\beta4$, are associated with increased metastatic potential [115]. It has been shown that estrogen/ERα increases the expression of integrin $\alpha5\beta1$ through the binding of ERα-Sp1 complex with ERE half-site in the $\alpha5$ gene, thus results in the maintenance of the stationary status of breast cancer cells [116]. Expression of ERβ also increases integrin $\alpha1$ and integrin $\beta1$ levels and enhances adhesion of breast cancer cells, leading to less cell migration [117]. Similarly, progestins diminish the expression of $\beta1$, $\beta4$, $\alpha2$, $\alpha3$, and $\alpha5$ integrin chains, resulting in the inhibition of T47-D cell migration [118].

5.3 *Role of p52Shc in Steroid-Regulated Cell Proliferation and Migration*

In addition to the classical role in mediating tyrosine kinase-activated pathways, p52Shc functions as a primary adaptor protein for mediating the mitogenic signals of steroids at the non-genomic level in human breast and prostate cancer cells [119, 120].

A direct involvement of p52Shc in breast cancer metastasis in transgenic mice that express polyomavirus middle T antigen with a mutated Shc-binding site has been demonstrated [121]. Polyomavirus middle T antigen couples with and activates signaling molecules, such as Src, Shc, and phosphatidylinositol 3-kinase (PI3K) for its oncogenic capacity. Importantly, in transgenic mice, which have metastatic tumors, the mutated p52Shc-binding site on middle T antigen had reverted to the wild type and regained its function, thus emphasizing the potential importance of the functional p52Shc in the process of metastasis in vivo [121]. In addition, it has been revealed that in integrin signaling, Shc recruitment to the actin-associated cytoskeleton is important [122, 123]. p52Shc potentiates integrin signaling, and integrin ligation results in the activation of non-receptor tyrosine kinases, such as Src, Fyn, and focal adhesion kinase (FAK), which phosphorylates p52Shc, leading to Ras activation and entering into the cell cycle [122, 123]. Besides, the SH3 domain of Fyn interacts with the proline-rich region in the CH1 domain of p52Shc [124] and the amino-terminal domain of p52Shc is shown to mediate the association of this adaptor protein to an actin-rich cellular fraction [124]. Additionally, a mutation of the PTB domain (S154P-p52Shc) abolishes integrin-induced p52Shc tyrosine phosphorylation where the SH2 domain of p52Shc is dispensable [125]. p52Shc phosphorylation by c-Src can be augmented when the PTB domain binds to phospholipids [126, 127]. These observations explain how the PTB domain localizes p52Shc to the membrane where it becomes phosphorylated by cytoskeleton-associated tyrosine kinases, which finally results in cell migration. It should be noted that these non-receptor tyrosine kinases, e.g., Src, closely interact with steroid hormone signaling pathways [20, 128]. The molecular mechanism by which steroids induce cell adhesion and/or migration via p52Shc requires further investigation.

6 Conclusions

Experimental and clinical data have demonstrated the importance of sex steroids and their receptors in the development and progression of breast cancer. The proper interference with sex steroid-initiated signaling is becoming a major target for breast cancer treatment. However, the effects of sex steroids on breast cancer metastasis remain controversial. This discrepancy may be related to the different breast experimental models used, to the complexities of sex steroids signaling, and to complicated molecular mechanisms of breast cancer cell migration and invasion. The development of animal models of different phenotypes of metastatic breast cancer would greatly facilitate to evaluate the effects of sex steroids on breast cancer metastasis. Moreover, further exploration on the molecular mechanisms of sex steroids on cell migration and invasion is needed. A deeper understanding of these complex areas will be of utmost importance for newer biologically-driven therapies to counteract breast cancer metastasis.

References

1. Henderson BE, Feigelson HS (2000) Hormonal carcinogenesis. Carcinogenesis 21:427–433
2. Alam SM, Rajendran M, Ouyang S, Veeramani S, Zhang L, Lin MF (2009) A novel role of Shc adaptor proteins in steroid hormone-regulated cancers. Endocr Relat Cancer 16:1–16
3. Kelsey JL, Gammon MD, John EM (1993) Reproductive factors and breast cancer. Epidemiol Rev 15:36–47
4. Verkooijen HM, Bouchardy C, Vinh-Hung V, Rapiti E, Hartman M (2009) The incidence of breast cancer and changes in the use of hormone replacement therapy: a review of the evidence. Maturitas 64:80–85
5. Russo J, Russo IH (2006) The role of estrogen in the initiation of breast cancer. J Steroid Biochem Mol Biol 102:89–96
6. Braun S, Auer D, Marth C (2009) The prognostic impact of bone marrow micrometastases in women with breast cancer. Cancer Invest 27:598–603
7. Fu XD, Giretti MS, Baldacci C, Garibaldi S, Flamini M, Sanchez AM, Gadducci A, Genazzani AR, Simoncini T (2008) Extra-nuclear signaling of progesterone receptor to breast cancer cell movement and invasion through the actin cytoskeleton. PLoS One 3:e2790
8. Janni W, Hepp P (2010) Adjuvant aromatase inhibitor therapy: outcomes and safety. Cancer Treat Rev 36:249–261
9. Collaborative Group on Hormonal Factors in Breast Cancer (1997) Breast cancer and hormone replacement therapy: collaborative reanalysis of data from 51 epidemiological studies of 52,705 women with breast cancer and 108,411 women without breast cancer. Lancet 350:1047–1059

10. DiSaia PJ (1996) Hormone replacement therapy in the gynecologic and breast cancer patient. Cancer Control 3:101–106
11. Fuqua SA (2001) The role of estrogen receptor in breast cancer metastasis. J Mammary Gland Biol Neoplasia 6:407–417
12. Poole AJ, Li Y, Kim Y, Lin SC, Lee WH, Lee EY (2006) Prevention of Brca1-mediated mammary tumorigenesis in mice by a progesterone antagonist. Science 314:1467–1470
13. Vanzulli SI, Soldati R, Meiss R, Colombo L, Molinolo AA, Lanari C (2005) Estrogen or antiprogestin treatment induces complete regression of pulmonary and axillary metastases in an experimental model of breast cancer progression. Carcinogenesis 26:1055–1063
14. Kato S, Pinto M, Carvajal A, Espinoza N, Monso C, Sadarangani A, Villalon M, Brosens JJ, White JO, Richer JK, Horwitz KB, Owen GI (2005) Progesterone increases tissue factor gene expression, procoagulant activity, and invasion in the breast cancer cell line ZR-75-1. J Clin Endocrinol Metab 90:1181–1188
15. Hyder SM, Chiappetta C, Stancel GM (2001) Pharmacological and endogenous progestins induce vascular endothelial growth factor expression in human breast cancer cells. Int J Cancer 92:469–473
16. Zhang Y, Ma B, Fan Q (2010) Mechanisms of breast cancer bone metastasis. Cancer Lett 292:1–7
17. Berridge MJ, Bootman MD, Lipp P (1998) Calcium–a life and death signal. Nature 395:645–648
18. Cutini P, Selles J, Massheimer V (2009) Cross-talk between rapid and long term effects of progesterone on vascular tissue. J Steroid Biochem Mol Biol 115:36–43
19. Rauschemberger MB, Selles J, Massheimer V (2008) The direct action of estrone on vascular tissue involves genomic and non-genomic action. Life Sci 82:115–123
20. Migliaccio A, Castoria G, Di Domenico M, de Falco A, Bilancio A, Lombardi M, Barone MV, Ametrano D, Zannini MS, Abbondanza C, Auricchio F (2000) Steroid-induced androgen receptor-oestradiol receptor beta-Src complex triggers prostate cancer cell proliferation. EMBO J 19:5406–5417
21. Kousteni S, Bellido T, Plotkin LI, O'Brien CA, Bodenner DL, Han L, Han K, DiGregorio GB, Katzenellenbogen JA, Katzenellenbogen BS, Roberson PK, Weinstein RS, Jilka RL, Manolagas SC (2001) Nongenotropic, sex-nonspecific signaling through the estrogen or androgen receptors: dissociation from transcriptional activity. Cell 104:719–730
22. Unni E, Sun S, Nan B, McPhaul MJ, Cheskis B, Mancini MA, Marcelli M (2004) Changes in androgen receptor nongenotropic signaling correlate with transition of LNCaP cells to androgen independence. Cancer Res 64:7156–7168
23. Ray P, Ghosh SK, Zhang DH, Ray A (1997) Repression of interleukin-6 gene expression by 17 beta-estradiol: inhibition of the DNA-binding activity of the transcription factors NF-IL6 and NF-kappa B by the estrogen receptor. FEBS Lett 409:79–85
24. Jakacka M, Ito M, Weiss J, Chien PY, Gehm BD, Jameson JL (2001) Estrogen receptor binding to DNA is not required for its activity through the nonclassical AP1 pathway. J Biol Chem 276:13615–13621
25. Safe S (2001) Transcriptional activation of genes by 17 beta-estradiol through estrogen receptor-Sp1 interactions. Vitam Horm 62:231–252
26. Fortunati N (1999) Sex hormone-binding globulin: not only a transport protein. What news is around the corner? J Endocrinol Invest 22:223–234
27. Rosner W, Hryb DJ, Khan MS, Nakhla AM, Romas NA (1999) Androgen and estrogen signaling at the cell membrane via G-proteins and cyclic adenosine monophosphate. Steroids 64:100–106
28. Fortunati N, Fissore F, Fazzari A, Becchis M, Comba A, Catalano MG, Berta L, Frairia R (1996) Sex steroid binding protein exerts a negative control on estradiol action in MCF-7 cells (human breast cancer) through cyclic adenosine 3′, 5′-monophosphate and protein kinase A. Endocrinology 137:686–692

29. Nakhla AM, Romas NA, Rosner W (1997) Estradiol activates the prostate androgen receptor and prostate-specific antigen secretion through the intermediacy of sex hormone-binding globulin. J Biol Chem 272:6838–6841
30. Armen TA, Gay CV (2000) Simultaneous detection and functional response of testosterone and estradiol receptors in osteoblast plasma membranes. J Cell Biochem 79:620–627
31. Kampa M, Papakonstanti EA, Hatzoglou A, Stathopoulos EN, Stournaras C, Castanas E (2002) The human prostate cancer cell line LNCaP bears functional membrane testosterone receptors that increase PSA secretion and modify actin cytoskeleton. FASEB J 16: 1429–1431
32. Kim HP, Lee JY, Jeong JK, Bae SW, Lee HK, Jo I (1999) Nongenomic stimulation of nitric oxide release by estrogen is mediated by estrogen receptor alpha localized in caveolae. Biochem Biophys Res Commun 263:257–262
33. Lu ML, Schneider MC, Zheng Y, Zhang X, Richie JP (2001) Caveolin-1 interacts with androgen receptor. A positive modulator of androgen receptor mediated transactivation. J Biol Chem 276:13442–13451
34. Lu Q, Pallas DC, Surks HK, Baur WE, Mendelsohn ME, Karas RH (2004) Striatin assembles a membrane signaling complex necessary for rapid, nongenomic activation of endothelial NO synthase by estrogen receptor alpha. Proc Natl Acad Sci U S A 101: 17126–17131
35. Song RX, Zhang Z, Santen RJ (2005) Estrogen rapid action via protein complex formation involving ERalpha and Src. Trends Endocrinol Metab 16:347–353
36. Lieberherr M, Grosse B (1994) Androgens increase intracellular calcium concentration and inositol 1, 4, 5-trisphosphate and diacylglycerol formation via a pertussis toxin-sensitive G-protein. J Biol Chem 269:7217–7223
37. Benten WP, Lieberherr M, Giese G, Wunderlich F (1998) Estradiol binding to cell surface raises cytosolic free calcium in T cells. FEBS Lett 422:349–353
38. Kelly MJ, Lagrange AH, Wagner EJ, Ronnekleiv OK (1999) Rapid effects of estrogen to modulate G protein-coupled receptors via activation of protein kinase A and protein kinase C pathways. Steroids 64:64–75
39. Estrada M, Espinosa A, Muller M, Jaimovich E (2003) Testosterone stimulates intracellular calcium release and mitogen-activated protein kinases via a G protein-coupled receptor in skeletal muscle cells. Endocrinology 144:3586–3597
40. Pierce KL, Premont RT, Lefkowitz RJ (2002) Seven-transmembrane receptors. Nat Rev Mol Cell Biol 3:639–650
41. Prossnitz ER, Arterburn JB, Smith HO, Oprea TI, Sklar LA, Hathaway HJ (2008) Estrogen signaling through the transmembrane G protein-coupled receptor GPR30. Annu Rev Physiol 70:165–190
42. Prossnitz ER, Arterburn JB, Sklar LA (2007) GPR30: A G protein-coupled receptor for estrogen. Mol Cell Endocrinol 265–266:138–142
43. Luttrell LM, Hawes BE, van Biesen T, Luttrell DK, Lansing TJ, Lefkowitz RJ (1996) Role of c-Src tyrosine kinase in G protein-coupled receptor- and Gbetagamma subunit-mediated activation of mitogen-activated protein kinases. J Biol Chem 271:19443–19450
44. Levin ER (2005) Integration of the extranuclear and nuclear actions of estrogen. Mol Endocrinol 19:1951–1959
45. Hammes SR, Levin ER (2007) Extranuclear steroid receptors: nature and actions. Endocr Rev 28:726–741
46. Meng TC, Lee MS, Lin MF (2000) Interaction between protein tyrosine phosphatase and protein tyrosine kinase is involved in androgen-promoted growth of human prostate cancer cells. Oncogene 19:2664–2677
47. Meyer G, Feldman EL (2002) Signaling mechanisms that regulate actin-based motility processes in the nervous system. J Neurochem 83:490–503
48. Kedrin D, van Rheenen J, Hernandez L, Condeelis J, Segall JE (2007) Cell motility and cytoskeletal regulation in invasion and metastasis. J Mammary Gland Biol Neoplasia 12:143–152

49. Yamazaki D, Kurisu S, Takenawa T (2005) Regulation of cancer cell motility through actin reorganization. Cancer Sci 96:379–386
50. Giretti MS, Simoncini T (2008) Rapid regulatory actions of sex steroids on cell movement through the actin cytoskeleton. Steroids 73:895–900
51. Giretti MS, Fu XD, De Rosa G, Sarotto I, Baldacci C, Garibaldi S, Mannella P, Biglia N, Sismondi P, Genazzani AR, Simoncini T (2008) Extra-nuclear signalling of estrogen receptor to breast cancer cytoskeletal remodelling, migration and invasion. PLoS One 3:e2238
52. Fu XD, Giretti MS, Goglia L, Flamini MI, Sanchez AM, Baldacci C, Garibaldi S, Sitruk-Ware R, Genazzani AR, Simoncini T (2008) Comparative actions of progesterone, medroxyprogesterone acetate, drospirenone and nestorone on breast cancer cell migration and invasion. BMC Cancer 8:166
53. Louvet-Vallee S (2000) ERM proteins: from cellular architecture to cell signaling. Biol Cell 92:305–316
54. Tsukita S, Yonemura S (1999) Cortical actin organization: lessons from ERM (ezrin/radixin/moesin) proteins. J Biol Chem 274:34507–34510
55. Sarrio D, Rodriguez-Pinilla SM, Dotor A, Calero F, Hardisson D, Palacios J (2006) Abnormal ezrin localization is associated with clinicopathological features in invasive breast carcinomas. Breast Cancer Res Treat 98:71–79
56. McGowan EM, Weinberger RP, Graham JD, Hill HD, Hughes JA, O'Neill GM, Clarke CL (2003) Cytoskeletal responsiveness to progestins is dependent on progesterone receptor A levels. J Mol Endocrinol 31:241–253
57. Ridley AJ, Allen WE, Peppelenbosch M, Jones GE (1999) Rho family proteins and cell migration. Biochem Soc Symp 65:111–123
58. Jiang P, Enomoto A, Takahashi M (2009) Cell biology of the movement of breast cancer cells: intracellular signalling and the actin cytoskeleton. Cancer Lett 284:122–130
59. Lu Q, Longo FM, Zhou H, Massa SM, Chen YH (2009) Signaling through Rho GTPase pathway as viable drug target. Curr Med Chem 16:1355–1365
60. Azios NG, Krishnamoorthy L, Harris M, Cubano LA, Cammer M, Dharmawardhane SF (2007) Estrogen and resveratrol regulate Rac and Cdc42 signaling to the actin cytoskeleton of metastatic breast cancer cells. Neoplasia 9:147–158
61. Chakravarty D, Nair SS, Santhamma B, Nair BC, Wang L, Bandyopadhyay A, Agyin JK, Brann D, Sun LZ, Yeh IT, Lee FY, Tekmal RR, Kumar R, Vadlamudi (2010) RK Extranuclear functions of ER impact invasive migration and metastasis by breast cancer cells. Cancer Res 70:4092–4101
62. Vadlamudi RK, Kumar R (2007) Functional and biological properties of the nuclear receptor coregulator PELP1/MNAR. Nucl Recept Signal 5:e004
63. Cheskis BJ, Greger J, Cooch N, McNally C, McLarney S, Lam HS, Rutledge S, Mekonnen B, Hauze D, Nagpal S, Freedman LP (2008) MNAR plays an important role in ERa activation of Src/MAPK and PI3K/Akt signaling pathways. Steroids 73:901–905
64. Nair SS, Mishra SK, Yang Z, Balasenthil S, Kumar R, Vadlamudi RK (2004) Potential role of a novel transcriptional coactivator PELP1 in histone H1 displacement in cancer cells. Cancer Res 64:6416–6423
65. Romer LH, Birukov KG, Garcia JG (2006) Focal adhesions: paradigm for a signaling nexus. Circ Res 98:606–616
66. van Nimwegen MJ, van de Water B (2007) Focal adhesion kinase: a potential target in cancer therapy. Biochem Pharmacol 73:597–609
67. Lark AL, Livasy CA, Dressler L, Moore DT, Millikan RC, Geradts J, Iacocca M, Cowan D, Little D, Craven RJ, Cance W (2005) High focal adhesion kinase expression in invasive breast carcinomas is associated with an aggressive phenotype. Mod Pathol 18:1289–1294
68. Luo M, Guan JL (2010) Focal adhesion kinase: a prominent determinant in breast cancer initiation, progression and metastasis. Cancer Lett 289:127–139
69. Fong YC, Liu SC, Huang CY, Li TM, Hsu SF, Kao ST, Tsai FJ, Chen WC, Chen CY, Tang CH (2009) Osteopontin increases lung cancer cells migration via activation of the alphavbeta3 integrin/FAK/Akt and NF-kappaB-dependent pathway. Lung Cancer 64:263–270

70. Hu XW, Meng D, Fang J (2008) Apigenin inhibited migration and invasion of human ovarian cancer A2780 cells through focal adhesion kinase. Carcinogenesis 29:2369–2376
71. Kaneda T, Sonoda Y, Ando K, Suzuki T, Sasaki Y, Oshio T, Tago M, Kasahara T (2008) Mutation of Y925F in focal adhesion kinase (FAK) suppresses melanoma cell proliferation and metastasis. Cancer Lett 270:354–361
72. van Nimwegen MJ, Verkoeijen S, van Buren L, Burg D, van de Water B (2005) Requirement for focal adhesion kinase in the early phase of mammary adenocarcinoma lung metastasis formation. Cancer Res 65:4698–4706
73. Luo M, Fan H, Nagy T, Wei H, Wang C, Liu S, Wicha MS, Guan JL (2009) Mammary epithelial-specific ablation of the focal adhesion kinase suppresses mammary tumorigenesis by affecting mammary cancer stem/progenitor cells. Cancer Res 69:466–474
74. Pylayeva Y, Gillen KM, Gerald W, Beggs HE, Reichardt LF, Giancotti FG (2009) Ras- and PI3K-dependent breast tumorigenesis in mice and humans requires focal adhesion kinase signaling. J Clin Invest 119:252–266
75. Lin VC, Ng EH, Aw SE, Tan MG, Bay BH (2000) Progesterone induces focal adhesion in breast cancer cells MDA-MB-231 transfected with progesterone receptor complementary DNA. Mol Endocrinol 14:348–358
76. Lin VC, Woon CT, Aw SE, Guo C (2003) Distinct molecular pathways mediate progesterone-induced growth inhibition and focal adhesion. Endocrinology 144:5650–5657
77. Fu XD, Goglia L, Sanchez AM, Flamini M, Giretti MS, Tosi V, Genazzani AR, Simoncini T (2010) Progesterone receptor enhances breast cancer cell motility and invasion via extranuclear activation of focal adhesion kinase. Endocr Relat Cancer 17:431–443
78. Azios NG, Dharmawardhane SF (2005) Resveratrol and estradiol exert disparate effects on cell migration, cell surface actin structures, and focal adhesion assembly in MDA-MB-231 human breast cancer cells. Neoplasia 7:128–140
79. Kublickiene K, Fu XD, Svedas E, Landgren BM, Genazzani AR, Simoncini T (2008) Effects in postmenopausal women of estradiol and medroxyprogesterone alone and combined on resistance artery function and endothelial morphology and movement. J Clin Endocrinol Metab 93:1874–1883
80. Ishida H, Wada K, Masuda T, Okura M, Kohama K, Sano Y, Nakajima A, Kogo M, Kamisaki Y (2007) Critical role of estrogen receptor on anoikis and invasion of squamous cell carcinoma. Cancer Sci 98:636–643
81. Bartholomew PJ, Vinci JM, DePasquale JA (1998) Decreased tyrosine phosphorylation of focal adhesion kinase after estradiol treatment of MCF-7 human breast carcinoma cells. J Steroid Biochem Mol Biol 67:241–249
82. Sanchez AM, Flamini MI, Baldacci C, Goglia L, Genazzani AR, Simoncini T (2010) Estrogen receptor-{alpha} promotes breast cancer cell motility and invasion via focal adhesion kinase and N-WASP. Mol Endocrinol 24:2114–2125
83. Matsumoto K, Nakamura T, Kramer RH (1994) Hepatocyte growth factor/scatter factor induces tyrosine phosphorylation of focal adhesion kinase (p125FAK) and promotes migration and invasion by oral squamous cell carcinoma cells. J Biol Chem 269: 31807–31813
84. Hsia DA, Mitra SK, Hauck CR, Streblow DN, Nelson JA, Ilic D, Huang S, Li E, Nemerow GR, Leng J, Spencer KS, Cheresh DA, Schlaepfer DD (2003) Differential regulation of cell motility and invasion by FAK. J Cell Biol 160:753–767
85. Reiske HR, Kao SC, Cary LA, Guan JL, Lai JF, Chen HC (1999) Requirement of phosphatidylinositol 3-kinase in focal adhesion kinase-promoted cell migration. J Biol Chem 274:12361–12366
86. Thamilselvan V, Craig DH, Basson MD (2007) FAK association with multiple signal proteins mediates pressure-induced colon cancer cell adhesion via a Src-dependent PI3K/Akt pathway. FASEB J 21:1730–1741
87. Bailly M, Macaluso F, Cammer M, Chan A, Segall JE, Condeelis JS (1999) Relationship between Arp2/3 complex and the barbed ends of actin filaments at the leading edge of carcinoma cells after epidermal growth factor stimulation. J Cell Biol 145:331–345

88. Higgs HN, Blanchoin L, Pollard TD (1999) Influence of the C terminus of Wiskott-Aldrich syndrome protein (WASp) and the Arp2/3 complex on actin polymerization. Biochemistry 38:15212–15222
89. Mullins RD, Heuser JA, Pollard TD (1998) The interaction of Arp2/3 complex with actin: nucleation, high affinity pointed end capping, and formation of branching networks of filaments. Proc Natl Acad Sci U S A 95:6181–6186
90. Takenawa T, Suetsugu S (2007) The WASP-WAVE protein network: connecting the membrane to the cytoskeleton. Nat Rev Mol Cell Biol 8:37–48
91. Wu X, Suetsugu S, Cooper LA, Takenawa T, Guan JL (2004) Focal adhesion kinase regulation of N-WASP subcellular localization and function. J Biol Chem 279:9565–9576
92. Mitra SK, Hanson DA, Schlaepfer DD (2005) Focal adhesion kinase: in command and control of cell motility. Nat Rev Mol Cell Biol 6:56–68
93. Flynn JF, Wong C, Wu JM (2009) Anti-EGFR therapy: mechanism and advances in clinical efficacy in breast cancer. J Oncol 2009:526963
94. Sabe H, Hashimoto S, Morishige M, Ogawa E, Hashimoto A, Nam JM, Miura K, Yano H, Onodera Y (2009) The EGFR-GEP100-Arf6-AMAP1 signaling pathway specific to breast cancer invasion and metastasis. Traffic 10:982–993
95. Kedrin D, Wyckoff J, Boimel PJ, Coniglio SJ, Hynes NE, Arteaga CL, Segall JE (2009) ERBB1 and ERBB2 have distinct functions in tumor cell invasion and intravasation. Clin Cancer Res 15:3733–3739
96. Cristofanilli M, Valero V, Mangalik A, Royce M, Rabinowitz I, Arena FP, Kroener JF, Curcio E, Watkins C, Bacus S, Cora EM, Anderson E, Magill PJ (2010) Phase II, randomized trial to compare anastrozole combined with gefitinib or placebo in postmenopausal women with hormone receptor-positive metastatic breast cancer. Clin Cancer Res 16:1904–1914
97. Filardo EJ, Quinn JA, Sabo E (2008) Association of the membrane estrogen receptor, GPR30, with breast tumor metastasis and transactivation of the epidermal growth factor receptor. Steroids 73:870–873
98. Fitzgibbons PL, Page DL, Weaver D, Thor AD, Allred DC, Clark GM, Ruby SG, O'Malley F, Simpson JF, Connolly JL, Hayes DF, Edge SB, Lichter A, Schnitt SJ (2000) Prognostic factors in breast cancer. College of american pathologists consensus statement 1999. Arch Pathol Lab Med 124:966–978
99. Pandey DP, Lappano R, Albanito L, Madeo A, Maggiolini M, Picard D (2009) Estrogenic GPR30 signalling induces proliferation and migration of breast cancer cells through CTGF. EMBO J 28:523–532
100. Ignatov A, Ignatov T, Roessner A, Costa SD, Kalinski T (2010) Role of GPR30 in the mechanisms of tamoxifen resistance in breast cancer MCF-7 cells. Breast Cancer Res Treat 123:87–96
101. Song RX, Barnes CJ, Zhang Z, Bao Y, Kumar R, Santen RJ (2004) The role of Shc and insulin-like growth factor 1 receptor in mediating the translocation of estrogen receptor alpha to the plasma membrane. Proc Natl Acad Sci U S A 101:2076–2081
102. Pietras RJ (2003) Interactions between estrogen and growth factor receptors in human breast cancer and the tumor-associated vasculature. Breast J 9:361–373
103. Song RX, Chen Y, Zhang Z, Bao Y, Yue W, Wang JP, Fan P, Santen RJ (2010) Estrogen utilization of IGF-1-R and EGF-R to signal in breast cancer cells. J Steroid Biochem Mol Biol 118:219–230
104. Migliaccio A, Castoria G, Di Domenico M, Ciociola A, Lombardi M, De Falco A, Nanayakkara M, Bottero D, De Stasio R, Varricchio L, Auricchio F (2006) Crosstalk between EGFR and extranuclear steroid receptors. Ann N Y Acad Sci 1089:194–200
105. Planas-Silva MD, Bruggeman RD, Grenko RT, Stanley Smith J (2006) Role of c-Src and focal adhesion kinase in progression and metastasis of estrogen receptor-positive breast cancer. Biochem Biophys Res Commun 341:73–81

106. Rahman MA, Senga T, Ito S, Hyodo T, Hasegawa H, Hamaguchi (2010) M S-nitrosylation at cysteine 498 of c-Src tyrosine kinase regulates nitric oxide-mediated cell invasion. J Biol Chem 285:3806–3814
107. Hinton CV, Avraham S, Avraham HK (2010) Role of the CXCR4/CXCL12 signaling axis in breast cancer metastasis to the brain. Clin Exp Metastasis 27:97–105
108. Ali S, Lazennec G (2007) Chemokines: novel targets for breast cancer metastasis. Cancer Metastasis Rev 26:401–420
109. Bendrik C, Dabrosin C (2009) Estradiol increases IL-8 secretion of normal human breast tissue and breast cancer in vivo. J Immunol 182:371–378
110. Lin Y, Huang R, Chen L, Li S, Shi Q, Jordan C, Huang RP (2004) Identification of interleukin-8 as estrogen receptor-regulated factor involved in breast cancer invasion and angiogenesis by protein arrays. Int J Cancer 109:507–515
111. Seeger H, Wallwiener D, Mueck AO (2006) Different effects of estradiol and various antiestrogens on TNF-alpha-induced changes of biochemical markers for growth and invasion of human breast cancerbreast cancer cells. Life Sci 78:1464–1468
112. Sengupta S, Schiff R, Katzenellenbogen BS (2009) Post-transcriptional regulation of chemokine receptor CXCR4 by estrogen in HER2 overexpressing, estrogen receptor-positive breast cancer cells. Breast Cancer Res Treat 117:243–251
113. Ruoslahti E, Reed JC (1994) Anchorage dependence, integrins, and apoptosis. Cell 77: 477–478
114. Hynes RO, Bader BL, Hodivala-Dilke K (1999) Integrins in vascular development. Braz J Med Biol Res 32:501–510
115. Desgrosellier JS, Cheresh DA (2010) Integrins in cancer: biological implications and therapeutic opportunities. Nat Rev Cancer 10:9–22
116. Sisci D, Middea E, Morelli C, Lanzino M, Aquila S, Rizza P, Catalano S, Casaburi I, Maggiolini M, Ando S 17beta-Estradiol enhances alpha(5) integrin subunit gene expression through ERalpha-Sp1 interaction and reduces cell motility and invasion of ERalpha-positive breast cancer cells. Breast Cancer Res Treat
117. Lindberg K, Strom A, Lock JG, Gustafsson JA, Haldosen LA, Helguero LA (2010) Expression of estrogen receptor beta increases integrin alpha1 and integrin beta1 levels and enhances adhesion of breast cancer cells. J Cell Physiol 222:156–167
118. McGowan EM, Saad S, Bendall LJ, Bradstock KF, Clarke CL (2004) Effect of progesterone receptor a predominance on breast cancer cell migration into bone marrow fibroblasts. Breast Cancer Res Treat 83:211–220
119. Stevenson LE, Ravichandran KS, Frackelton AR Jr (1999) Shc dominant negative disrupts cell cycle progression in both G0–G1 and G2-M of ErbB2-positive breast cancer cells. Cell Growth Differ 10:61–71
120. Lee MS, Igawa T, Lin MF (2004) Tyrosine-317 of p52(Shc) mediates androgen-stimulated proliferation signals in human prostate cancer cells. Oncogene 23:3048–3058
121. Webster MA, Hutchinson JN, Rauh MJ, Muthuswamy SK, Anton M, Tortorice CG, Cardiff RD, Graham FL, Hassell JA, Muller WJ (1998) Requirement for both Shc and phosphatidylinositol 3′ kinase signaling pathways in polyomavirus middle T-mediated mammary tumorigenesis. Mol Cell Biol 18:2344–2359
122. McGlade J, Cheng A, Pelicci G, Pelicci PG, Pawson T (1992) Shc proteins are phosphorylated and regulated by the v-Src and v-Fps protein-tyrosine kinases. Proc Natl Acad Sci U S A 89:8869–8873
123. Wary KK, Mariotti A, Zurzolo C, Giancotti FG (1998) A requirement for caveolin-1 and associated kinase Fyn in integrin signaling and anchorage-dependent cell growth. Cell 94:625–634
124. Thomas D, Bradshaw RA (1997) Differential utilization of ShcA tyrosine residues and functional domains in the transduction of epidermal growth factor-induced mitogen-activated protein kinase activation in 293T cells and nerve growth factor-induced neurite outgrowth in PC12 cells. Identification of a new Grb2.Sos1 binding site. J Biol Chem 272:22293–22299

125. Collins LR, Ricketts WA, Yeh L, Cheresh D (1999) Bifurcation of cell migratory and proliferative signaling by the adaptor protein Shc. J Cell Biol 147:1561–1568
126. Zhou MM, Ravichandran KS, Olejniczak EF, Petros AM, Meadows RP, Sattler M, Harlan JE, Wade WS, Burakoff SJ, Fesik SW (1995) Structure and ligand recognition of the phosphotyrosine binding domain of Shc. Nature 378:584–592
127. Sato K, Gotoh N, Otsuki T, Kakumoto M, Aoto M, Tokmakov AA, Shibuya M, Fukami Y (1997) Tyrosine residues 239 and 240 of Shc are phosphatidylinositol 4, 5-bisphosphate-dependent phosphorylation sites by c-Src. Biochem Biophys Res Commun 240:399–404
128. Guo Z, Dai B, Jiang T, Xu K, Xie Y, Kim O, Nesheiwat I, Kong X, Melamed J, Handratta VD, Njar VC, Brodie AM, Yu LR, Veenstra TD, Chen H, Qiu Y (2006) Regulation of androgen receptor activity by tyrosine phosphorylation. Cancer Cell 10:309–319

Unraveling the Role of GPER in Breast Cancer

Rosamaria Lappano and Marcello Maggiolini

Abstract The G protein-coupled estrogen receptor-1 (GPER, formerly called GPR30) has been recently involved in the multifaceted transduction pathways through which estrogens induce diverse biological responses as well as pathological processes, including cancer development and progression. In this regard, it has been shown that not only estrogens but also antiestrogens binding to and activating the GPER-dependent signaling elicit stimulatory effects in hormone-dependent tumors like breast cancer. In accordance with these findings, GPER expression was associated with worse clinical features commonly used to assess the progression of breast malignancies, such as the detection of distant metastases. On the basis of diverse studies demonstrating the potential role of GPER in mediating the stimulatory action of estrogens in breast tumor, GPER may be considered as a valuable target toward novel therapeutic strategies against the development of breast cancer. Furthermore, the promiscuous activity exerted by antiestrogens, which act as GPER agonists and antagonists of the nuclear estrogen receptors, addresses the need of new selective estrogen receptor inhibitors.

Keywords GPER · Signaling · Breast cancer · Agonists · Antagonists

Abbreviations

AP-1	activating protein-1
cAMP	cyclic AMP
cDNA	complementary DNA
EGFR	Epidermal Growth Factor Receptor

R. Lappano · M. Maggiolini (✉)
Department of Pharmaco-Biology, University of Calabria, Rende, CS, Italy
e-mail: marcellomaggiolini@yahoo.it

R. Lappano
e-mail: rosamaria3@interfree.it

G. Castoria and A. Migliaccio (eds.), *Advances in Rapid Sex-Steroid Action*,
DOI: 10.1007/978-1-4614-1764-4_7, © Springer Science+Business Media, LLC 2012

ERK	extracellular signal-regulated kinase
MAPK	mitogen-activated protein kinase
NF-κB	Nuclear Factor-κB
OHT	4-hydroxytamoxifen
ROS	Reactive Oxygen Species
Sp-1	stimulating factor-1

Contents

1 Introduction

Breast cancer is the most frequently diagnosed cancer in women [1]. Worldwide, it is estimated that more than one million women are diagnosed with breast cancer every year [2]. Additionally, breast cancer incidence rates have been reported to be increasing by up to 5% per year in many populations in developing countries [3, 4]. Despite recent advances in its diagnosis and treatment with adjuvant therapies, breast cancer represents 14% of female cancer deaths and 20% of all female malignancies, remaining the second leading cause of cancer death in women globally [2, 5].

Estrogens are a group of steroid hormones which regulate many physiological processes, including reproduction, bone formation, cardiovascular and central nervous system functions [6]. Moreover, a wide number of studies have demonstrated that an excessive and/or prolonged exposure to estrogens play a key role in the development and progression of breast cancer [7–9]. The biological effects elicited by estrogens are mainly mediated by the classical estrogen receptors (ERα and ERβ), which belong to the nuclear receptor superfamily of transcription factors [7]. In the absence of ligands, monomeric ERs are complexed with heat-shock proteins (Hsp90 and Hsp70) by a multi-protein chaperone machinery formed specifically with the ligand binding domain (LBD) [10]. Upon ligand binding to the LBD and the subsequent Hsp dissociation, ERs undergo a conformational change triggering the receptor homodimerization and the interaction with the estrogen responsive elements (EREs) located within the promoter regions of target genes [11]. Ligand-bound ERs can also influence the transcription of genes whose promoters do not harbor EREs by interacting with other transcription factors such as AP-1-responsive elements, Sp-1 (GC-rich Sp-1 motifs) and NF-κB [12–14]. ER function requires the recruitment of transcriptional regulators, such as coactivators and corepressors, which contribute to the transcription and the accessibility of target gene promoters [15]. In addition, ER activity can occur even in a ligand-independent fashion, particularly through growth factor-dependent signaling [16–18]. A large body of evidence has demonstrated the main role elicited by ERα in mediating the stimulatory action of estrogens in breast cancer development [19]. In this regard, it has been shown that ERα represents one of the most important markers toward the responsiveness to antiestrogen treatment as well as breast cancer outcomes [20, 21]. Nevertheless, in ER-positive breast tumors de novo and acquired resistance to antiestrogen therapy often occur, as observed by using the selective estrogen receptor modulator (SERM) tamoxifen [21, 22]. These observations together with major clinical benefits of the aromatase inhibitors [23] have suggested that additional factors (e.g. receptors) and signaling mechanisms may be involved in the stimulatory action of estrogens as well as in the failure of antiestrogen therapy in breast cancer.

2 GPER Signaling in Breast Cancer

In the last years, numerous studies have suggested that a member of the 7-transmembrane G protein-coupled receptor family mediates estrogen signals in a wide number of normal and cancer cells [24]. In particular, the G protein-coupled estrogen receptor-1 (GPER, formerly called GPR30), has emerged as a key mediator of estrogen action in hormone-responsive tumors like breast cancer [24, 25]. GPER was cloned in 1997 as a cDNA of a gene mapped to chromosome 7p22 and was found abundantly expressed in breast cancer cells as well as in samples of primary breast carcinomas [26]. A few years later, the functional role elicited by GPER was investigated by Filardo and coworkers [27]. Interestingly, the rapid ERK1/2 phosphorylation induced by 17β-estradiol (E2) was shown to occur through GPER in ER-negative breast cancer cells. The ERK1/2 activation by E2 was consequent to the G$\beta\gamma$ subunit-dependent transactivation of the epidermal growth factor (EGF) receptor through the cleavage and the release of heparan-bound EGF (HB-EGF) by metalloproteinases (MMPs) [27] (Fig. 1). In this respect, it has been recently shown that integrin $\alpha5\beta1$ is involved in the EGFR transactivation by ligand-activated GPER as it interacts with and then converts fibronectin (FN) from a soluble plasma protein into an insoluble fibrillar structure in the extracellular matrix (ECM) [28]. This process previously known as FN matrix assembly [29] involves a number of intracellular signaling pathways that promote cellular adhesion, haptotaxis and survival [30–32]. In breast cancer cells, GPER coordinates the estrogen-induced FN matrix assembly and growth factor release which lead to the activation of integrin $\alpha5\beta1$ [28] (Fig. 1). Hence, the integrin-ECM interactions and the local growth factor release mediated by GPER

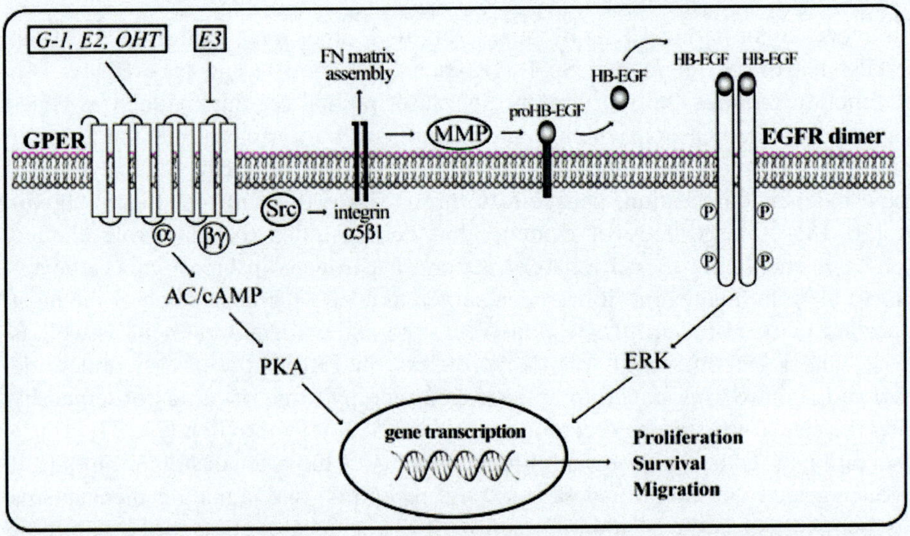

Fig. 1 Schematic GPER signaling in breast cancer cells. Estrogens and antiestrogens bind to and activate the GPER. The ligand binding leads to G protein complex dissociation into $G\alpha s$ and $G\beta\gamma$ proteins, which trigger two distinct cascade events. $G\alpha s$ through adenylyl cyclase induces the increase of cAMP and the activation of protein kinase A-dependent transduction pathway (PKA). $G\beta\gamma$ causes calcium mobilization (not shown) and the activation of diverse effectors like PI3K-signaling, Src-like kinases and integrin $\alpha 5\beta 1$, which in turn induce the fibronectin matrix (FN) assembly and the metalloproteinase (MMP)-dependent release of membrane-tethered proHB-EGF. Then, the ligand-activated Epidermal Growth Factor Receptor (EGFR) stimulates the ERK signaling cascade which triggers gene transcription and relevant biological responses as the proliferation, migration and survival of breast cancer cells

represent cellular events critical to the survival of normal ductal epithelia and tumor cells that invade the local parenchyma or seed distant sites. On the basis of these findings, GPER has been suggested to ensure cellular survival during estrus cycle-dependent remodeling of the mammary gland.

The increasing evidence on the potential of GPER in mediating estrogen signaling has entailed a great number of studies with the aim to characterize the molecular mechanisms involved in its signal transduction and functions. For instance, GPER was required for the estrogen-induced stimulation of adenylyl cyclase and cAMP-mediated inhibition of the EGFR/ERK pathway in GPER-positive breast cancer cells [33]. Moreover, in breast cancer cells the ER antagonists tamoxifen and ICI 182,780 induced rapid signaling events through GPER similar to estrogens [27, 33]. Cumulatively, these findings indicated a key function of GPER in breast cancer biology suggesting that in ER-negative but GPER-positive breast tumors which do not respond favorably to antiestrogen therapy [21], both estrogens and antiestrogens stimulate growth effects via GPER and growth factor-dependent signals. On the basis of the unresponsiveness of one in four patients with ER-positive tumors to antiestrogens [21], the existence of an alternative mediator of estrogen action provided a new mechanism by which antiestrogens can induce the proliferation of hormone-dependent cancer cells, including the growth and survival of breast carcinoma cells.

In recent years, diverse studies have demonstrated that the activation of GPER signaling regulates a number of genes involved in the progression of breast malignancies. For instance, in ER-negative breast cancer cells, E2 and two major phytoestrogens, genistein and quercetin, induced in a GPER- dependent manner the rapid up-regulation of *c-fos*, which is a transcription factor involved in many biological processes including cell growth, differentiation and cellular transformation [24]. In addition, estrogens as well as the selective GPER ligand G-1 [34] stimulated gene transcription and the proliferation of ER-negative breast cancer cells through the GPER/EGFR/ERK transduction signaling [35]. Likewise, GPER activation by E2 and the ER antagonist 4-hydroxytamoxifen (OHT) generated in ER-negative breast cancer cells a valuable transcription factor network [36]. In particular, the most strongly induced gene, the connective tissue growth factor (CTGF), was shown to be involved in the proliferation and migration of ER-negative breast cancer cells stimulated by E2 or OHT through the GPER-dependent pathway [36]. Interestingly, the aforementioned findings were also demonstrated in carcinoma-associated fibroblasts derived from breast cancer biopsies [37], suggesting that GPER may play a stimulatory action also in the tumor microenvironment which has been largely involved in the progression of malignancies toward aggressive biological features [38].

As it concerns the distribution pattern, GPER was localized at the endoplasmic reticulum in different cell lines [39], on the plasma membrane of breast cancer cells [40] also associated with cytokeratin intermediate filaments [41]. In further studies, GPER showed different intracellular distributions [42, 43] and a nuclear localization in cancer associated fibroblasts (CAFs) obtained from breast tumor biopsies [37]. These observations address the need of additional investigations to ascertain whether GPER may elicit different biological functions depending on its cellular localization.

3 Binding Specificity and Biological Characterization of GPER Ligands

The first evidence on the binding characteristics of GPER ligands was provided by Thomas and coworkers in 2005 [44]. For instance, E2 as well as the ER antagonists OHT and ICI 182,780 showed a strong binding affinity for GPER. These findings, corroborating the aforementioned studies regarding the stimulatory actions elicited by antiestrogens may have important implications for the progression and the treatment of breast cancer. In contrast to E2, estriol (E3) was shown to act as a GPER antagonist in ER-negative breast cancer cells [45]. This finding indicates that estrogenic compounds can exert stimulatory effects through both the classical ERs and GPER as observed with E2; however, an opposite biological activity can be also elicited through these receptors, as reported for E3. Further compounds exerting an estrogen-like activity in cancer cells, such as diverse environmental contaminants, were investigated for their potential capability to bind to and activate GPER. For instance, bisphenol A (BPA) as GPER ligand increased the cAMP levels and stimulated c-fos transcription by activating the GPER/EGFR/ERK transduction cascade in breast cancer cells [46, 47]. Several studies have shown that the herbicide atrazine may exhibit an estrogen-like activity without binding to the classical ERs [48, 49]. Even though this endocrine disruptor exhibited a low binding affinity for GPER, rapid ERK1/2 phosphorylation and c-fos expression were induced in a GPER-dependent manner by atrazine in breast cancer cells [47, 48, 50]. Recently, it was demonstrated that also cadmium through GPER stimulates cAMP production, ERK activation and the proliferation of ER-negative breast cancer cells [51]. In addition to the environmental contaminants, diverse phytoestrogens like genistein, quercetin and tectoridin activated the GPER transduction pathway [52, 53], although only genistein displayed a high binding affinity for GPER [47]. Moreover, genistein was recently shown to induce through a GPER/Src/ERK-dependent pathway the transcription of acid ceramidase (ASAH1), which regulates the intracellular concentration of two sphingolipid metabolites, ceramide and sphingosine-1-phosphate, both involved in cell proliferation, migration, angiogenesis and tumor chemo-resistance [54].

The identification of the selective GPER ligands, the agonist G-1 and the antagonist G-15 [34, 55], which failed to bind to and regulate the classical ERs, allowed the characterization of the biological activity mediated by GPER. In particular, G-1 was of fundamental importance in order to reveal the key role elicited by GPER in mediating the estrogen signaling in breast cancer cells. For instance, in ER-negative breast cancer cells G-1 like E2 triggered through the GPER/EGFR transduction pathway stimulatory effects such as ERK phosphorylation, the up-regulation of the two major GPER-target genes c-fos and CTGF as well as cell proliferation [35]. Moreover, G-1 increased in breast cancer cells the current amplitude of voltage-gated Na(+) channels (VGSCs), which enhances several types of cellular behavior that would be involved in the metastatic cancer progression [56]. Next, G-1 stimulated in ER-negative breast cancer cells through GPER, the expression of the estrogen-related receptor α (ERRα) [57], and elicited exclusively through GPER, the cytosolic Ca(2+), increase in both ER-negative and ER-positive breast cancer cells [58].

4 Implication of GPER in the Resistance to Antiestrogen Therapy

GPER has been recently involved in the failure of antiestrogen treatment in breast cancer. For instance, both E2 and ICI 182,780 activating the GPER/ERK transduction pathway rapidly inhibited the transforming growth factor (TGF)-β mediated activity, which acts as a tumor suppressor in breast cancer cells [59]. These findings well fit with the observation that the down-regulation of TGF-β signaling network is associated with the resistance to antiestrogens in breast cancer [60]. Afterward, OHT-resistant breast cancer cells exhibited an enhanced sensitivity to E2 and G-1 with respect to the parental cells [61]. In particular, in cancer cells showing OHT resistance these ligands induced ERK phosphorylation and growth effects through the GPER/EGFR-mediated signaling [61]. The inhibitory effects exerted by OHT in parental breast cancer cells were lost by the continuous treatment with G-1 and the inhibition of the GPER/EGFR signaling restored the repressive action exerted by OHT [61]. In addition, the treatment with E2 in both parental and tamoxifen-resistant breast cancer cells up-regulated GPER expression, which additionally increased the sensitivity to G-1 exposure, particularly in the tamoxifen-resistant cells [61]. Overall, these data provided evidence on the potential cooperation between GPER and EGFR in the development, at least in part, of tamoxifen failure. The evaluation of the functional cross-talk between these two receptors toward the regulation of GPER expression contributed to better understanding the molecular mechanisms involved in the estrogen-induced progression of hormone-sensitive tumors and the resistance to antiestrogens in breast cancer. For instance, ligand-dependent EGFR activation up-regulated GPER expression in ER-negative breast cancer cells [62]. Hence, GPER increase upon exposure to EGF was suggested as an additional mechanism by which this growth factor may engage estrogenic signals in the stimulation of ER-negative breast cancer cells. In addition, EGFR ligands were shown to up-regulate GPER expression by activating the EGFR/ERK pathway in ER-positive and tamoxifen-resistant breast cancer cells [63]. These findings suggested that ligand-activated EGFR may contribute to tamoxifen resistance, at least in part, by up-regulating GPER which in turn facilitates the action of estrogens. As it concerns the role of the classical ERs, initial evidence showed that the GPER/EGFR signaling mediates gene expression changes and growth effects in ER-negative breast cancer cells [52]. Recently, it has been also demonstrated that GPER and ERα cooperate in mediating the action of estrogens in ER-positive and tamoxifen-resistant breast cancer cells as well as in ovarian and endometrial tumor cells [35, 63].

The importance of the EGFR transduction pathway in regulating GPER expression has been also extended to the biological responses to hypoxia, which is considered a key feature of the tumor microenvironment as well as a hallmark of cancer growth, resistance to chemotherapy and decreased survival of patients [64]. In this regard, the hypoxia-inducible factor HIF-1α, which is well recognized as a major factor involved in the adaptation to hypoxic conditions, was shown to mediate the up-regulation of GPER and CTGF protein levels upon exposure to hypoxia in ER-negative breast cancer cells. In particular, the hypoxia-dependent transcription of GPER required the ROS-induced activation of EGFR/ERK transduction pathway in both breast cancer cells and cardiomyocytes. Remarkably, the apoptotic response to hypoxia was prevented through GPER in breast cancer cells treated with estrogens [64]. On the basis of these data, the hypoxia-induced expression of GPER may be included among the mechanisms potentially involved in the anti-apoptotic effects elicited by estrogens in tumor cells exposed to low oxygen tension.

5 GPER as a Biological Marker in Breast Carcinomas

GPER has been recently considered as a valuable biomarker and therapeutic target in breast cancer. In 2006, Filardo and coworkers explored the expression of GPER in breast carcinomas in association with other well known histopathologic markers of disease, including ERα, progesterone receptor (PR) and EGFR/HER-2 [25]. In this immunohistochemical study 361 breast carcinomas (321 invasive and 40 intraductal tumors) and 12 controls obtained from breast reduction surgery were examined. All normal controls were positive for GPER, ERα and PR, whereas the expression of GPER varied in breast tumors: 62% (199 of 321) of invasive tumors and 42% (17 of 40) of intraductal tumors resulted positive. A co-distribution pattern of ERα and GPER was observed in 43% (139 of 321) of invasive breast tumors, whereas in 19% (61 of 321) of the tumors analyzed neither ERα nor GPER were detected, indicating a significant but incomplete association between the expression of both receptors. GPER expression did not correlate with PR in primary tumors from patients with invasive ductal tumors, whereas PR expression was more than twice as common in tumors that coexpressed ERα and GPER compared with breast tumors that produced ERα but not GPER. Unlike ERα, which varied inversely with tumor size and HER-2/neu, the overexpression of GPER was significantly associated with tumor size and the presence of distant metastases. In line with the ability of GPER to transactivate EGFR through the release of heparan-bound EGF in breast cancer cells, GPER expression directly varied with HER-2/neu expression [25]. These findings highlighted the biological significance of GPER in human breast cancer as strongly supported by its association with the risk of developing metastatic disease, which is a variable clearly reflecting breast tumor progression as well as influencing the therapeutic strategies.

In a further study, GPER expression did not show any correlation with age, lymph node metastasis, lymph-vascular invasion, grade and stage in tumor samples of 118 Taiwanese patients with infiltrating ductal carcinoma (IDC) and 27 non-tumor mammary tissues [65]. In particular, GPER expression was found down-regulated in IDC respect to normal mammary tissues, positively correlated with ERα and PR but not associated with HER-2/neu expression. The discrepancy in the results obtained by the aforementioned studies may be consequent to the use of different experimental approaches. Filardo and coworkers employed immunohistochemistry to assess GPER expression exclusively in epithelial tumor cells [25], whereas in the later investigation GPER expression was detected by evaluating total RNA without isolating epithelial tumor cells [65]. In 2010, the role of GPER was also investigated in relation to other biomarkers and the prognosis in 88 primary inflammatory breast cancer (IBC) patients [66]. GPER over-expression was found associated with an improved overall survival in ER-positive IBC patients. Moreover, no correlation was observed between GPER and HER-2 expression as well as between GPER and EGFR expression. These findings were explained by the authors considering the intrinsic nature of IBC tumors, which are thought to be metastatic at the onset of the disease

[67, 68]. On the basis of these observations, it was suggested that agents targeting GPER could also be useful as novel therapeutic approaches in IBC patients.

Numerous genome-wide association studies have identified a number of gene polymorphisms affecting breast cancer susceptibility [69–73]. In this context, a recent genotype-phenotype association study examined three GPER single nucleotide polymorphisms (SNPs) with regard to breast cancer risk and characteristics [74]. Genotype and allele frequencies of these SNPs were compared in 257 women with sporadic breast cancer and 247 healthy women. The first SNP was located in the promoter region of the GPER gene, the second in the 5′-untranslated region, whereas the third is a missense SNP in coding exon 1. The polymorphism in the 5′-region was hypothesized to alter GPER expression, while the missense exon-SNP to affect the GPER protein structure and function. The comparison of the breast cancer cases and the control group with regard to the SNP allele, genotype and haplotype frequencies did not show significant differences [74]. Of note, an association of GPER SNPs with tumor size, grading, nodal status and progesterone receptor (PR) status was shown, whereas no connection of any of the GPER SNPs to the HER-2/neu status was demonstrated in patients studied. Overall, further evaluations on the relation between the SNP genotypes considered and GPER expression and function are required toward a better understanding of this issue in estrogen signaling and the progression of breast cancer.

6 Conclusions

The discovery of GPER as a novel mediator of estrogen actions has amplified the biological routes that may be engaged by these hormones. The increasing number of publications on GPER has allowed a more comprehensive evaluation of the molecular mechanisms through which estrogens can function either in the presence or absence of the classical ERs. Moreover, the connection of GPER to breast cancer has been well corroborated by the results obtained in a wide number of investigations. In particular, the biological relevance of GPER in breast carcinomas has been highlighted by the strong association of GPER expression with diverse clinical-pathological parameters that are commonly used to assess tumor progression. Based on such correlations, GPER overexpression may be considered as a predictor of aggressive breast tumors. In addition, the regulation and function of GPER have been also involved in the resistance to antiestrogen treatment in breast cancer patients. This may be not surprising as several studies have shown that antiestrogens can act as GPER agonists leading to cell proliferation in different tumor types, including breast cancer. Hence, the inhibition of the GPER-mediated signaling could be also considered as a potential target to overcome the resistance to antiestrogens in malignant cells. A further characterization of the biological functions exerted by GPER as well as a better knowledge on the molecular mechanisms involved in the stimulatory network triggered through the cross-talk between GPER and key signaling molecules like EGFR and the classical ERs, would allow the discovery of new pharmacological tools targeting breast cancer progression.

Acknowledgments This work was supported by Associazione Italiana per la Ricerca sul Cancro (AIRC, project n. 8925/2009; http://www.airc.it/) and Ministero dell'Università e Ricerca Scientifica e Tecnologica (MIUR; http://www.istruzione.it/).

References

1. Coughlin SS, Ekwueme DU (2009) Breast cancer as a global health concern. Cancer Epidemiol 33:315–318
2. Parkin DM, Fernández LM (2006) Use of statistics to assess the global burden of breast cancer. Breast J 12(Suppl 1):S70–S80
3. Stewart B, Kleihues PE (2003) World Cancer Report. IARC Press, Lyon
4. IARC Working Group on the Evaluation of Cancer-Preventive Strategies. IARC handbooks of cancer prevention (2002) Vol. 7: breast cancer screening. Lyon: Oxford University Press
5. Jemal A, Siegel R, Xu J, CA Ward E (2010) Cancer statistics, 2010. Cancer J Clin 60:277–300
6. Hall JM, Couse JF, Korach KS (2001) The multifaceted mechanisms of estradiol and estrogen receptor signaling. J Biol Chem 276:36869–36872
7. Ascenzi P, Bocedi A, Marino M (2006) Structure-function relationship of estrogen receptor alpha and beta: impact on human health. Mol Aspects Med 27:299–402
8. Hankinson SE, Colditz GA, Willett WC (2004) Towards an integrated model for breast cancer etiology: the lifelong interplay of genes, lifestyle, and hormones. Breast Cancer Res 6:213–218
9. Pearce ST, Jordan VC (2004) The biological role of estrogen receptor alpha and beta in cancer. Crit Rev Oncol Hematol 50:3–22
10. Pratt WB, Galigniana MD, Morishima Y, Murphy PJ (2004) Role of molecular chaperones in steroid receptor action. Essays Biochem 40:41–58
11. Sanchez R, Nguyen D, Rocha W, White JH, Mader S (2002) Diversity in the mechanisms of gene regulation by estrogen receptor. Bioessays 24:244–254
12. Kalaitzidis D, Gilmore TD (2005) Transcription factor cross-talk: the estrogen receptor and NF-kappaB. Trends Endocrinol Metab 16:46–52
13. Kushner PJ, Agard DA, Greene GL, Scanlan TS, Shiau AK, Uht RM, Webb P (2000) Estrogen receptor pathways to AP-1. J Steroid Biochem Mol Biol 74:311–317
14. Saville B, Wormke M, Wang F, Nguyen T, Enmark E, Kuiper G, Gustafsson JA, Safe S (2000) Ligand-, cell-, and estrogen receptor subtype (alpha/beta)-dependent activation at GC-rich (Sp1) promoter elements. J Biol Chem 275:5379–5387
15. Klinge CM (2000) Estrogen receptor interaction with co-activators and co-repressors. Steroids 65:227–251
16. Lannigan DA (2003) Estrogen receptor phosphorylation. Steroids 68:1–9
17. Kato S (2001) Estrogen receptor-mediated cross-talk with growth factor signaling pathways. Breast Cancer 8:3–9
18. Levin ER (2002) Cellular functions of plasma membrane estrogen receptors. Steroids 67:471–475
19. Deroo BJ, Korach KS (2006) Estrogen receptors and human disease. J Clin Invest 116:561–570
20. Conzen SD (2008) Minireview: nuclear receptors and breast cancer. Mol Endocrinol 22:2215–2228
21. Wittliff JL (1984) Steroid-hormone receptors in breast cancer. Cancer 53:630–643

22. Katzenellenbogen BS, Montano MM, Ekena K, Herman ME, McInerney EM (1997) William L. McGuire memorial lecture. antiestrogens: mechanisms of action and resistance in breast cancer. Breast Cancer Res Treat 44:23–38
23. Howell A (2005) New developments in the treatment of postmenopausal breast cancer. Trends Endocrinol Metab 16:420–428
24. Maggiolini M, Picard D (2010) The unfolding stories of GPR30, a new membrane-bound estrogen receptor. J Endocrinol 204:105–114
25. Filardo EJ, Graeber CT, Quinn JA, Resnick MB, Giri D, DeLellis RA, Steinhoff MM, Sabo E (2006) Distribution of GPR30, a seven membrane-spanning estrogen receptor, in primary breast cancer and its association with clinicopathologic determinants of tumor progression. Clin Cancer Res 12:6359–6366
26. Carmeci C, Thompson DA, Ring HZ, Francke U, Weigel RJ (1997) Identification of a gene (GPR30) with homology to the G-protein-coupled receptor superfamily associated with estrogen receptor expression in breast cancer. Genomics 45:607–617
27. Filardo EJ, Quinn JA, Bland KI, Frackelton AR Jr (2000) Estrogen-induced activation of Erk-1 and Erk-2 requires the G protein-coupled receptor homolog, GPR30, and occurs via trans-activation of the epidermal growth factor receptor through release of HB-EGF. Mol Endocrinol 14:1649–1660
28. Quinn JA, Graeber CT, Frackelton AR Jr, Kim M, Schwarzbauer JE, Filardo EJ (2009) Coordinate regulation of estrogen-mediated fibronectin matrix assembly and epidermal growth factor receptor transactivation by the G protein-coupled receptor, GPR30. Mol Endocrinol 23:1052–1064
29. Mao Y, Schwarzbauer JE (2005) Stimulatory effects of a three-dimensional microenvironment on cell-mediated fibronectin fibrillogenesis. J Cell Sci 118:4427–4436
30. Somanath PR, Kandel ES, Hay N, Byzova TV (2007) Akt1 signaling regulates integrin activation, matrix recognition, and fibronectin assembly. J Biol Chem 282:22964–22976
31. Yang RS, Tang CH, Ling QD, Liu SH, Fu WM (2002) Regulation of fibronectin fibrillogenesis by protein kinases in cultured rat osteoblasts. Mol Pharmacol 61:1163–1173
32. Wierzbicka-Patynowski I, Schwarzbauer JE (2002) Regulatory role for SRC and phosphatidylinositol 3-kinase in initiation of fibronectin matrix assembly. J Biol Chem 277:19703–19708
33. Filardo EJ, Quinn JA, Frackelton AR Jr, Bland KI (2002) Estrogen action via the G protein-coupled receptor, GPR30: stimulation of adenylyl cyclase and cAMP-mediated attenuation of the epidermal growth factor receptor-to-MAPK signaling axis. Mol Endocrinol 16:70–84
34. Bologa CG, Revankar CM, Young SM, Edwards BS, Arterburn JB, Kiselyov AS, Parker MA, Tkachenko SE, Savchuck NP, Sklar LA, Oprea TI, Prossnitz ER (2006) Virtual and biomolecular screening converge on a selective agonist for GPR30. Nat Chem Biol 2:207–212
35. Albanito L, Madeo A, Lappano R, Vivacqua A, Rago V, Carpino A, Oprea TI, Prossnitz ER, Musti AM, Andò S, Maggiolini M (2007) G protein-coupled receptor 30 (GPR30) mediates gene expression changes and growth response to 17beta-estradiol and selective GPR30 ligand G-1 in ovarian cancer cells. Cancer Res 67:1859–1866
36. Pandey DP, Lappano R, Albanito L, Madeo A, Maggiolini M, Picard D (2009) Estrogenic GPR30 signalling induces proliferation and migration of breast cancer cells through CTGF. EMBO J 28:523–532
37. Madeo A, Maggiolini M (2010) Nuclear alternate estrogen receptor GPR30 mediates 17beta-estradiol-induced gene expression and migration in breast cancer-associated fibroblasts. Cancer Res 70:6036–6046
38. Albini A, Sporn MB (2007) The tumour microenvironment as a target for chemoprevention. Nature Rev Cancer 7:139–147
39. Revankar CM, Cimino DF, Sklar LA, Arterburn JB, Prossnitz ER (2005) A transmembrane intracellular estrogen receptor mediates rapid cell signaling. Science 307:1625–1630
40. Filardo E, Quinn J, Pang Y, Graeber C, Shaw S, Dong J, Thomas P (2007) Activation of the novel estrogen receptor G protein-coupled receptor 30 (GPR30) at the plasma membrane. Endocrinology 148:3236–3245

41. Sandén C, Broselid S, Cornmark L, Andersson K, Daszkiewicz-Nilsson J, Mårtensson UE, Olde B, Leeb-Lundberg LM (2011) G protein-coupled estrogen recepto 1/G protein-coupled receptor 30 localizes in the plasma membrane and traffics intracellularly on cytokeratin intermediate filaments. Mol Pharmacol 79:400–410
42. Sakamoto H, Matsuda K, Hosokawa K, Nishi M, Morris JF, Prossnitz ER, Kawata M (2007) Expression of G protein-coupled receptor-30, a G protein-coupled membrane estrogen receptor, in oxytocin neurons of the rat paraventricular and supraoptic nuclei. Endocrinology 148:5842–5850
43. Funakoshi T, Yanai A, Shinoda K, Kawano MM, Mizukami Y (2006) G protein-coupled receptor 30 is an estrogen receptor in the plasma membrane. Biochem Biophys Res Commun 346:904–910
44. Thomas P, Pang Y, Filardo EJ, Dong J (2005) Identity of an estrogen membrane receptor coupled to a G protein in human breast cancer cells. Endocrinology 146:624–632
45. Lappano R, Rosano C, De Marco P, De Francesco EM, Pezzi V, Maggiolini M (2010) Estriol acts as a GPR30 antagonist in estrogen receptor-negative breast cancer cells. Mol Cell Endocrinol 320:162–170
46. Dong S, Terasaka S, Kiyama R (2011) Bisphenol A induces a rapid activation of Erk1/2 through GPR30 in human breast cancer cells. Environ Pollut 159:212–218
47. Thomas P, Dong J (2006) Binding and activation of the seven-transmembrane estrogen receptor GPR30 by environmental estrogens: a potential novel mechanism of endocrine disruption. J Steroid Biochem Mol Biol 102:175–179
48. Roberge M, Hakk H, Larsen G (2004) Atrazine is a competitive inhibitor of phosphodiesterase but does not affect the estrogen receptor. Toxicol Lett 154:61–68
49. Tennant MK, Hill DS, Eldridge JC, Wetzel LT, Breckenridge CB, Stevens JT (1994) Chloro-s-triazine antagonism of estrogen action: limited interaction with estrogen receptor binding. J Toxicol Environ Health 43:197–211
50. Albanito L, Lappano R, Madeo A, Chimento A, Prossnitz ER, Cappello AR, Dolce V, Abonante S, Pezzi V, Maggiolini M (2008) G-protein-coupled receptor 30 and estrogen receptor-alpha are involved in the proliferative effects induced by atrazine in ovarian ancer cells. Environ Health Perspect 116:1648–1655
51. Yu X, Filardo EJ, Shaikh ZA (2010) The membrane estrogen receptor GPR30 mediates cadmium-induced proliferation of breast cancer cells. Toxicol Appl Pharmacol 245:83–90
52. Maggiolini M, Vivacqua A, Fasanella G, Recchia AG, Sisci D, Pezzi V, Montanaro D, Musti AM, Picard D, Andò S (2004) The G protein-coupled receptor GPR30 mediates c-fos up-regulation by 17beta-estradiol and phytoestrogens in breast cancer cells. J Biol Chem 279:27008–27016
53. Kang K, Lee SB, Jung SH, Cha KH, Park WD, Sohn YC, Nho CW (2009) Tectoridin, a poor ligand of estrogen receptor alpha, exerts its estrogenic effects via an ERK-dependent pathway. Mol Cells 27:351–357
54. Lucki NC, Sewer MB (2011) Genistein stimulates MCF-7 breast cancerbreast cancer cell growth by inducing acid ceramidase (ASAH1) gene expression. J Biol Chem. doi:10.1074/jbc.M110.195826
55. Dennis MK, Burai R, Ramesh C, Petrie WK, Alcon SN, Nayak TK, Bologa CG, Leitao A, Brailoiu E, Deliu E, Dun NJ, Sklar LA, Hathaway HJ, Arterburn JB, Oprea TI, Prossnitz ER (2009) In vivo effects of a GPR30 antagonist. Nat Chem Biol 5:421–427
56. Fraser SP, Ozerlat-Gunduz I, Onkal R, Diss JK, Latchman DS, Djamgoz MB (2010) Estrogen and non-genomic upregulation of voltage-gated Na(+) channel activity in MDA-MB-231 human breast cancer cells: role in adhesion. J Cell Physiol 224:527–539
57. Li Y, Birnbaumer L, Teng CT (2010) Regulation of ERRalpha gene expression by estrogen receptor agonists and antagonists in SKBR3 breast cancer cells: differential molecular mechanisms mediated by g protein-coupled receptor GPR30/GPERGPER-1. Mol Endocrinol 24:969–980
58. Ariazi EA, Brailoiu E, Yerrum S, Shupp HA, Slifker MJ, Cunliffe HE, Black MA, Donato AL, Arterburn JB, Oprea TI, Prossnitz ER, Dun NJ, Jordan VC (2010) The G protein-coupled

receptor GPR30 inhibits proliferation of estrogen receptor-positive breast cancer cells. Cancer Res 70:1184–1194
59. Kleuser B, Malek D, Gust R, Pertz HH, Potteck H (2008) 17-Beta-estradiol inhibits transforming growth factor-beta signaling and function in breast cancer cells via activation of extracellular signal-regulated kinase through the G protein-coupled receptor 30. Mol Pharmacol 74:1533–1543
60. Yoo YA, Kim YH, Kim JS, Seo JH (2008) The functional implications of Akt activity and TGF-beta signaling in tamoxifen-resistant breast cancer. Biochim Biophys Acta 1783:438–447
61. Ignatov A, Ignatov T, Roessner A, Costa SD, Kalinski T (2010) Role of GPR30 in the mechanisms of tamoxifen resistance in breast cancer MCF-7 cells. Breast Cancer Res Treat 123:87–96
62. Albanito L, Sisci D, Aquila S, Brunelli E, Vivacqua A, Madeo A, Lappano R, Pandey DP, Picard D, Mauro L, Andò S, Maggiolini M (2008) Epidermal growth factor induces G protein-coupled receptor 30 expression in estrogen receptor-negative breast cancer cells. Endocrinology 149:3799–3808
63. Vivacqua A, Lappano R, De Marco P, Sisci D, Aquila S, De Amicis F, Fuqua SA, Andò S, Maggiolini M (2009) G protein-coupled receptor 30 expression is up-regulated by EGF and TGF alpha in estrogen receptor alpha-positive cancer cells. Mol Endocrinol 23:1815–1826
64. Recchia AG, De Francesco EM, Vivacqua A, Sisci D, Panno ML, Andò S, Maggiolini M (2011) The G protein-coupled receptor 30 is up-regulated by Hypoxia-inducible factor-1{alpha} (HIF-1{alpha}) in breast cancer cells and cardiomyocytes. J Biol Chem 286:10773–10782
65. Kuo WH, Chang LY, Liu DL, Hwa HL, Lin JJ, Lee PH, Chen CN, Lien HC, Yuan RH, Shun CT, Chang KJ, Hsieh FJ (2007) The interactions between GPR30 and the major biomarkers in infiltrating ductal carcinoma of the breast in an Asian population. Taiwan J Obstet Gynecol 46:135–145
66. Arias-Pulido H, Royce M, Gong Y, Joste N, Lomo L, Lee SJ, Chaher N, Verschraegen C, Lara J, Prossnitz ER, Cristofanilli M (2010) GPR30 and estrogen receptor expression: new insights into hormone dependence of inflammatory breast cancer. Breast Cancer Res Treat 123:51–58
67. Charafe-Jauffret E, Tarpin C, Viens P, Bertucci F (2008) Defining the molecular biology of inflammatory breast cancer. Semin Oncol 35:41–50
68. Ventura AC, Merajver SD (2008) Genetic determinants of aggressive breast cancer. Annu Rev Med 59:199–212
69. Ahmed S et al (2009) Newly discovered breast cancer susceptibility loci on 3p24 and 17q23.2. Nat Genet 41:585–590
70. Easton DF et al (2007) Genome-wide association study identifies novel breast cancer susceptibility loci. Nature 447:1087–1093
71. Gold B, Kirchhoff T, Stefanov S, Lautenberger J, Viale A, Garber J, Friedman E, Narod S, Olshen AB, Gregersen P, Kosarin K, Olsh A, Bergeron J, Ellis NA, Klein RJ, Clark AG, Norton L, Dean M, Boyd J, Offit K (2008) Genome-wide association study provides evidence for a breast cancer risk locus at 6q22.33. Proc Natl Acad Sci U S A 105:4340–4345
72. Hunter DJ et al (2007) A genome-wide association study identifies alleles in FGFR2 associated with risk of sporadic postmenopausal breast cancer. Nat Genet 39:870–874
73. Thomas G et al (2009) A multistage genome-wide association study in breast cancer identifies two new risk alleles at 1p11.2 and 14q24.1 (RAD51L1). Nat Genet 41:579–584
74. Giess M, Lattrich C, Springwald A, Goerse R, Ortmann O, Treeck O (2010) GPR30 gene polymorphisms are associated with progesterone receptor status and histopathological characteristics of breast cancer patients. J Steroid Biochem Mol Biol 118:7–12

Nongenomic Actions of Estrogens and Xenoestrogens Affecting Endocrine Cancer Cells

Cheryl S. Watson, Dragoslava Zivadinovic, Yow-Jiun Jeng, Rebecca A. Alyea, Terumi Midoro-Horiuti, Randall Goldblum and Anannya Banga

Abstract Estrogens act via multiple membrane-associated receptors (α, β, and GPR30) to mediate diverse rapid signaling cascades affecting functional endpoints in both normal and cancer cells. The mitogen-activated protein kinases are a summative signaling node that integrates upstream signaling cascades into responses for major functional cellular outcomes such as proliferation, migration, differentiation, and death. These responses are complex; they oscillate with time, as well as fluctuate up and down with increasing ligand concentration (hormesis). Nonphysiologic estrogenic compounds also use these receptors and signaling systems, but do so imperfectly, causing disruptions to both the phasing and dose-responsiveness of physiologic estrogens. Disruptions to the signaling of different physiologic estrogens could cause life stage-specific tissue malfunctions or cancer vulnerabilities.

Keywords Nongenomic · Estrogens · Nonmonotonic · Breast cancer · Pituitary · Neurons · Xenoestrogens · Immune system · Membrane estrogen receptors · Ligand mixtures

Abbreviations

BPA	bisphenol A
Ca++	calcium
E1	estrone
E2	estradiol

C. S. Watson (✉) · D. Zivadinovic · Y.-J. Jeng · R. A. Alyea · A. Banga
Department of Biochemistry and Molecular Biology, University of Texas Medical Branch, Galveston, TX 77555, USA
e-mail: cswatson@utmb.edu

T. Midoro-Horiuti · R. Goldblum
Department of Pediatrics, University of Texas Medical Branch, Galveston, TX 77555, USA

G. Castoria and A. Migliaccio (eds.), *Advances in Rapid Sex-Steroid Action*,
DOI: 10.1007/978-1-4614-1764-4_8, © Springer Science+Business Media, LLC 2012

E3	estriol
ER	estrogen receptor
ERK	extracellular regulated kinase
JUNK	Jun-kinase
MAPK	mitogen-activated protein kinase
mERs	membrane estrogen receptors
mERα	membrane ERα
NHANES	National Health and Nutrition Examination Survey

Contents

1 Introduction

Cells, including cancer cells, first respond to hormones by rapidly triggering signaling cascades, that if sustained, eventually prompt the cell to retool (become more differentiated) or proliferate, requiring synthesis of new macromolecules. Both these early and late phases are important parts of the cellular response to new conditions (represented by changes in developmental stages, reproductive tasks, etc.,). The first decades of investigations into hormonal responses of cells focused on the permanent retooling of cells for differentiation or proliferative responses, and usually involved measurements of gene and protein expression. More recently an expanded repertoire of responsive cell lines, a rich library of specific antibodies, new more sensitive assays, and other experimental tools have made it practical to re-explore the rapid cellular signaling phase that begins the process of cellular adaptation to a new hormonal status. We have focused on these early responses to a wide variety of estrogens and the receptor subpopulations that mediate them.

Membrane-resident estrogen receptors (mERs) on uterine epithelial cells were first suggested some 40 years ago, by virtue of their binding to estrogens anchored to fibers [1]. Since then, there have been many more detections and descriptions of extranuclear ERs and nongenomic actions in estrogen-responsive cancer cell types [2–4]. Here we review the mER features we have found to be similar or contrasting, mainly between breast cancer, pituitary cancer, and pheochromocytoma cells that we have studied. We will also summarize the estrogen-initiated signaling abilities of mERs (such as different pathway engagement and hormesis) and review what is known about the types of mERs expressed in different tissues. Finally, we will describe the effects that physiologic estrogens have in comparison to nonphysiologic estrogens. These can be endocrine disruptors that contaminate environments and expose humans and animals to their effects, or they can be naturally occurring dietary (plant) estrogens. Their interference with the actions of endogenous estrogens has important implications for both normal and cancer cell behavior.

2 Receptors and the Signaling Responses and Functions Associated with Them

There are currently three main types of estrogen receptors (ERs): the classical ER proteins α and β, and the relatively newly described GPR30 (also called GPER) which is a 7-transmembrane receptor typical of those whose signaling is coupled to G proteins [5], and which may be coupled in its actions to an ERα 36KD splice variant [6]. Although GPR30 is exclusively a membrane protein (either in the cell or endoplasmic reticulum membrane) [7, 8], the ERs α and β can be located either in the nucleus (bound to chromatin) or in the plasma membrane (or other non-nuclear sites) [9] where they are tethered to membrane rafts of specialized lipid composition [10–12] by lipid post-translational modifications [13].

For breast cancers, the protein identity and cellular status (quantity, location) of ERs is a critically important clinical marker for choosing effective treatments for patients. In the past only the nuclear versions, mainly of ERα, have been viewed as important in deciding estrogen-dependence, and thus in choosing therapeutic agents such as anti-estrogens and aromatase inhibitors vs. chemotherapy. However, as we continue to learn more about membrane forms of ERs and the specific responses linked to their early effects, it will be prudent to look for other therapeutic opportunities for affecting these alternative signaling pathways for patients with endocrine cancers.

We demonstrated that cultured breast cancer cells selected for expressing high levels of mERα had a greater cAMP-protein kinase A response leading to cell death at higher administered E_2 concentrations [14]. This is consistent with estrogen-induced killing behavior of some other breast cancer cell sublines which may express mERs [15–18]. Some estrogens can selectively activate other kinase pathways affecting therapeutic apoptosis. We recently observed an estrogen-induced JNK kinase activation in pituitary cells [19] and breast cancer cells (Banga and Watson, unpublished data); activation of this kinase is often associated with the apoptotic death pathway. The activation of these alternative cancer cell-killing pathways has yet to be systematically exploited, despite the findings many years ago that a subset of breast cancers could actually be successfully treated with high doses of estrogens, as opposed to estrogen ablative techniques [20]. However, in order to take advantage of these selective activities via mERs, we will have to understand them more thoroughly. But it is possible that the signaling pathways leading to cell death could be therapeutically harnessed via these receptors.

The GPR30 has been shown to inhibit the actions caused by ERα in breast cancer cells [21]. We have found similar actions in pituitary and pheochromocytoma tumor cells where use of selective ligands for GPR30 and ERβ inhibited ERα-driven cell proliferation and differentiated responses of these cells such as ERK activation and dopamine transport [22, 23]. A similar story about ERβ opposition of ERα-driven responses has been told in a variety of female reproductive tissues [24, 25]. It will be interesting to see if GPR30 generally fills a similar role. However, in tissues where ERβ or GPR30 predominate, the rules for these stimulations vs. inhibitions will have to be more thoroughly investigated. For instance, in prostate gland and cancers of that tissue, ERβ is the dominant estrogen receptor [26]. We found [22], as have others [27] that when present or activated alone (e.g. via selective ligands), ERβ becomes the driver of estrogen-induced actions in some tissues. There may be lessons there for the estrogen-based therapeutics for late stage cancers of prostate or other tissues that express predominantly a receptor other than ERα, such as certain regions of the brain [28].

3 Time-Oscillating Responses

MAPK responses typically oscillate with time as has been shown by many investigators, including those in our own lab [12, 29, 30]. After initial response triggering by estrogens at the membrane, the signaling pathway journeys are variant in timing for different estrogens. To illustrate this, Fig. 1 displays four examples of responses to different estrogens in MCF-7 breast cancer cells: two endogenous (17β- and 17α-E_2) and two nonphysiolgic (the dietary phytoestrogen coumestrol and the pesticide endosulfan). Each rapidly triggers an ERK response that oscillates, as is typical. However, these responses to different estrogens differ from one another in both amplitude and phasing. 17α-E_2 has a delayed and muted response compared to 17β-E_2. Endosulfan causes a very large and rapidly peaking activation of ERK, followed by an equally dramatic dephosphorylation, and recovery. Coumestrol causes an early activation peak similar in size to that caused by 17β-E_2, but then after only a brief dephosphorylation phase, again activates to sustained high levels for an extended time (similar to the sustained response we have seen previously in pituitary tumor cells) [29]. These differences in phasing are perhaps part of the reason that functional outcomes for these estrogens differ. Many of the mechanisms discussed below for hormesis (nonmonotonic dose responses) can also be used to explain oscillating responses with time.

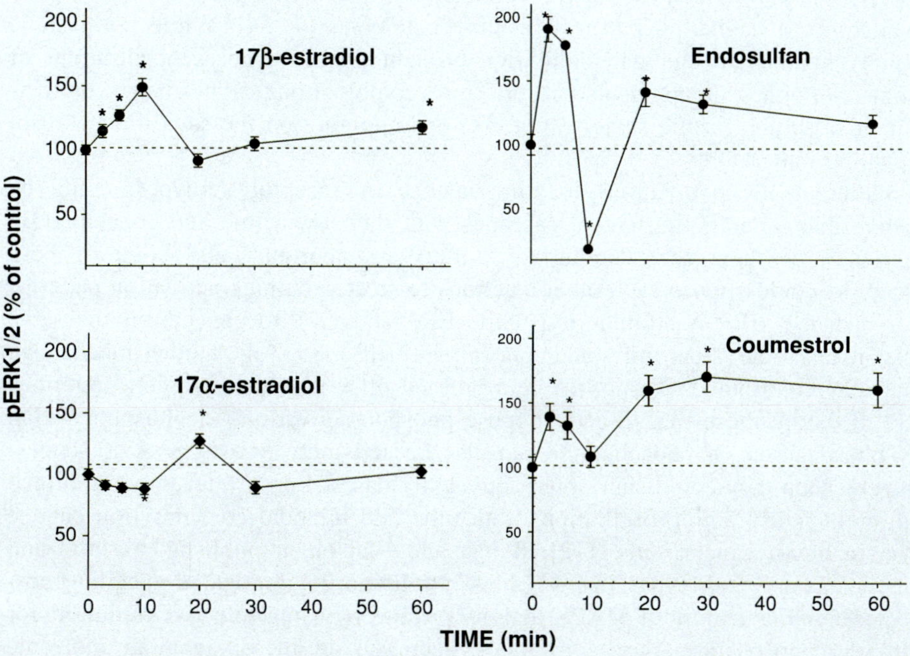

Fig. 1 Different estrogens activate/deactivate ERK with different time-phasing characteristics and efficacies in MCF-7 breast cancer cells. Cells that had been selected for high expression levels of mERα were plated at 4,000 cells/well, withdrawn from serum hormones (2–3 days) in medium containing 1% 4x charcoal-stripped serum, and then treated with hormones and xenoestrogens in the same medium. Estrogens were administerd at the following dose optima for these responses: 17β-estradiol at 1 pM, endosulfan at 1 pM, 17α-estradiol at 10 nM, and coumestrol at 1 nM. All the experiments were repeated at least three times with 24 replicates/experiment; the averaged values ± SE are presented; asterisks indicate significant differences ($p < 0.05$) from vehicle controls. The left panels for α and ß estradiol are reproduced [12] with permission, and the detailed methods for these measurements are described in the cited work

4 Hormesis-Nonmonotonic Responses

Estrogens are both useful and dangerous. With too little estrogenic activity, a species cannot reproduce. However, too much estrogenic activity, or imperfect mimicry of estrogenic activity (as is possible with xenoestrogens) can cause some responsive organs to malfunction or develop cancers. Therefore, estrogens must be very tightly regulated, and multiple cellular mechanisms may have evolved to ensure prevention of overstimulation and its harmful consequences. Hormesis is defined as a hormonal response in which a response plateau is not reached and sustained, but instead the response declines at higher concentrations [31]. In some cases responses can also be inhibited at intermediate doses when a wide range of doses is tested [32]. Estrogens activate a myriad of signaling cascades collectively in many tissues, but also initiate multiple signals in the same individual tissues/cell types [33]. The pathways used are dictated by which ERs are engaged and the availability of signaling partners in those cell types [4, 34]. While hormesis is usually invoked to elucidate inhibition brought on by higher concentrations of single hormones, it could also result from combinations of hormones or their mimetics acting via the same receptor(s) or impinging on the same downstream signaling integrators.

Different ER populations, or the balance of receptor subtypes, could be responsible for initiating signal cascades with their own time and concentration optima, as we have seen comparing pituitary and neuronal cells. Some of these receptors could oppose each other's actions to create complex activation patterns. For instance, ERα is stimulatory, while ERβ and GPR30 can inhibit the same responses at equivalent times and concentrations [22, 35, 36]. Another mechanism that may contribute to responses being turned off at intermediate concentrations and times are those that directly oppose phospho-activation—dephosphorylation by phosphatases. If phosphatases can also be activated by estrogens or xenoestrogens, then they could shut down activated kinases shortly after they are turned on, perhaps explaining oscillations with time and bimodal concentration curves. We, in breast cancer cells ([12], Banga and Watson, unpublished results) and others in many cell types [37–41] have preliminarily implicated specific phosphatases in this feature of MAPK activity profiles by using selective inhibitors for different phosphatase classes to block decreases in these signaling molecule activations.

Non-monotonic MAPK responses may fluctuate up and down with increasing concentration for other reasons. In trying to understand the control mechanisms that shut down estrogenic responses at selective concentrations (and times), our own data suggested that many different parallel signaling pathways (probed with pathway-selective inhibitors at different times) feed into the estrogen-activated ERK response and travel at different speeds down their individual cascades [29]. These signaling streams, arriving either early or late—or being induced by low or high concentrations of estrogens or xenoestrogens—could sum to an oscillating pattern. Because there are quite a few different estrogens, their composite actions must be considered, and of course, more than two pathways can participate, resulting in an even more complex summation (oscillations or even in apparent sustained activations). Hormonal influences can also be "blended" or summed with actions caused by other important cellular regulators that also funnel upstream signals into downstream MAPK "nodes" (see Fig. 2).

Each activation or deactivation by upstream kinases and phosphatases ratchets the final level of MAPK phosphorylation up or down. The resultant activity level of the integrator MAPK then goes on to dispense decisions to downstream cellular machineries that coordinately manage major cellular fates, including: proliferation (or inappropriate proliferation/malignant transformation), migration, differentiation, or death.

Nonmonotonic dose curves are typically described as V-, U-, upside down U-, or J-shaped. Because we assess such wide ranges of concentrations in our relatively high throughput cultured cell-based assays, we think we see a more

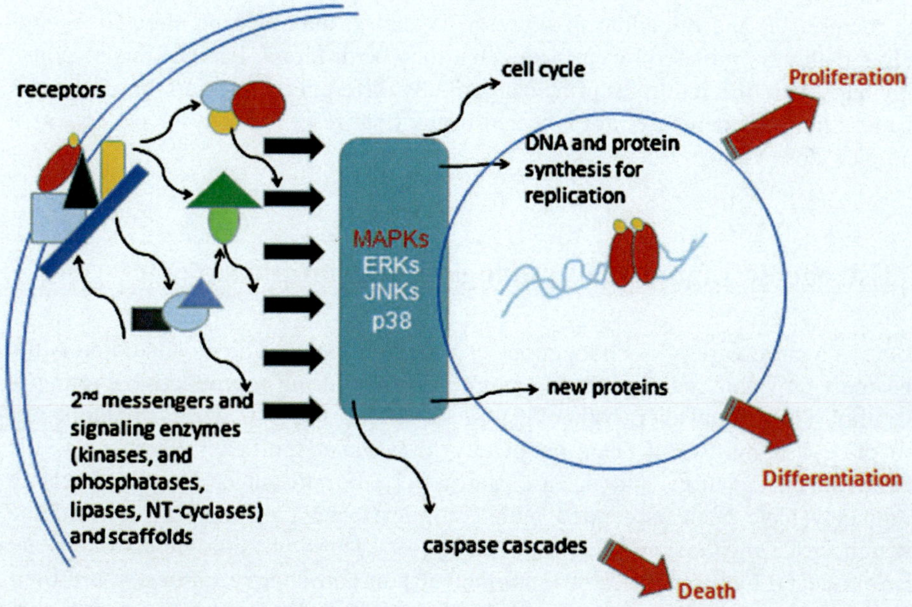

Fig. 2 Signaling leading to global functional responses in cells. Steroid receptors (yellow liganded red oval at the membrane) interact with a variety of signaling proteins (various colored shapes), generating messages, and altering enzyme activities. Many of these activities culminate in activation of MAPKs, which then can lead to cell proliferation (altering activation of cell cycle proteins and causing production of new DNA and proteins), differentiation (the production of new proteins for an altered function), or cell death (by initiating caspase cascades or other forms of active cell death mechanisms). MAPKs collect the upstream information by summing the level and type of activation, and then orchestrate downstream effects that become major cell outcomes

complete picture. We often see M-shaped curves [42] that we think consist of combinations of these other reported shapes. Most reported dose curves cover only a fraction of the range that our assays do, and would therefore represent only a portion of the M shape. We have produced many such non-classical concentration-response curves in our assessment of the ERK response in our selected MCF-7 breast cancer cells that robustly express mERα [12, 14], see Fig. 1. We have also seen this phenomenon in several responses of pituitary cells (PRL release, ERK activation, other MAPK activations) to a variety of estrogens [29, 32, 43], and in pheochromocytoma cells [22, 44] responding to a variety of estrogens via a combination of mERs (α, β, and GPR30).

We have examined several other factors that may contribute to our complex M-shaped dose response curves for a variety of responses. Because actions of estrogens at the membrane via mERs can simultaneously initiate a web of signaling cascades, the consideration of these multiple pathways adds complexity. An example is prolactin release from pituitary tumor cells [45], which really consists of several cellular responses that all contribute to the release of the peptide from the cell. Fusion of the secretory vesicle with the membrane is likely triggered by Ca^{++} increases [46]. However, the docking and travel of secretory vesicles to the membrane, and reloading of secretory vesicles, may also be affected by signaling pathways initiated by estrogens that may be different. Parts of this response may happen at different rates or be triggered by different concentrations. The sums of these multiple pathways are invested in the final response that we observe as a complex dose curve.

5 Estrogenic Ligands: Physiologic and Non-physiologic

There is a large variety of endogenous estrogenic ligands. The most studied is the one most prevalent and potent at genomic actions during reproductive cycling—estradiol (E_2). However, other estrogens ((E_1) highest at postmenopause; estriol (E_3), highest during late pregnancy) may have significant effects on tissue development, function, and disease states [47]. For instance, low E_3 levels in pregnancy have been associated with complications of eclampsia [48] and the incidence of Down's syndrome in offspring [49]. These physiologic estrogens are also produced by aromatases in a number of nonreproductive tissues where their effects may extend beyond reproductive functions [50]. One example is that E_3 has protective effects against the development of arthritis in certain experimental models [51], as has been known previously for E_2. Effects in brain, bone, cardiovascular system, and many other tissues may be affected differentially by all three of these endogenous estrogenic compounds during different life stages; therefore, loss or enhancement of these effects due to interference by xenoestrogenic compounds could affect human health in a large number of tissues. We found that these estrogens all act potently via nongenomic signaling pathways [30]. The prominent presence of these different physiologic estrogens during different life stages suggests that disruption of their actions might cause disease processes for women that are life stage-specific.

We are facing ever-increasing incidences of chronic diseases that cannot be explained by other factors, and are probably influenced by our environment and the chemicals to which we are exposed. Some diseases (e.g. infertility, diabetes, asthma, cancer) are likely to be influenced by actions of nonphysiological estrogens (xenoestrogens) acting as endocrine disruptors by imperfectly mimicking physiologic estrogens [52–56]. Bisphenol A (BPA) levels now can be correlated directly to different measures of sperm dysfunction (levels, motility, morphology) [57], and the National Health and Nutrition Examination Survey (NHANES) database records that 93% of Americans have levels of detectable urinary BPA [58]. These are levels that if reflective of active unconjugated levels, are comparable to those which can affect various physiologic systems. Many new compounds are being adopted for various industrial and consumer uses [59] and soon it will become very difficult to keep up with the potential health threats posed if we do not begin to decode the chemical structural features of estrogens that contribute to these actions.

We must also devise efficient ways to determine how they act on signaling systems as mixtures, where there is a potential for additive or even synergistic impacts [60].

We recently determined that several classes of xenoestrogens were also rapid and potent activators of membrane-initiated signaling mechanisms and resulting functional responses [61–63] in pituitary tumor cells, (reviewed in [64]). We ranked these compounds according to chemical characteristics (lipophillicity/carbon chain length, substitution of a phenol group), which in some cases could be correlated with their response levels (e.g. PRL release, Ca^{++} oscillation frequency, or MAP kinase activity) [61, 64]. We demonstrated correlations (either positive or negative) depending upon the type of signaling involved [64]. The story is still unfolding about how xenoestrogens signal differently via the web of available signaling pathways to eventually affect diverse functions. We will have to survey a variety of estrogens and endpoints to begin to assemble a complete picture of how estrogens use these mechanisms to either promote normal functioning (therapeutic) or disrupt normal signals and their downstream functions.

6 Responses to Ligand Mixtures

Nonphysiologic xenoestrogens contaminate humans and animals on top of an already endogenous level of estrogens. Xenoestrogens themselves also contaminate our environment in complex mixtures because of their various uses, so we must begin to understand how all these compounds, endogenous and exogenous, act simultaneously in mixtures to alter endocrine functions and cell behavior in both normal and cancer cells. Sensitive, quantitative, and relatively high throughput assays are needed to study xenoestrogen mixture effects, because there are so many potential physiologic and nonphysiologic estrogen combinations. Different combinations may interact differently, and could be more threatening to specific life stages (e.g. pregnancy, development). Their often nonmonotonic dose-response characteristics make it necessary to study wide ranges of concentrations (instead of single or limited doses with extrapolations) to compare different estrogens to each other.

We recently challenged pituitary cells [35, 65] and pheochromocytoma cells [44] responding to individual physiologic estrogens with xenoestrogens. We found overall that these compounds, as expected, showed striking non-monotonic dose relationships. Interestingly, the more potent a xenoestrogen is in eliciting a response, the better its ability to disrupt responses induced by endogenous estrogens. We saw this effect on both signaling responses and for functional endpoints [23, 66]. Xenoestrogens also caused re-phasing of the ERK activations elicited by physiological estrogens, which is likely to disrupt the kinetics of normal signaling cascades. One can see that xenoestrogens could have this effect from the phasing differences shown in Fig. 1. Combinations of physiologic estrogens with xenoestrogens cause even more pronounced phasing disruptions. Because all three physiologic estrogens that we have studied can be disrupted by the actions of xenoestrogens, it is likely that these contaminants differentially affect estrogenic functioning at different life stages (such as pregnancy, fertility, development, and aging).

7 Developmental and Immune System Effects, Affecting Cancer

Endogenous production of estrogens generally rises throughout development until sexual maturity, and the type of estrogen or its metabolites change even after maturity. Therefore, estrogens as important mediators of developmental change are also affected by the actions of xenoestrogens. Disruptions of developmental processes can impact a variety of tissue and organ systems, and can have a significant impact on both childhood and subsequent adult diseases.

Our studies of the immune system illustrate how developmental effects of xenoestrogens might influence associated disease risks later in life. Allergic airway diseases are more common in females than in males during early adulthood. Therefore, we examined the effects of estrogens and xenoestrogen pollutants on mast cell/basophil cell lines and on primary bone marrow-derived mast cells, all of which naturally express ERα, but not ERβ. Both physiological concentrations of E_2, and xenoestrogens at low concentrations, caused the release of allergic mediators (β-hexosaminidase, leukotrienes) except in cells derived from ERα knockout mice. These responses were at least partially mediated by estrogen-induced uptake of extracellular Ca^{++} [67, 68]. The rapidity of these responses suggests that they are mediated through nongenomic mechanisms. These studies were extended to an animal model of childhood asthma. When mouse pups were exposed to the xenoestrogen BPA transferred from their dams, they developed allergic asthma, as manifested by increased production of IgE antibodies to mildly sensitizing immunization, and airway inflammation and hyper-responsiveness [52]. This example of xenoestrogen exposure during a critical period of development strongly suggests that cells of the developing immune system can respond to xenoestrogens with disease-promoting consequences. Other cells of the immune system express ERs [69], and are also likely to be affected. If those cells are ones involved in resisting the development and expansion of cancer cells, then there are likely to be consequences for this disease also, and for many different tissues.

8 Summary

Our studies are contributing to the understanding of the endocrine basis of xenoestrogen disruptions that lead to diseases or disease predispositions in humans and animals. By understanding how specific small lipophilic molecules imperfectly mimic physiologic estrogens in cellular signaling pathways, we are helping to establish criteria to justify restrictions of their levels or the elimination of such compounds in manufacturing and consumer products. By studying the chemical structures of xenoestrogens that cause disruptions, we also hope to predict which substitute compounds would avoid such health risks, hopefully preventing more harmful compounds from being incorporated into product development and manufacturing processes. Prevention of toxin-based disasters, would not only benefit health, but also generate large cost savings to consumer industries that must retool with acceptable substitutes, and eliminate the need to judge and compensate for exposures to dangerous precursors, products, or byproduct metabolites of xenoestrogens.

Acknowledgments We acknowledge the following funding sources over the last decade for support of our work discussed here: DOD Breast Cancer Initiative (DAMD17-01-1-0418); NIH (ES010987, ES015292, ES006676); American Institute for Cancer Research (06A126); NIH training grants (T32 ES07254, T32 DA07287); the UTMB Center for Addiction Research; the UTMB Sealy Memorial Endowment Fund; and the UTMB Clinical and Translational Science Award UL1RR029876.Permissions to use previously published materials: We have used two figure panels from previously published work [12] and we authorize its use here according to the rules set forth by BioMed Central on its Web Site. BMC articles are licensed by their respective authors for use and distribution subject to citation of the original source in accordance with the Open Access license.

References

1. Pietras RJ, Szego CM (1977) Specific binding sites for oestrogen at the outer surfaces of isolated endometrial cells. Nature 265:69–72
2. Castoria G, Migliaccio A, D'Amato L, Di SR, Ciociola A, Lombardi M, Bilancio A, Di Domenico M, de Falco A, Auricchio F (2008) Integrating signals between cAMP and MAPK pathways in breast cancer. Front Biosci 13:1318–1327
3. Watson CS (2003) The identities of membrane steroid receptors…and other proteins mediating nongenomic steroid action. Kluwer Academic Publishers, Boston
4. Watson CS, Gametchu B (2003) Proteins of multiple classes participate in nongenomic steroid actions. Exp Biol Med 228:1272–1281
5. Thomas P, Alyea R, Pang Y, Peyton C, Dong J, Berg AH (2010) Conserved estrogen binding and signaling functions of the G protein-coupled estrogen receptor 1 (GPER) in mammals and fish. Steroids 75:595–602
6. Kang L, Zhang X, Xie Y, Tu Y, Wang D, Liu Z, Wang ZY (2010) Involvement of estrogen receptor variant ER-α36, not GPR30, in nongenomic estrogen signaling. Mol Endocrinol 24:709–721
7. Filardo EJ, Quinn JA, Frackelton AR, Bland KI (2002) Estrogen action via the G protein-coupled receptor, GPR30: stimulation of adenylyl cyclase and cAMP-mediated attenuation of the epidermal growth factor receptor-to-MAPK signaling axis. Mol Endocrinol 16:70–84
8. Revankar CM, Cimino DF, Sklar LA, Arterburn JB, Prossnitz ER (2005) A transmembrane intracellular estrogen receptor mediates rapid cell signaling. Science 307:1625–1630
9. Giraldi T, Giovannelli P, Di Donato M, Castoria G, Migliaccio A, Auricchio F (2010) Steroid signaling activation and intracellular localization of sex steroid receptors. J Cell Commun Signal 4:161–172
10. Chambliss KL, Shaul PW (2002) Rapid activation of endothelial NO synthase by estrogen: evidence for a steroid receptor fast-action complex (SRFC) in caveolae. Steroids 67:413–419

11. Razandi M, Oh P, Pedram A, Schnitzer J, Levin ER (2002) ERs associate with and regulate the production of caveolin: implications for signaling and cellular actions. Mol Endocrinol 16:100–115
12. Zivadinovic D, Watson CS (2005) Membrane estrogen receptor-alpha levels predict estrogen-induced ERK1/2 activation in MCF-7 cells. Breast Cancer Res 7:R130–R144
13. Pedram A, Razandi M, Sainson RC, Kim JK, Hughes CC, Levin ER (2007) A conserved mechanism for steroid receptor translocation to the plasma membrane. J Biol Chem 282:22278–22288
14. Zivadinovic D, Gametchu B, Watson CS (2005) Membrane estrogen receptor-α levels in MCF-7 breast cancer cells predict cAMP and proliferation responses PMCID:15642158. Breast Cancer Res 7:R101–R112
15. Kushner PJ, Hort E, Shine J, Baxter JD, Greene GL (1990) Construction of cell lines that express high levels of the human estrogen receptor and are killed by estrogens. Mol Endocrinol 4:1465–1473
16. Maximov PY, Lewis-Wambi JS, Jordan VC (2009) The paradox of oestradiol-induced breast cancer cell growth and apoptosis. Curr Signal Transduct Ther 4:88–102
17. Razandi M, Pedram A, Greene GL, Levin ER (1999) Cell membrane and nuclear estrogen receptors (ERs) originate from a single transcript: Studies of ERα and ERβ expressed in chinese hamster ovary cells. Mol Endocrinol 13:307–319
18. Song RX, Santen RJ, Kumar R, Adam L, Jeng MH, Masamura S, Yue W (2002) Adaptive mechanisms induced by long-term estrogen deprivation in breast cancer cells. Mol Cell Endocrinol 193:29–42
19. Jeng YJ, Watson CS (2009) Proliferative and anti-proliferative effects of dietary levels of phytoestrogens in rat pituitary GH3/B6/F10 cells—the involvement of rapidly activated kinases and caspases. BMC Cancer 9:334
20. Carter AC, Sedransk N, Kelley RM, Ansfield FJ, Ravdin RG, Talley RW, Potter NR (1977) Diethylstilbestrol: recommended dosages for different categories of breast cancer patients. Report of the cooperative breast cancer group. JAMA 237:2079–2085
21. Ariazi EA, Brailoiu E, Yerrum S, Shupp HA, Slifker MJ, Cunliffe HE, Black MA, Donato AL, Arterburn JB, Oprea TI, Prossnitz ER, Dun NJ, Jordan VC (2010) The G protein-coupled receptor GPR30 inhibits proliferation of estrogen receptor-positive breast cancer cells. Cancer Res 70:1184–1194
22. Alyea RA, Laurence SE, Kim SH, Katzenellenbogen BS, Katzenellenbogen JA, Watson CS (2008) The roles of membrane estrogen receptor subtypes in modulating dopamine transporters in PC-12 cells. J Neurochem 106:1525–1533
23. Jeng YJ, Watson CS (2011) Combinations of physiologic estrogens with xenoestrogens alter ERK phosphorylation profiles in rat pituitary cells. Environ Health Perspect 119:104–112
24. Hall JM, McDonnell DP (1999) The estrogen receptor β-isoform (ERβ) of the human estrogen receptor modulates ERα transcriptional activity and is a key regulator of the cellular response to estrogens and antiestrogens. Endocr 140:5566–5578
25. Paech K, Webb P, Kuiper GGJM, Nilsson S, Gustafsson J-Å, Kushner PJ, Scanlan TS (1997) Differential ligand activation of estrogen receptors ERa and ERb at AP1 sites. Science 227:1508–1510
26. Kuiper GG, Enmark E, Pelto-Huikko M, Nilsson S, Gustafsson J-Å (1996) Cloning of a novel estrogen receptor expressed in rat prostate and ovary. Proc Natl Acad Sci USA 93:5925–5930
27. Hewitt SC, Deroo BJ, Korach KS (2005) Signal transduction. A new mediator for an old hormone? Science 307:1572–1573
28. Morissette M, Le SM, D'Astous M, Jourdain S, Al SS, Morin N, Estrada-Camarena E, Mendez P, Garcia-Segura LM, Di PT (2008) Contribution of estrogen receptors alpha and beta to the effects of estradiol in the brain. J Steroid Biochem Mol Biol 108:327–338
29. Bulayeva NN, Watson CS (2004) Xenoestrogen-induced ERK-1 and ERK-2 activation via multiple membrane-initiated signaling pathways. Environ Health Perspect 112:1481–1487
30. Watson CS, Jeng YJ, Kochukov MY (2008) Nongenomic actions of estradiol compared with estrone and estriol in pituitary tumor cell signaling and proliferation. FASEB J 22:3328–3336

31. Calabrese EJ (2010) Hormesis is central to toxicology, pharmacology and risk assessment. Hum Exp Toxicol 29:249–261
32. Watson CS, Norfleet AM, Pappas TC, Gametchu B (1999) Rapid actions of estrogens in GH3/B6 pituitary tumor cells via a plasma membrane version of estrogen receptor-alpha. Steroids 64:5–13
33. Watson CS, Gametchu B (1999) Membrane-initiated steroid actions and the proteins that mediate them. Proc Soc Exp Biol Med 220:9–19
34. Belcheva MM, Coscia CJ (2002) Diversity of G protein-coupled receptor signaling pathways to ERK/MAP kinase. Neurosignals 11:34–44
35. Jeng YJ, Watson CS (2010) Combinations of physiologic estrogens with xenoestrogensxenoestrogens alter ERK phosphorylation profiles in rat pituitary cells. Environ Health Perspect. doi:10.1289/ehp.1002512
36. Jeng YJ, Watson CS (2011) Combinations of physiologic estrogens with xenoestrogens alter ERK phosphorylation profiles in rat pituitary cells. Environ Health Perspect 119:104–112
37. Bermudez O, Marchetti S, Pages G, Gimond C (2008) Post-translational regulation of the ERK phosphatase DUSP6/MKP3 by the mTOR pathway. Oncogene 27:3685–3691
38. Boutros T, Chevet E, Metrakos P (2008) Mitogen-activated protein (MAP) kinase/MAP kinase phosphatase regulation: roles in cell growth, death, and cancer. Pharmacol Rev 60:261–310
39. Hayashi Y, Sanada K, Fukada Y (2001) Circadian and photic regulation of MAP kinase by Ras- and protein phosphatase-dependent pathways in the chick pineal gland. FEBS Lett 491:71–75
40. Wang Z, Zhang B, Wang M, Carr BI (2005) Cdc25A and ERK interaction: EGFR-independent ERK activation by a protein phosphatase Cdc25A inhibitor, compound 5. J Cell Physiol 204:437–444
41. Yu LG, Packman LC, Weldon M, Hamlett J, Rhodes JM (2004) Protein phosphatase 2A, a negative regulator of the ERK signaling pathway, is activated by tyrosine phosphorylation of putative HLA class II-associated protein I (PHAPI)/pp32 in response to the antiproliferative lectin, jacalin. J Biol Chem 279:41377–41383
42. Watson CS, Norfleet AM, Pappas TC, Gametchu B (1999) Rapid actions of estrogens in GH_3/B6 pituitiary tumor cells via a plasma membrane version of estrogen receptor-aplha. Steroids 64:5–13
43. Jeng YJ, Kochukov MY, Watson CS (2009) Membrane estrogen receptor-alpha-mediated nongenomic actions of phytoestrogens in GH3/B6/F10 pituitary tumor cells. J Mol Signal 4:2
44. Alyea RA, Watson CS (2009) Differential regulation of dopamine transporter function and location by low concentrations of environmental estrogens and 17β-estradiol. Environ Health Perspect 117:778–783
45. Bulayeva NN, Wozniak A, Lash LL, Watson CS (2005) Mechanisms of membrane estrogen receptor-{alpha}-mediated rapid stimulation of Ca2+ levels and prolactin release in a pituitary cell line. Am J Physiol Endocrinol Metab 288:E388–E397
46. Burgoyne RD, Morgan A (2003) Secretory granule exocytosis. Physiol Rev 83:581–632
47. Greenspan FS, Gardner DG (2004) Basic and clinical endocrinology, 7th edn. Lange Medical Books, McGraw Hill, New York
48. Shenhav S, Gemer O, Volodarsky M, Zohav E, Segal S (2003) Midtrimester triple test levels in women with severe preeclampsia and HELLP syndrome. Acta Obstet Gynecol Scand 82:912–915
49. Chard T, Macintosh MC (1995) Screening for down's syndrome. J Perinat Med 23:421–436
50. Meinhardt U, Mullis PE (2002) The essential role of the aromatase/p450arom. Semin Reprod Med 20:277–284
51. Jansson L, Holmdahl R (2001) Enhancement of collagen-induced arthritis in female mice by estrogen receptor blockage. Arthritis Rheum 44:2168–2175
52. Midoro-Horiuti T, Tiwari R, Watson CS, Goldblum RM (2010) Maternal bisphenol a exposure promotes the development of experimental asthma in mouse pups. Environ Health Perspect 118:273–277

53. Nadal A, Alonso-Magdalena P, Soriano S, Quesada I, Ropero AB (2009) The pancreatic beta-cell as a target of estrogens and xenoestrogens: implications for blood glucose homeostasis and diabetes. Mol Cell Endocrinol 304:63–68
54. Soto AM, Vandenberg LN, Maffini MV, Sonnenschein C (2008) Does breast cancer start in the womb? Basic Clin Pharmacol Toxicol 102:125–133
55. Talsness CE, Andrade AJ, Kuriyama SN, Taylor JA, vom Saal FS (2009) Components of plastic: experimental studies in animals and relevance for human health. Philos Trans R Soc Lond B Biol Sci 364:2079–2096
56. Vandenberg LN, Maffini MV, Sonnenschein C, Rubin BS, Soto AM (2009) Bisphenol-A and the great divide: a review of controversies in the field of endocrine disruption. Endocr Rev 30:75–95
57. Li DK, Zhou Z, Miao M, He Y, Wang J, Ferber J, Herrinton LJ, Gao E, Yuan W (2011) Urine bisphenol-A (BPA) level in relation to semen quality. Fertil Steril 95:625–630
58. Stahlhut RW, Welshons WV, Swan SH (2009) Bisphenol A data in NHANES suggest longer than expected half-life, substantial nonfood exposure, or both. Environ Health Perspect 117:784–789
59. Thompson RC, Moore CJ, vom Saal FS, Swan SH (2009) Plastics, the environment and human health: current consensus and future trends. Philos Trans R Soc Lond B Biol Sci 364:2153–2166
60. Kortenkamp A (2008) Low dose mixture effects of endocrine disrupters: implications for risk assessment and epidemiology. Int J Androl 31:233–240
61. Kochukov MY, Jeng Y-J, Watson CS (2009) Alkylphenol xenoestrogens with varying carbon chain lengths differentially and potently activate signaling and functional responses in GH_3/B_6/F10 somatomammotropes. Env Health Perspect 117:723–730
62. Watson CS, Alyea RA, Jeng YJ, Kochukov MY (2007) Nongenomic actions of low concentration estrogens and xenoestrogens on multiple tissues PMCID:17601655. Mol Cell Endocrinol 274:1–7
63. Watson CS, Bulayeva NN, Wozniak AL, Alyea RA (2007) Xenoestrogens are potent activators of nongenomic estrogenic responses. Steroids 72:124–134
64. Watson CS, Jeng YJ, Kochukov MY (2010) Nongenomic signaling pathways of estrogen toxicity. Toxicol Sci 115:1–11
65. Jeng YJ, Kochukov MY, Watson CS (2010) Combinations of physiologic estrogens with xenoestrogens alter calcium and kinase responses, prolactin release, and membrane estrogen receptor trafficking in rat pituitary cells. BMC Environ Health 9:61
66. Jeng YJ, Kochukov M, Watson CS (2010) Combinations of physiologic estrogens with xenoestrogens alter calcium and kinase responses, prolactin release, and membrane estrogen receptor trafficking in rat pituitary cells. Environ Health 9:61
67. Narita S, Goldblum RM, Watson CS, Brooks EG, Estes DM, Curran EM, Midoro-Horiuti T (2007) Environmental estrogens induce mast cell degranulation and enhance IgE-mediated release of allergic mediators. Environ Health Perspect 115:48–52
68. Zaitsu M, Narita S, Lambert KC, Grady JJ, Estes DM, Curran EM, Brooks EG, Watson CS, Goldblum RM, Midoro-Horiuti T (2007) Estradiol activates mast cellsmast cells via a non-genomic estrogen receptor-alpha and calcium influx PMCID:17084457. Mol Immunol 44:1987–1995
69. Cunningham M, Gilkeson G (2011) Estrogen receptors in immunity and autoimmunity. Clin Rev Allergy Immunol 40:66–73

Part II
Prostate Cancer

Differential Functions of Stromal and Epithelial Androgen Receptor in Prostate Cancer Before and After Castration Resistant Stage

S. Lee, K.-P. Lai, S. Yeh and C. Chang

Abstract Androgen receptor (AR) has been the center of prostate cancer (PCa) therapy for decades, so androgen deprivation therapy (ADT) to suppress androgens binding to AR has become the major therapeutic option. However, the ADT is initially effective on blocking tumor growth, but eventually fails, leading to a stage of castration resistant prostate cancer and more advanced metastatic stage. The failure might be due to the nonspecific targeting of androgen/AR signaling without considering the tumor stage or cell types comprising the tumor microenvironment. The recent accumulating evidences indicate that the AR role is different in early (positive role) and advanced metastatic stage of PCa (suppressive role). In addition, AR was shown to act as a tumor promoter in luminal epithelial and stromal cells, but as a suppressor in basal and stem/progenitor/intermediate cells. Therefore, targeting androgen/AR signaling can suppress one type of tumor at a specific stage, but may lead to undesired more aggressive tumors. Accordingly, a combined therapy targeting both tumor stages and different cell types in the tumor microenvironment should be considered. Recently, several promising anti-androgen and anti-AR drugs have been developed and their efficiency is being tested. So, the combination therapy strategy to target metastatic tumors and other types of cells together with the new drugs targeting androgen/AR signaling might overcome the current failure of the

S. Lee · K.-P. Lai· S. Yeh · C. Chang (✉)
Department of Urology and Pathology, George Whipple Laboratory for Cancer Research, University of Rochester, Rochester, NY, USA
e-mail: chang@urmc.rochester.edu

S. Lee
e-mail: Soook_lee@urmc.rochester.edu

K.-P. Lai
e-mail:Kuopao_lai@urmc.rochester.edu

S. Yeh
e-mail: Shuyuan_yeh@urmc.rochester.edu

G. Castoria and A. Migliaccio (eds.), *Advances in Rapid Sex-Steroid Action*,
DOI: 10.1007/978-1-4614-1764-4_9, © Springer Science+Business Media, LLC 2012

ADT method and bring in more efficient therapy to battle PCa. This chapter describes the AR role in different tumor stages and cell types, and discusses the better therapeutic approaches with more effective outcome.

Keywords Androgen receptor · Epithelium · Stroma · CRPC · Combination therapy

Contents

1 Introduction

The androgen receptor (AR) plays an important role in the development and progression of prostate cancer (PCa). Ever since the first observation by Huggins and Hodges [1] that PCa progression is influenced by androgen actions and the cloning of human AR by Chang et al. [2], extensive studies have been focused on revealing the mechanism of AR action and targeting androgen/AR signaling. Therefore, the androgen deprivation therapy (ADT) to suppress androgens binding to AR has become the major therapeutic option for advanced PCa [3]. The ADT is initially effective on blocking tumor growth, but eventually fails, leading to a stage of castration resistant PCa (CRPC).

Androgens function mainly through testosterone [4] and 5α-dihydrotestosterone (DHT), the more active androgen that is produced from testosterone by 5α-reductase reaction [5, 6]. In CRPC patients, the serum level of androgen drops to an almost undetectable level, but prostate tissue androgen level does not drop to that low a level. Mizokami et al. [7] showed that the adrenal androgen, androstenediol, level in PCa tissue after CRPC is 1–3 nM and this adrenal androgen can transactivate AR. Titus et al. [8, 9] also demonstrated similar testosterone and DHT levels in CRPC tissues. Androgens were also suggested to act as anti-apoptotic factors in PCa cells [10].

AR expresses persistently in most cells of the CRPC [11–14] and several mechanisms were suggested to be involved in the transactivation of AR at the CRPC stage. One of the mechanisms is the gene amplification and amino acid substitutions in the AR gene that are detected at a high frequency in recurrent tumors. These changes confer a growth advantage to the tumor cells due to hypersensitivity of AR at the low castrated level of androgens [8]. The altered AR ligand specificity toward antiandrogens, adrenal androgens, and non-androgen steroids could lead to an increased AR transactivity in CRPC [7]. Additional mechanisms involve activation of AR by peptide growth factors [15] or cytokines [16, 17] via other cellular pathways [18–21]. Some other molecules like cellular prostatic acid phosphatase [22] and prostate leucine zipper [23] were suggested to activate AR at even less than 0.1 nM androgen level. AR phosphorylation by src tyrosine kinase was reported to be increased in CRPC [24]. Mechanisms of cross-talk of signaling pathways with AR have been suggested [25, 26] and possible cross-talk with G protein coupled receptor has also been suggested [27]. In addition, in CRPC, spliced forms of AR lacking the ligand binding domain (LBD), (AR3, AR4, and AR5) were found [28]. Those shorter splicing forms are constitutively active at castrated condition and do not have androgen or anti-androgen effects on their transactivation [28, 29]. The expression of AR3 was found in tumor PCa tissues of malignant PCa patients, yet the amount is relatively low and the result from Watson et al. [29] suggested that the growth promoting activity of AR3 needs the full-length of AR.

In addition to the above mechanisms, AR transactivation could be modulated by various coregulators [30, 31]. After elucidation of the first AR co-activators, ARA70 [32, 33], many coregulators, either co-activators or co-repressors, have been reported to influence AR transcription [34–37]. The interplay between Her2/Neu, AR, and the AR coregulator was also demonstrated [38]. Those co-activators interact with AR, but generally do not bind to ARE or the genomic sequence DNA. The detailed mechanisms of some AR co-regulator actions have not been elucidated clearly, but most of them could be considered to remodel or affect the chromatin structure [39, 40].

The PCa cells are comprised of cytokeratin (CK) 8-positive luminal epithelial cells, and some CK5-positive intermediate and stem/progenitor (S/P) cells [41]. Recent reports suggest that the CK5-positive S/P or CK5-positive intermediate cells increase after castration/ADT [42, 43], and in PCa tissues of the castration resistant stage [44]. The AR role in these CK5-positive S/P or intermediate cells in PCa initiation and progression remains unknown.

The environment of PCa tumors contains other types of cells [45]. Besides malignant transformed cancer cells, tumors are surrounded by many non-malignant cell types including fibroblasts, endothelial cells, and infiltrating immune cells and these composite structures build the extracellular matrix (ECM). The ECM and the non-malignant stromal cells of the tumors are defined as the "tumor stroma" [46]. The effect of AR on the epithelia as related to PCa initiation and progression has been extensively studied in the last few decades, but relatively few studies have been done to elucidate the AR role in stroma. Since the importance of interactions of stromal cells and epithelial cells has been raised significantly, a clarification of the AR role in this interaction should be addressed.

Current therapies focus on targeting the proliferation-stimulating function of AR. ADT with either surgical or chemical castration usually results in a response, but after an average of 12–24 months [47], the tumors recur and no longer respond to ADT. Human clinical data suggest that ADT may be effective for PCa patients only in selective prostate tumor cells and within short time periods, beyond which tumors will progress into the castration resistant stage with more aggressive metastases. Moreover, several studies have indicated that androgen replacement (supplement) therapy (ART) of selected patients with CRPC led to improved quality of life without any adverse effect on their cancer progression for a considerable follow-up duration [48–50]. Some of the selected patients even displayed a decrease in their serum prostate specific antigen (PSA) levels after ART, indicating that there might be reduced cancer progression. These clinical studies also suggest that PCa patients have differential responses to androgen/AR signals. However, the reasons why there are differential responses to androgen/AR signals in different PCa patients remain unclear at present. This could be due to the differential AR roles in various cell types and tumor stages.

This chapter focuses on discussion of differential roles of AR in many types of cells that may contribute to PCa progression to androgen independence and distant metastases.

2 Epithelial AR Role in PCa

2.1 *Epithelial AR Role in In Vitro PCa Cell Line Studies (Growth vs. Invasion)*

For decades, human PCa cell lines have been used in in vitro tests to study the molecular nature of PCa, but it should be noted the AR role in proliferation and metastatic ability of these cell lines are distinctively different and thus it is questionable whether using a single PCa cell line in experimentation is sufficient to make a plausible conclusion.

The androgen-dependent (sensitive) LNCaP cells (CK5-negative, CK8/18-positive) [51] express a mutant AR (T877A) [52] and for cell proliferation they require androgen/AR signaling. With changes of the androgen/AR signal, LNCaP cells may behave differentially depending upon the cell culture condition or passage number. When AR level was knocked down by siRNA [53–55] or antisense oligonucleotides [56], apoptosis was induced and proliferation was suppressed. Similar AR knockdown effects on inhibition of tumor growth were also observed in xenograft mouse models [57]. Together, these results suggest that AR functions as a key survival factor for androgen sensitive LNCaP cells. However, when the androgen-independent sublines were developed from long-term androgen deprivation culture, the androgen/AR signaling does not function as a stimulator or survival factor and the higher androgen/AR signals might suppress cell proliferation [58–60]. Moreover, the responsiveness of the LNCaP cells to androgen/AR signaling might be different among cells from the same xenograft tissue [61]. Collectively, AR might function as a cell survival factor, stimulator, or suppressor in LNCaP cells depending on the culture condition, cell environment, or passage number.

Among PCa cell lines, PC3 cells are characterized as CK5- and CK8/18-positive [51], and are widely used as a CRPC cell line model for numerous studies. PC3 cells are androgen-insensitive and lack expression of AR protein [51]. In order to study the role of AR in CRPC, several laboratories generated AR expressing PC3 cells [62–66]. When functional human AR was expressed in PC3 cells, cell proliferation was either slightly promoted or repressed depending on different expression levels of the AR protein due to promoter differences. However, when AR expressing PC3 cells (PC3/AR+) were orthotopically injected into mice, they form smaller primary tumors as compared to parental PC3 cells [64]. It was also found that AR negatively regulates invasion and metastasis of PC3 cells. Niu et al. [67] injected PC3 vector control cells and PC3/AR+ cells into the tibia of athymic nude mice and detected that the tumors of PC3/AR+ cells were less aggressive and less invasive than the tumors of PC3/vector control cells. Similarly when these cells were injected into anterior prostates of nude mice, PC3/AR+ cells developed less metastatic lymph nodes than PC3/vector control cells. Together, the roles of AR in PC3 cells challenged the classical concept that the AR functions as a stimulator in prostate tumor growth and metastasis.

Another AR negative prostate cancer cell line, DU145, also belongs to the CK5- and CK8-positive basal intermediate type of PCa cells [31]. It was postulated that methylation of the AR promoter prevents the AR expression in DU145 cells [68]. The effect of AR on the growth of DU145 cells remains controversial [69, 70], and Nagakawa et al. [71] reported that the AR might negatively regulate the invasion capability of DU145 cells. Since PC3 and DU145 cells are basal intermediate-like tumor cells, the AR effect in these two cell lines might be different from other PCa cells (this will be further discussed in Sect. 2. 3).

CWR22rv1 cells (characterized as CK5-negative and CK8/18-positive) were derived from a recurrent tumor, following ADT of a CWR22 xenograft [72]. They express two forms of AR, intact and a cleaved form of AR, AR3 [28]. Although CWR22rv1 cells express a functional AR, these cells' survival is androgen-independent and their proliferation is slightly increased upon androgenic stimulation. Together, the proliferation of CWR22rv1 cells is slightly increased upon AR expression, but their metastatic ability was reduced with AR expression [67].

2.2 *Epithelial AR Role in PCa Mouse Model Studies (Initiation vs. Metastasis)*

In investigating AR role in epithelial cells specifically, genetically engineered cre-LoxP gene knockout is a timely strategy [73]. First, the mice lacking AR in prostate luminal epithelial cells were generated by mating floxAR mice with probasin-cre (prostate epithelial specific AR knockout mouse, pes-ARKO) [74]. The initial characterization has found that prostate luminal epithelial AR sustains the luminal cells to maintain infolding, promotes cell differentiation, but inhibits proliferation. A rescue experiment has been conducted by mating the pes-ARKO mice with the PB-ARt857a transgenic mice. The data clearly showed that the luminal epithelial AR cells are critical for those functions. The second cre-loxP ARKO mouse line was established by Kato et al. [75]. Furthermore, there is another ARKO mouse model developed by Walters et al. [76], but it was reported that the mice that were developed with exon 3 deleted AR genes continue to express AR protein with LBD.

The pes-ARKO mice were then crossed with transgenic adenocarcinoma (TRAMP) mice to generate pes-ARKO-TRAMP mouse model [67], which is a mouse PCa model lacking AR in epithelium and the tumor development and progression has been extensively studied. The pes-ARKO derivative of Pten mutant (Pb-Cre^{+}; Pten$^{L/L}$) has also been developed [77]. It was shown that the deletion of AR in the epithelium promotes the proliferation of these Pten-null cancer cells by activation of the Akt signal.

The pes-ARKO-TRAMP mice spontaneously develop tumors, and the knockout of epithelial AR is progressive (starts at 6 weeks). These mice develop larger primary tumors and die earlier than wild type (wt)-TRAMP littermate controls [67]. The prostate tumors of pes-ARKO mice showed that knocking out of epithelial AR might lead to decreased number of secretory luminal epithelial cells. These results suggested that epithelial AR might function as a survival factor in luminal epithelial cells.

The AR signals in prostate cancer epithelial cells also affect the invasiveness of PCa. In the pes-ARKO-TRAMP mice [67], the size of metastatic tumors in pelvic lymph nodes (PLN) was shown to be larger than those from wt control mice at 24 weeks of age. In addition, more PCa metastatic foci were observed within the livers of pes-ARKO-TRAMP mice than in wt type control mice. The data from pes-ARKO-TRAMP mice and its wt control mice suggest that the epithelial AR can suppress tumor growth and metastasis.

AR-negative PLN metastatic tumors, isolated from pes-ARKO-TRAMP mice, were more invasive than those from TRAMP mice. Restoration of AR expression in pes-ARKO-TRAMP primary cells by AR cDNA transfection could reduce their invasion to PLN in orthotopic mouse PCa model. Together, those data further support the notion that the epithelial AR functions as a suppressor of prostate tumor invasion and metastasis.

2.3 *AR Role in CK5-Positive vs. CK8-Positive PCa Cells*

It is generally agreed [41, 78, 79] that the S/P cells in PCa are CD133-positive, CK5-positive, and integrin-positive and could differentiate into transit amplifying cells/intermediate cells (p63-positive, integrin-positive, CD133-negative, CK5-positive, and CK8-positive) to final well differentiated epithelial luminal cells

(CD133-, CK5-negative, CK8-positive). Interestingly, a recent report indicated that the PCa S/P cells could also originate from luminal epithelial cells and then differentiate into epithelial basal cells [80].

After ADT/castration, CK5-positive cells increase. Immunostaining data of PCa patients at the hormone refractory stage revealed that CK5-positive cells increased from 29 to 75% [44]. The CK5-positive S/P cells were also shown increased after castration in mouse PCa model [81]. When the expressions of stem cell markers were examined in intact and castrated mice with LNCaP cells xenografts and in TRAMP mice, it was shown that stem cell marker stained cells increased significantly after castration compared to the intact mice [81], suggesting that CK5-positive S/P cells increase after castration. This increase was also shown in pes-ARKO-PTEN mice model [67]. The sca-1 positively stained cells were increased in these mice after castration [43]. Considering that metastatic tumors increased after patients received ADT [82], the increase in CK5-positive cells seemed to be correlated with higher metastatic potential of PCa cells.

Earlier report showed a significantly lower expression of AR in intermediate type tumors [83]. However, it is unclear whether the low level of AR is essential in maintaining and proliferation of these CK5-positive cells. Recently, Niu et al. [67] showed expansion of CK5-positive cells in pes-ARKO-TRAMP mice, implying that depletion of AR expression acts in favor of proliferation of CK5-positive cells. The suppressive role of AR in CK5-positive basal epithelial and intermediate cells was also reported in normal prostatic development [84].

3 Stromal AR Role in PCa

In normal human prostate, the stroma is constituted mainly of smooth muscle cells expressing AR-whereas in prostatic carcinoma, the tumor stroma is constituted mainly of fibroblastic and myofibroblastic cells [85], suggesting that cell-transition changes have occurred in both the stroma and the epithelia during tumorigenesis.

Cunha et al. [86] earlier showed that stroma cells can modulate the differentiation pattern of normal prostate epithelial cells and are critical for normal tissue development and disease processes, such as development of PCa. The recent result of Niu et al. [84] further indicate the importance of stromal-epithelial interaction in normal prostatic development. In addition to the normal developmental process, many studies indicate that stromal-epithelial interaction is also important in initiation and progression of PCa [87, 88].

AR expression is less prominent in stromal cells than in epithelial cells, but they are functional. When the immortalized stromal cell lines, WPMY-1 and PS-30, and primary stromal cells were tested for the effect of androgen on their growth, it was shown that they do not require androgen for their growth, but the growth of WPMY-1 cells was slightly increased with androgen [89]. This finding indicates that unlike epithelial cells, prostate stromal cells are relatively insensitive to androgen stimulation and deprivation.

3.1 Stromal AR Effect on Epithelial AR Activity

Cano et al. [88] showed reciprocal interaction of stromal and epithelial cells in regulating the AR activity by demonstrating that stromal cells enhanced the transcriptional activity of AR in prostate epithelial cells and in turn, epithelial cells enhanced the AR activity in the stromal cells. They also isolated stromal cells from benign prostate tissues and cancer associated prostate tissues and investigated the AR-mediated transcriptional activity. It was shown that cancer associated stromal cells exhibited lower AR transactivity compared to cells in benign tissues. They explained this by different recruitment patterns of AR coregulators in the transcriptional complex. This reduced AR transactivity in cancer associated stroma further reduced the transactivity of AR in epithelial cells. Therefore it was speculated that the stromal AR of benign tissue activates epithelial AR activity, but in cancer the stromal AR down-regulates epithelial AR activity and this could contribute to PCa cells having higher metastatic potential. The finding that stromal AR level was decreased in androgen-independent cancer [90] also supports this hypothesis. However, the exact correlation between AR transactivation and metastatic potential of PCa cells needs to be studied further.

3.2 Stromal AR Effect on Metastatic Potential of PCa

3.2.1 In Vitro Stromal-Epithelial Co-Culture System

In vitro co-culture system was used to study AR roles in stromal cells effects on PCa growth. Niu et al. [67] used the immortalized human prostate stromal cells, WPMY-1, as the stromal cell source. These cells express functional AR and secrete paracrine growth factors. When they tested the invasion of PC3 cells in the absence and presence of stromal WPMY-1 cells, it was found that the invasion potential of PC3 cells was enhanced when stromal cells were present [67]. The stromal AR can promote epithelial cell invasion through the secretion of various growth factors, chemokines, or cytokines. Tanner et al. [91] WPMY-1 cells with expression level similar to LNCaP cells and then used WPMY-1 conditioned medium to treat LNCaP cells. They found significant increase in LNCaP cell growth suggesting cross-talk between stromal-epithelial cells. They also categorized highly effected gene expressions in AR overexpressing WPMY-1 cells upon DHT treatment and found androgen/AR expression changes resulted in up-regulation of factors involved in their paracrine action.

Regarding the AR role in stromal cells effects on invasion of PCa cells, there are conflicting results. Niu et al. [67] found that stromal AR promoted invasion of PCa cells in their co-culture system of WPMY-1 and PC3 cells. When PC3 cells were co-cultured with WPMY-1 cells, the knockdown of AR in WPMY-1 cells resulted in less invasive potential of PC3 cells [67]. However, in contrast, Li et al. [90] revealed that two human stromal cell lines lacking AR increased the invasion ability of PC3 cells, which suggests negative regulation of stromal AR in mediating PCa growth and invasion. As Niu et al. [67] also reported that stromal AR plays a supportive role in PCa invasion in their orthotopic implantation experiment using WPMY-1 cells and PCa epithelial cells, it is favorably believed that the stromal AR plays a supportive role in cancer cell invasion.

Stromal cells are also reported to be involved in the regulation of epithelial cells morphology and integrity by sending paracrine signals to the epithelial cells [92]. Stromal cells can increase adhesion of epithelial cells [92], however, how AR in stromal cells is involved in this process is unknown.

3.2.2 In Vivo Cre-LoxP Stromal ARKO Mouse Model

In addition to in vitro studies, Niu et al. [67] also performed in vivo studies by co-inoculating PC3 with WPMY-1 cells orthotopically into nude mice after manipulation of AR expression in WPMY-1 cells. It was shown that PC3 cells produced smaller primary and PLN metastatic tumors when combined with WPMY-1-ARsi than with WPMY-1-v cells.

The inducible ARKO mice of TRAMP (ind-ARKO-TRAMP) [93] have been generated to assess the consequence of simultaneous knockdown of both the stromal and epithelial AR. The knockout of AR in ind-ARKO-TRAMP mice is mediated by Mx1-Cre, which is interferon inducible and can be activated by injection of polyinosinic-polycytidic acid to induce endogenous interferon and thus activate the Cre recombinase action in various tissues including prostate. In these ind-ARKO-TRAMP mice, 50% of AR knockout in stroma and 60% of ARKO in epithelium were observed compared to the control mice. Compared to pes-ARKO-TRAMP mice, these inducible mice showed smaller metastatic tumors indicating that the stromal AR may have more dominant functions during PCa progression.

In addition to PCa models, Yu et al. [94] developed the smooth muscle selective AR knockout (SM-ARKO) mouse model and tested for effects on epithelial cells proliferation, apoptosis, and differentiation. They found that the proliferation of epithelial was decreased, but had little effect on apoptosis and differentiation. The data were further supported by FSP-ARKO (another stromal fibroblast selective AR knockout mouse model) by the same group [95]. They also showed altered prostate epithelium development when AR was knocked out in stromal fibroblasts.

3.2.3 Stromal AR Role in BPH as Compared to PCa

When the expression levels of AR in normal, BPH, and PCa tissues were examined, it was found that the AR level was similar in normal and BPH, but higher in PCa tissues [96]. However, the nuclear location of AR was higher in BPH and PCa compared to the normal tissues [97] indicating a positive role of AR in progression

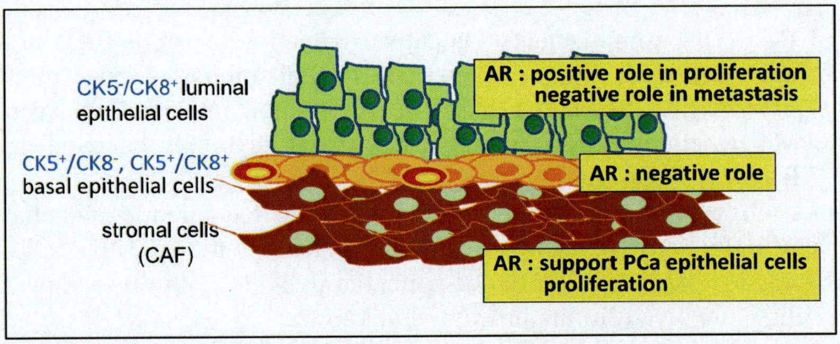

Fig. 1 In PCa, AR plays a positive role in proliferation of luminal epithelial cells. However, AR plays a negative role in growth of CK5-positive cells. The AR in stromal cells may promote PCa growth, but down-regulates AR signaling in epithelial cells, in turn, results in PCa cells with higher metastatic potential

of normal to BPH tissues, and further into PCa. There have been attempts to target androgen/AR signaling to treat BPH clinically. It was shown that the inhibitor of DHT synthesizing enzyme, 5α-reductase, retarded the progression of BPH and reduced the symptoms of BPH [98, 99].

3.2.4 Stromal AR Role Effects on S/P Cells

Liao et al. [100] isolated a stem cell population from the Pten deletion mouse tumors and investigated their spheroid forming efficiency in the co-culture system with cancer associated fibroblasts (CAFs) and found that the spheroid forming ability was enhanced when co-cultured with CAFs. When they further performed xenograft experiments, it was found that PCa stem cells resulted in more tumor-like histopathologies, which suggests a possible role of cancer associated stromal in initiation of stem originated tumors. However, the stromal AR role in this process remains unknown. On the other hand, Vander Griend et al. [101] suggested the possibility that cell-autonomous intracellular AR signaling drives the growth of human PCa initiating cells.

3.3 Stromal AR Role in Epithelial-Mesenchymal Transition (EMT)

Epithelial tumor cells lose cell polarity and cell-junction proteins (E-cadherin and β-catenin) and at the same time acquire protein mesenchymal cell markers such as N-cadherin and vimentin. During this process, the signaling associated with mesenchymal cells becomes activated, which facilitates epithelial cells migration and ultimately leads to metastases. EMT can be activated by soluble factors such as transforming growth factor β [102]. The involvement of androgen and AR in the EMT process has been studied by Zhu et al. [103], who found an inverse correlation between EMT and AR expression level, which is consistent with the earlier notion that AR down-regulation accelerates migration/invasion potential of epithelial cells [67]. Considering that mesenchymal cells possess stem cell characteristics and high metastatic potential, the observed suppressive role of AR in the EMT process is not surprising.

In summary, the AR role in proliferation of each cell type and how they affect each other's proliferation and invasion ability of PCa cells are described in Fig. 1.

4 Therapeutic Approaches Targeting Differential Roles of AR

Targeting the proliferation-stimulating role of AR has been at the center of PCa therapy, and the established and under-developed treatments for PCa focused on targeting androgen/AR. Those strategies include anti-androgen therapy, blocking of androgen production, inhibiting AR nuclear transport, and degradation of AR. The anti-androgen therapy includes the use of the AR antagonists, bicalutamide, flutamide, or nilutamide. These treatments showed reduction of symptoms and reduced serum PSA level, however, cannot completely regress and control PCa. The use of inhibitors of steroid synthesizing enzymes to block the synthesis of androgens in the adrenal gland and tumor tissues is relatively new. The enzymes that are involved in biosynthesis of steroids and use of drugs to block those steroid synthesis pathways are well discussed in the recent review paper by Massard and Fizazi [104]. For example, Abiraterone inhibits CYP17 (cytochrome P450-17) enzyme and is in the last stage of clinical trials. Several new compounds targeting AR were developed and are currently being evaluated. They are orteronel (TAK-700) and MDV3100. TAK-700 are a nonsteroidal inhibitor of 17, 20-lyse and the last stages of clinical trials are ongoing [105]. MDV3100 [106] is a novel AR antagonist that binds to the AR more avidly than bicalutamide and showed no agonist activity compared to bicalutamide. However, recent data presented in the 2011 SUO/SBUR spring Meeting raised the issue that this therapy reduces tumor volume, but might promote the PCa metastasis. These above discussed strategies focus on targeting the LBD of AR, however, an additional small molecule targeting AR amino-terminal domain (NTD) has been developed by Andersen et al. [107]. The advantage of using this drug is to avoid mutations in the LBD and expression of constitutively active AR splicing variants. Another promising drug is ASC-J9®, an AR degrading compound showing AR specificity and no toxicity [108–110]. Although it is not in prostate cancer related clinical trials yet, the long-term administration of ASC-J9® did not show adverse effects when tested in

TRAMP mouse PCa model (Li et al., manuscript in press). Also the long-term treatment of ASC-J9® will not affect the male mouse fertility [108].

The effectiveness of drug treatments mentioned above proves that targeting AR even in CRPC is working, however, so far, there is no successful case reported to stop both tumor growth and metastasis completely. This could be due to the differential AR roles in different tumor stages as we discussed in earlier sections. Even in the same mouse model the AR role was shown differentially in various cell types and different tumor stages. Therefore, it is essential to develop a combination treatment strategy to effectively target both stages of PCa.

4.1 Targeting Stromal/Luminal Epithelial AR with ASC-J9®

As previously mentioned (Sect. 2.3), the in vivo study with pes-ARKO-TRAMP mice found that the AR knockout in total epithelium led to the increase in CK5-positive cells and this increase, in turn, resulted in increased PCa metastasis. Therefore, Lai et al. (unpublished, manuscript submitted) used a strategy to degrade AR selectively in stromal and luminal epithelial cells only. This was possible by using ASC-J9® since this drug targets AR via interruption of AR and AR coregulators that are mainly expressed in PCa stromal and/or luminal epithelial cells. The in vivo study using different mouse models, such as $Pten^{+/-}$, TRAMP, and castrated nude mice xenografted with castration resistant LNCaP cells, showed that this drug effectively degrades AR in selective cells to suppress PCa progression at early androgen-dependent and later androgen-independent castration resistant stages. Mechanistic dissection showed that ASC-J9® could promote AR degradation via the proteasome degradation pathway to enhance the AR-Mdm2 complex, which resulted in AR becoming more vulnerable to be degraded by proteases. The consequences of such ASC-J9®-induced AR degradation might then lead to reductions of androgens binding to AR, AR N–C terminal interaction, and AR nuclear translocation that results in suppression of AR transactivation and AR-mediated PCa growth.

4.2 Combination Therapy of (1) Targeting Differential AR Roles in Different Tumor Stages and (2) Targeting Differential AR Roles in Various Cell Types

Earlier, Lin et al. [111] applied this concept using different passage numbers of LNCaP cells. As mentioned in Sect. 2.1, AR roles in LNCaP cells of earlier passage (promotive) and late passage (suppressive) are opposite and PI3K/Akt signaling was suggested to be critical in late passage LNCaP cells, therefore they targeted different signaling to block differential roles of AR in LNCaP cells of two types (early and late passage cells). This concept was further shown by Miyamoto et al. [112] suggesting a

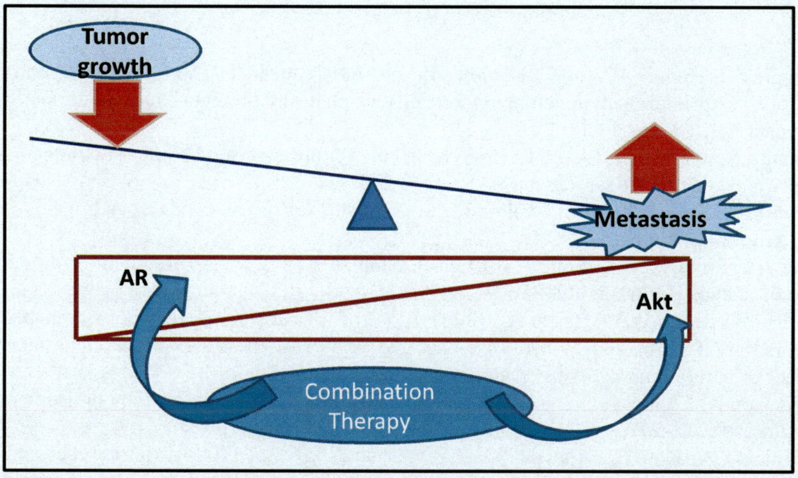

Fig. 2 A strategy of combination therapy targeting two stages, PCa tumor growth and metastasis. ADT either by anti-androgen or AR degrading therapy will down-regulate androgen/AR signaling, which, in turn, would result in PCa cells with higher metastatic potential. A combination therapy targeting AR signaling (by inhibiting AR role in initiation and early castration resistant stages) and targeting metastasis (by inhibiting AR role in the metastatic stage) is shown. This figure is modified from our previously published paper [111]

combination therapy of targeting Akt, cyclooxygenase-2, and matrix metalloproteinase-9 pathways together with classical ADT to battle PCa. Moreover, this concept is further supported by recent reports by Carver et al. [113] suggesting the reciprocal feed-back regulation of PI3K/Akt and AR signaling. They found that AR inhibition activates Akt signaling and PI3K/Akt inhibition, in turn, activates AR activation. Together, in order to target both the earlier and later metastatic stage of PCa, it seems essential to target both stages of PCa as illustrated in Fig. 2.

We also need to consider differential AR roles in various cell types comprising the TME. All studies involving AR role in epithelial, stromal, and CK5-positive cells mentioned above indicated differential AR roles in each cell type. For example, at early stages of PCa when tumors are dependent predominantly on luminal epithelial AR and stromal AR, ADT would result in regression of tumors, but ADT would affect the fate of other types of cells because of the suppressor function of AR on other types of CK5-positive cells such as S/P and intermediate cells, thereby would result in undesired expansion of more tumorigenic populations and eventual failure of ADT. The AR functions in other components comprising the PCa TME, such as infiltrating macrophages and endothelial cells, are not revealed yet, but their possible differential AR roles should also be considered in developing effective therapies to battle PCa.

Taken together, developing a strategy depending on one angle only will result in blocking of one direction of PCa, but would bring in undesirable outcomes, so it is essential to develop a strategy to target differential clinicopathological roles of AR in each tumor stage and each cell type in the TME to battle PCa efficiently.

References

1. Huggins C, Hodges CV (1972) Studies on prostatic cancer. I. The effect of castration, of estrogen and androgen injection on serum phosphatases in metastatic carcinoma of the prostate. CA Cancer J Clin 22:232–240
2. Chang CS, Kokontis J, Liao ST (1988) Molecular cloning of human and rat complementary DNA encoding androgen receptors. Science 240:324–326
3. Griffiths K, Denis LJ (2000) Exploitable mechanisms for the blockade of androgenic action. Prostate Suppl 10:43–51
4. Roy AK, Lavrovsky Y, Song CS, Chen S, Jung MH et al (1999) Regulation of androgen action. Vitam Horm 55:309–352
5. Shimazaki J, Kurihara H, Ito Y, Shida K (1965) Testosterone metabolism in prostate; formation of androstan-17-beta-ol-3-one and androst-4-ene-3, 17-dione, and inhibitory effect of natural and synthetic estrogens. Gunma J Med Sci 14:313–325
6. Anderson KM, Liao S (1968) Selective retention of dihydrotestosterone by prostatic nuclei. Nature 219:277–279
7. Mizokami A, Koh E, Fujita H, Maeda Y, Egawa M et al (2004) The adrenal androgen androstenediol is present in prostate cancer tissue after androgen deprivation therapy and activates mutated androgen receptor. Cancer Res 64:765–771
8. Titus MA, Schell MJ, Lih FB, Tomer KB, Mohler JL (2005) Testosterone and dihydrotestosterone tissue levels in recurrent prostate cancer. Clin Cancer Res 11: 4653–4657
9. Titus MA, Gregory CW, Ford OH 3rd, Schell MJ, Maygarden SJ et al (2005) Steroid 5alpha-reductase isozymes I and II in recurrent prostate cancer. Clin Cancer Res 11:4365–4371
10. Huang H, Muddiman DC, Tindall DJ (2004) Androgens negatively regulate forkhead transcription factor FKHR (FOXO1) through a proteolytic mechanism in prostate cancer cells. J Biol Chem 279:13866–13877
11. Sadi MV, Walsh PC, Barrack ER (1991) Immunohistochemical study of androgen receptors in metastatic prostate cancer. Comparison of receptor content and response to hormonal therapy. Cancer 67:3057–3064
12. Mohler JL, Chen Y, Hamil K, Hall SH, Cidlowski JA et al (1996) Androgen and glucocorticoid receptors in the stroma and epithelium of prostatic hyperplasia and carcinoma. Clin Cancer Res 2:889–895
13. Hobisch A, Culig Z, Radmayr C, Bartsch G, Klocker H et al (1996) Androgen receptor status of lymph node metastases from prostate cancer. Prostate 28:129–135
14. van der Kwast TH, Schalken J, Ruizeveld de Winter JA, van Vroonhoven CC, Mulder E et al (1991) Androgen receptors in endocrine-therapy-resistant human prostate cancer. Int J Cancer 48:189–193
15. Kung HJ, Evans CP (2009) Oncogenic activation of androgen receptor. Urol Oncol 27: 48–52
16. Lee SO, Chun JY, Nadiminty N, Lou W, Gao AC (2007) Interleukin-6 undergoes transition from growth inhibitor associated with neuroendocrine differentiation to stimulator accompanied by androgen receptor activation during LNCaP prostate cancer cell progression. Prostate 67:764–773
17. Lee SO, Lou W, Nadiminty N, Lin X, Gao AC (2005) Requirement for NF-(kappa)B in interleukin-4-induced androgen receptor activation in prostate cancer cells. Prostate 64: 160–167
18. Desai SJ, Ma AH, Tepper CG, Chen HW, Kung HJ (2006) Inappropriate activation of the androgen receptor by nonsteroids: involvement of the src kinase pathway and its therapeutic implications. Cancer Res 66:10449–10459
19. Ishiguro H, Akimoto K, Nagashima Y, Kojima Y, Sasaki T et al (2009) aPKClambda/iota promotes growth of prostate cancer cells in an autocrine manner through transcriptional activation of interleukin-6. Proc Natl Acad Sci U S A 106:16369–16374

20. Cabrespine A, Guy L, Chollet P, Debiton E, Bay JO (2004) Molecular mechanisms involved in hormone resistance of prostate cancer. Bull Cancer 91:747–757
21. Hammacher A, Thompson EW, Williams ED (2005) Interleukin-6 is a potent inducer of S100P, which is up-regulated in androgen-refractory and metastatic prostate cancer. Int J Biochem Cell Biol 37:442–450
22. Chuang TD, Chen SJ, Lin FF, Veeramani S, Kumar S et al (2010) Human prostatic acid phosphatase, an authentic tyrosine phosphatase, dephosphorylates ErbB-2 and regulates prostate cancer cell growth. J Biol Chem 285:23598–23606
23. Zhang D, He D, Xue Y, Wang R, Wu K et al (2011) PrLZ protects prostate cancer cells from apoptosis induced by androgen deprivation via the activation of Stat3/Bcl-2 pathway. Cancer Res 71:2193–2202
24. Guo Z, Dai B, Jiang T, Xu K, Xie Y et al (2006) Regulation of androgen receptor activity by tyrosine phosphorylation. Cancer Cell 10:309–319
25. El Sheikh SS, Domin J, Abel P, Stamp G, Lalani el N (2003) Androgen-independent prostate cancer: potential role of androgen and ErbB receptor signal transduction crosstalk. Neoplasia 5:99–109
26. Leotoing L, Manin M, Monte D, Baron S, Communal Y et al (2007) Crosstalk between androgen receptor and epidermal growth factor receptor-signalling pathways: a molecular switch for epithelial cell differentiation. J Mol Endocrinol 39:151–162
27. Montalvo L, Carmena MJ, Solano RM, Clemente C, Roman ID et al (2000) Effect of flutamide-induced androgen-receptor blockade on adenylate cyclase activation through G-protein coupled receptors in rat prostate. Cell Signal 12:311–316
28. Guo Z, Yang X, Sun F, Jiang R, Linn DE et al (2009) A novel androgen receptor splice variant is up-regulated during prostate cancer progression and promotes androgen depletion-resistant growth. Cancer Res 69:2305–2313
29. Watson PA, Chen YF, Balbas MD, Wongvipat J, Socci ND et al (2010) Constitutively active androgen receptor splice variants expressed in castration-resistant prostate cancer require full-length androgen receptor. Proc Natl Acad Sci U S A 107:16759–16765
30. Heinlein CA, Chang C (2002) Androgen receptor (AR) coregulators: an overview. Endocr Rev 23:175–200
31. Rahman M, Miyamoto H, Chang C (2004) Androgen receptor coregulators in prostate cancer: mechanisms and clinical implications. Clin Cancer Res 10:2208–2219
32. Yeh S, Chang C (1996) Cloning and characterization of a specific coactivator, ARA70, for the androgen receptor in human prostate cells. Proc Natl Acad Sci U S A 93:5517–5521
33. Yeh S, Miyamoto H, Chang C (1997) Hydroxyflutamide may not always be a pure antiandrogen. Lancet 349:852–853
34. Onate SA, Tsai SY, Tsai MJ, O'Malley BW (1995) Sequence and characterization of a coactivator for the steroid hormone receptor superfamily. Science 270:1354–1357
35. Voegel JJ, Heine MJ, Zechel C, Chambon P, Gronemeyer H (1996) TIF2, a 160 kDa transcriptional mediator for the ligand-dependent activation function AF-2 of nuclear receptors. EMBO J 15:3667–3675
36. Nagy L, Kao HY, Chakravarti D, Lin RJ, Hassig CA et al (1997) Nuclear receptor repression mediated by a complex containing SMRT, mSin3A, and histone deacetylase. Cell 89:373–380
37. Alland L, Muhle R, Hou H Jr, Potes J, Chin L et al (1997) Role for N-CoR and histone deacetylase in Sin3-mediated transcriptional repression. Nature 387:49–55
38. Yeh S, Lin HK, Kang HY, Thin TH, Lin MF et al (1999) From HER2/Neu signal cascade to androgen receptor and its coactivators: a novel pathway by induction of androgen target genes through MAP kinase in prostate cancer cells. Proc Natl Acad Sci U S A 96:5458–5463
39. Spencer TE, Jenster G, Burcin MM, Allis CD, Zhou J et al (1997) Steroid receptor coactivator-1 is a histone acetyltransferase. Nature 389:194–198
40. Fu M, Wang C, Reutens AT, Wang J, Angeletti RH et al (2000) p300 and p300/cAMP-response element-binding protein-associated factor acetylate the androgen receptor at sites governing hormone-dependent transactivation. J Biol Chem 275:20853–20860

41. Litvinov IV, De Marzo AM, Isaacs JT (2003) Is the Achilles' heel for prostate cancer therapy a gain of function in androgen receptor signaling? J Clin Endocrinol Metab 88: 2972–2982
42. Tang DG, Patrawala L, Calhoun T, Bhatia B, Choy G et al (2007) Prostate cancer stem/progenitor cells: identification, characterization, and implications. Mol Carcinog 46:1–14
43. Lawson DA, Zong Y, Memarzadeh S, Xin L, Huang J et al (2010) Basal epithelial stem cells are efficient targets for prostate cancer initiation. Proc Natl Acad Sci U S A 107:2610–2615
44. van Leenders GJ, Aalders TW, Hulsbergen-van de Kaa CA, Ruiter DJ, Schalken JA (2001) Expression of basal cell keratins in human prostate cancer metastases and cell lines. J Pathol 195:563–570
45. Patrawala L, Calhoun-Davis T, Schneider-Broussard R, Tang DG (2007) Hierarchical organization of prostate cancer cells in xenograft tumors: the CD44 + alpha2beta1 + cell population is enriched in tumor-initiating cells. Cancer Res 67:6796–6805
46. Sund M, Kalluri R (2009) Tumor stroma derived biomarkers in cancer. Cancer Metastasis Rev 28:177–183
47. DeVita VT Jr, Canellos GP (2011) Hematology in 2010: new therapies and standard of care in oncology. Nat Rev Clin Oncol 8:67–68
48. Mathew P (2008) Prolonged control of progressive castration-resistant metastatic prostate cancer with testosterone replacement therapy: the case for a prospective trial. Ann Oncol 19:395–396
49. Meacham RB (2003) Androgen replacement therapy: treatment advances and clinical implications. Rev Urol 5:245–247
50. Morris MJ, Huang D, Kelly WK, Slovin SF, Stephenson RD et al (2009) Phase 1 trial of high-dose exogenous testosterone in patients with castration-resistant metastatic prostate cancer. Eur Urol 56:237–244
51. van Bokhoven A, Varella-Garcia M, Korch C, Johannes WU, Smith EE et al (2003) Molecular characterization of human prostate carcinoma cell lines. Prostate 57:205–225
52. Veldscholte J, Ris-Stalpers C, Kuiper GG, Jenster G, Berrevoets C et al (1990) A mutation in the ligand binding domain of the androgen receptor of human LNCaP cells affects steroid binding characteristics and response to anti-androgens. Biochem Biophys Res Commun 173:534–540
53. Yang Q, Fung KM, Day WV, Kropp BP, Lin HK (2005) Androgen receptor signaling is required for androgen-sensitive human prostate cancer cell proliferation and survival. Cancer Cell Int 5:8
54. Compagno D, Merle C, Morin A, Gilbert C, Mathieu JR et al (2007) SIRNA-directed in vivo silencing of androgen receptor inhibits the growth of castration-resistant prostate carcinomas. PLoS One 2:e1006
55. Liao X, Tang S, Thrasher JB, Griebling TL, Li B (2005) Small-interfering RNA-induced androgen receptor silencing leads to apoptotic cell death in prostate cancer. Mol Cancer Ther 4:505–515
56. Eder IE, Culig Z, Ramoner R, Thurnher M, Putz T et al (2000) Inhibition of LncaP prostate cancer cells by means of androgen receptor antisense oligonucleotides. Cancer Gene Ther 7:997–1007
57. Eder IE, Hoffmann J, Rogatsch H, Schafer G, Zopf D et al (2002) Inhibition of LNCaP prostate tumor growth in vivo by an antisense oligonucleotide directed against the human androgen receptor. Cancer Gene Ther 9:117–125
58. Joly-Pharaboz MO, Soave MC, Nicolas B, Mebarki F, Renaud M et al (1995) Androgens inhibit the proliferation of a variant of the human prostate cancer cell line LNCaP. J Steroid Biochem Mol Biol 55:67–76
59. Kokontis JM, Hay N, Liao S (1998) Progression of LNCaP prostate tumor cells during androgen deprivation: hormone-independent growth, repression of proliferation by androgen, and role for p27Kip1 in androgen-induced cell cycle arrest. Mol Endocrinol 12:941–953

60. Joly-Pharaboz MO, Ruffion A, Roch A, Michel-Calemard L, Andre J et al (2000) Inhibition of growth and induction of apoptosis by androgens of a variant of LNCaP cell line. J Steroid Biochem Mol Biol 73:237–249
61. Soto AM, Lin TM, Sakabe K, Olea N, Damassa DA et al (1995) Variants of the human prostate LNCaP cell line as tools to study discrete components of the androgen-mediated proliferative response. Oncol Res 7:545–558
62. Litvinov IV, Antony L, Dalrymple SL, Becker R, Cheng L et al (2006) PC3, but not DU145, human prostate cancer cells retain the coregulators required for tumor suppressor ability of androgen receptor. Prostate 66:1329–1338
63. Yuan S, Trachtenberg J, Mills GB, Brown TJ, Xu F et al (1993) Androgen-induced inhibition of cell proliferation in an androgen-insensitive prostate cancer cell line (PC-3) transfected with a human androgen receptor complementary DNA. Cancer Res 53:1304–1311
64. Altuwaijri S, Wu CC, Niu YJ, Mizokami A, Chang HC et al (2007) Expression of human AR cDNA driven by its own promoter results in mild promotion, but not suppression, of growth in human prostate cancer PC-3 cells. Asian J Androl 9:181–188
65. Shen R, Sumitomo M, Dai J, Harris A, Kaminetzky D et al (2000) Androgen-induced growth inhibition of androgen receptor expressing androgen-independent prostate cancer cells is mediated by increased levels of neutral endopeptidase. Endocrinology 141: 1699–1704
66. Xu XF, Zhou SW, Zhang X, Ye ZQ, Zhang JH et al (2006) Prostate androgen-regulated gene: a novel potential target for androgen-independent prostate cancer therapy. Asian J Androl 8:455–462
67. Niu Y, Altuwaijri S, Lai KP, Wu CT, Ricke WA et al (2008) Androgen receptor is a tumor suppressor and proliferator in prostate cancer. Proc Natl Acad Sci U S A 105: 12182–12187
68. Chlenski A, Nakashiro K, Ketels KV, Korovaitseva GI, Oyasu R (2001) Androgen receptor expression in androgen-independent prostate cancer cell lines. Prostate 47:66–75
69. Litvinov IV, Vander Griend DJ, Antony L, Dalrymple S, De Marzo AM et al (2006) Androgen receptor as a licensing factor for DNA replication in androgen-sensitive prostate cancer cells. Proc Natl Acad Sci U S A 103:15085–15090
70. Scaccianoce E, Festuccia C, Dondi D, Guerini V, Bologna M et al (2003) Characterization of prostate cancer DU145 cells expressing the recombinant androgen receptor. Oncol Res 14:101–112
71. Nagakawa O, Akashi T, Hayakawa Y, Junicho A, Koizumi K et al (2004) Differential expression of integrin subunits in DU-145/AR prostate cancer cells. Oncol Rep 12:837–841
72. Sramkoski RM, Pretlow TG 2nd, Giaconia JM, Pretlow TP, Schwartz S et al (1999) A new human prostate carcinoma cell line, 22Rv1. In Vitro Cell Dev Biol Anim 35:403–409
73. Yeh S, Tsai MY, Xu Q, Mu XM, Lardy H et al (2002) Generation and characterization of androgen receptor knockout (ARKO) mice: an in vivo model for the study of androgen functions in selective tissues. Proc Natl Acad Sci U S A 99:13498–13503
74. Wu CT, Altuwaijri S, Ricke WA, Huang SP, Yeh S et al (2007) Increased prostate cell proliferation and loss of cell differentiation in mice lacking prostate epithelial androgen receptor. Proc Natl Acad Sci U S A 104:12679–12684
75. Matsumoto T, Takeyama K, Sato T, Kato S (2005) Study of androgen receptor functions by genetic models. J Biochem 138:105–110
76. Walters KA, Allan CM, Jimenez M, Lim PR, Davey RA et al (2007) Female mice haploinsufficient for an inactivated androgen receptor (AR) exhibit age-dependent defects that resemble the AR null phenotype of dysfunctional late follicle development, ovulation, and fertility. Endocrinology 148:3674–3684
77. Mulholland DJ, Tran LM, Li Y, Cai H, Morim A et al (2011) Cell autonomous role of PTEN in regulating castration-resistant prostate cancer growth. Cancer Cell 19:792–804
78. Verhagen AP, Ramaekers FC, Aalders TW, Schaafsma HE, Debruyne FM et al (1992) Colocalization of basal and luminal cell-type cytokeratins in human prostate cancer. Cancer Res 52:6182–6187

79. Collins AT, Habib FK, Maitland NJ, Neal DE (2001) Identification and isolation of human prostate epithelial stem cells based on alpha(2)beta(1)-integrin expression. J Cell Sci 114:3865–3872
80. Wang X, Kruithof-de Julio M, Economides KD, Walker D, Yu H et al (2009) A luminal epithelial stem cell that is a cell of origin for prostate cancer. Nature 461:495–500
81. Tang Y, Hamburger AW, Wang L, Khan MA, Hussain A (2009) Androgen deprivation and stem cell markers in prostate cancers. Int J Clin Exp Pathol 3:128–138
82. Kleeberger W, Bova GS, Nielsen ME, Herawi M, Chuang AY et al (2007) Roles for the stem cell associated intermediate filament nestin in prostate cancer migration and metastasis. Cancer Res 67:9199–9206
83. Yu DJ, Tang YQ, Shi YF, Wang YC, Zhuo J et al (2010) Proportion of intermediate epithelial cells and human prostate cancer. Zhonghua Nan Ke Xue 16:1063–1067
84. Niu Y, Wang J, Shang Z, Huang SP, Shyr CR et al (2011) Increased CK5/CK8-positive intermediate cells with stromal smooth muscle cell atrophy in the mice lacking prostate epithelial androgen receptor. PLoS One 6:e20202
85. Cunha GR, Hayward SW, Wang YZ, Ricke WA (2003) Role of the stromal microenvironment in carcinogenesis of the prostate. Int J Cancer 107:1–10
86. Cunha GR, Ricke W, Thomson A, Marker PC, Risbridger G et al (2004) Hormonal, cellular, and molecular regulation of normal and neoplastic prostatic development. J Steroid Biochem Mol Biol 92:221–236
87. Barclay WW, Woodruff RD, Hall MC, Cramer SD (2005) A system for studying epithelial-stromal interactions reveals distinct inductive abilities of stromal cells from benign prostatic hyperplasia and prostate cancer. Endocrinology 146:13–18
88. Cano P, Godoy A, Escamilla R, Dhir R, Onate SA (2007) Stromal-epithelial cell interactions and androgen receptor-coregulator recruitment is altered in the tissue microenvironment of prostate cancer. Cancer Res 67:511–519
89. Sun X, He H, Xie Z, Qian W, Zhau HE et al (2010) Matched pairs of human prostate stromal cells display differential tropic effects on LNCaP prostate cancer cells. In Vitro Cell Dev Biol Anim 46:538–546
90. Li Y, Li CX, Ye H, Chen F, Melamed J et al (2008) Decrease in stromal androgen receptor associates with androgen-independent disease and promotes prostate cancer cell proliferation and invasion. J Cell Mol Med 12:2790–2798
91. Tanner MJ, Welliver RC Jr, Chen M, Shtutman M, Godoy A et al (2011) Effects of androgen receptor and androgen on gene expression in prostate stromal fibroblasts and paracrine signaling to prostate cancer cells. PLoS One 6:e16027
92. Chambers KF, Pearson JF, Aziz N, O'Toole P, Garrod D et al (2011) Stroma regulates increased epithelial lateral cell adhesion in 3D culture: a role for actin/cadherin dynamics. PLoS One 6:e18796
93. Niu Y, Altuwaijri S, Yeh S, Lai KP, Yu S et al (2008) Targeting the stromal androgen receptor in primary prostate tumors at earlier stages. Proc Natl Acad Sci U S A 105: 12188–12193
94. Yu S, Zhang C, Lin CC, Niu Y, Lai KP et al (2011) Altered prostate epithelial development and IGF-1 signal in mice lacking the androgen receptor in stromal smooth muscle cells. Prostate 71:517–524
95. Yu S, Yeh CR, Niu Y, Chang HC, Tsai YC et al. (2011) Altered prostate epithelial development in mice lacking the androgen receptor in stromal fibroblasts. Prostate
96. Zeng R, Liu ZY, Sun YH, Xu CL, Gao X et al (2010) Expressions of the androgen receptor in normal prostate, benigh prostatic hyperplasia and prostate cancer. Zhonghua Nan Ke Xue 16:967–972
97. Salazar EL, Mercado E, Calzada L (2005) Prostatic cancer/benign prostatic hypertrophy. Subcellular distribution of estradiol/androgen receptors. Arch Androl 51:135–139
98. Andriole G, Bruchovsky N, Chung LW, Matsumoto AM, Rittmaster R et al (2004) Dihydrotestosterone and the prostate: the scientific rationale for 5alpha-reductase inhibitors in the treatment of benign prostatic hyperplasia. J Urol 172:1399–1403

99. Clark RV, Hermann DJ, Cunningham GR, Wilson TH, Morrill BB et al (2004) Marked suppression of dihydrotestosterone in men with benign prostatic hyperplasia by dutasteride, a dual 5alpha-reductase inhibitor. J Clin Endocrinol Metab 89:2179–2184
100. Liao CP, Adisetiyo H, Liang M, Roy-Burman P (2010) Cancer-associated fibroblasts enhance the gland-forming capability of prostate cancer stem cells. Cancer Res 70:7294–7303
101. Vander Griend DJ, D'Antonio J, Gurel B, Antony L, Demarzo AM et al (2010) Cell-autonomous intracellular androgen receptor signaling drives the growth of human prostate cancer initiating cells. Prostate 70:90–99
102. Odero-Marah VA, Wang R, Chu G, Zayzafoon M, Xu J et al (2008) Receptor activator of NF-kappaB ligand (RANKL) expression is associated with epithelial to mesenchymal transition in human prostate cancer cells. Cell Res 18:858–870
103. Zhu ML, Kyprianou N (2010) Role of androgens and the androgen receptor in epithelial-mesenchymal transition and invasion of prostate cancer cells. FASEB J 24:769–777
104. Massard C, Fizazi K (2011) Targeting continued androgen receptor signaling in prostate cancer. Clin Cancer Res 17:3876–3883
105. Chu FM, Picus J, Fracasso PM, Dreicer R, Lang Z et al (2011) A phase 1, multicenter, open-label study of the safety of two dose levels of a human monoclonal antibody to human alpha(v) integrins, intetumumab, in combination with docetaxel and prednisone in patients with castrate-resistant metastatic prostate cancer. Invest New Drugs 29:674–679
106. Tran C, Ouk S, Clegg NJ, Chen Y, Watson PA et al (2009) Development of a second-generation antiandrogen for treatment of advanced prostate cancer. Science 324:787–790
107. Andersen RJ, Mawji NR, Wang J, Wang G, Haile S et al (2010) Regression of castrate-recurrent prostate cancer by a small-molecule inhibitor of the amino-terminus domain of the androgen receptor. Cancer Cell 17:535–546
108. Yang Z, Chang YJ, Yu IC, Yeh S, Wu CC et al (2007) ASC-J9 ameliorates spinal and bulbar muscular atrophy phenotype via degradation of androgen receptor. Nat Med 13:348–353
109. Lai JJ, Lai KP, Chuang KH, Chang P, Yu IC et al (2009) Monocyte/macrophage androgen receptor suppresses cutaneous wound healing in mice by enhancing local TNF-alpha expression. J Clin Invest 119:3739–3751
110. Wu MH, Ma WL, Hsu CL, Chen YL, Ou JH et al (2010) Androgen receptor promotes hepatitis B virus-induced hepatocarcinogenesis through modulation of hepatitis B virus RNA transcription. Sci Transl Med 2:32ra35
111. Lin HK, Hu YC, Yang L, Altuwaijri S, Chen YT et al (2003) Suppression versus induction of androgen receptor functions by the phosphatidylinositol 3-kinase/Akt pathway in prostate cancer LNCaP cells with different passage numbers. J Biol Chem 278:50902–50907
112. Miyamoto H, Altuwaijri S, Cai Y, Messing EM, Chang C (2005) Inhibition of the Akt, cyclooxygenase-2, and matrix metalloproteinase-9 pathways in combination with androgen deprivation therapy: potential therapeutic approaches for prostate cancer. Mol Carcinog 44:1–10
113. Carver BS, Chapinski C, Wongvipat J, Hieronymus H, Chen Y et al (2011) Reciprocal feedback regulation of PI3K and androgen receptor signaling in PTEN-deficient prostate cancer. Cancer Cell 19:575–586

Role of Androgens and Androgen Receptor in Prostate Cancer: Genomic and Non-Genomic Actions

Sara Marchiani, Lara Tamburrino, Monica Muratori, Lorella Bonaccorsi, Gianni Forti and Elisabetta Baldi

Abstract Prostate cancer (PCa) is the most common malignancy in western countries, representing the second leading cause of death. Androgen deprivation therapy (ADT) represents a good therapeutic tool for the treatment of PCa patients, but after an initial period of remission, the disease progresses towards an androgen-independent (AI) state. While in androgen-dependent (AD) stage the roles of androgens and their receptor (AR) are fully described in AI, they are yet a matter of research and discussion. Consolidated evidence demonstrates that, beside the well characterized genomic effects of AR, the non-classic ones contribute to PCa development and progression. In this chapter, we summarize the main non-classic androgen pathways and their involvement in the main phases of PCa. All these studies demonstrate that AR is a crucial factor both in pathogenesis development and progression of PCa; its rapid effects are integrated with the genomic ones to

S. Marchiani · L. Tamburrino · M. Muratori · L. Bonaccorsi · G. Forti · E. Baldi (✉)
Department of Clinical Physiopathology, Sexual Medicine and Andrology Unit, Center of Excellence for Research, Transfer and High Education 'DeNothe', University of Florence, Viale Pieraccini 6, 50139 Florence, Italy
e-mail: e.baldi@dfc.unifi.it

S. Marchiani
e-mail: sara.marchiani@unifi.it

L. Tamburrino
e-mail: lara.tamburrino@unifi.it

M. Muratori
e-mail: monica@dfc.unifi.it; muratori@dfc.unifi.it

L. Bonaccorsi
e-mail: lorella.bonaccorsi@unifi.it

G. Forti
e-mail: g.forti@dfc.unifi.it

G. Castoria and A. Migliaccio (eds.), *Advances in Rapid Sex-Steroid Action*,
DOI: 10.1007/978-1-4614-1764-4_10,

mediate the complexity of the receptor signalling. In such a scenario, taking into account not only the classic mechanisms leading to AR activation, but also the non-classic ones should be helpful to find new potential therapeutic targets for treatment of PCa.

Keywords Prostate cancer · Androgen receptor · Genomic and non genomic signalling

Abbreviations

AD	androgen-dependent
ADT	androgen-deprivation therapy
AI	androgen-independent
AR	androgen receptor
DHT	dihydrotestosterone
EGF	epidermal growth factor
EGFR	EGF receptor
ERK	extracellular-regulated kinase
GFs	growth factors
GPR30	G-protein coupled receptor
Hsp27	heat shock protein 27
IGF	insulin-like growth factor
IL-6	interleukin-6
KGF	keratinocyte growth factor
m-TOR	mammalian target of rapamycin
MAPK	mitogen activated protein kinases
MEK-1	mitogen-activated kinase
NED	neuroendocrine differentiation
PCa	prostate cancer
PDGF	platelet-derived growth factor
PIN	prostatic intraepithelial neoplasia
PI3-K	phosphatidylinositol-3-kinase
TKRs	tyrosine kinase receptors

Contents

1 Introduction

Prostate cancer (PCa) develops primarily in men over fifty and is the most common type of cancer in western countries' male population [1], representing the second leading cause of cancer death. In most cases (about 2/3), PCa is slow-growing, symptom-free, and, since men with this condition are old, they often die of causes unrelated to it. In about 30% of cases, however, PCa is more aggressive, fast developing and leading to death of the patient. Current treatment options for clinically localized or locally advanced PCa include radical prostatectomy, radiation therapy, brachytherapy, cryotherapy, or "watchful waiting". If PCa is not organ confined at the diagnosis, androgen deprivation therapy (ADT) represents a good tool to treat patients. However, after an initial period of remission the disease progresses towards an androgen-independent (AI) state leading to uncontrolled spread. At this point, only palliative treatments are substantially possible. The lack of clinical options of treatment for metastatic PCa reflects our poor understanding of the molecular and cellular mechanisms that underlie the progression of the disease from an androgen-dependent (AD) to an androgen-refractory state.

During foetal and adult life, prostate development, growth and differentiation are regulated both directly and indirectly by androgens and their receptors (androgen receptor, AR) [2–4]. At least in its initial phases, PCa is AD for its growth (as demonstrated by the efficacy of ADT). An early role for AR in the pathogenesis of PCa is also suggested by recent studies demonstrating the formation of *TMPRSS2-ERG* fusions, a chromosomal rearrangement leading to AR-dependent expression of ERG, an ETS transcription factor, in a significant percentage of PCas [5, 6]. The role of androgens and AR in AI stages of PCa is less clear. There is evidence that re-expression of AR into AI-PCa cell lines restores an androgen controlled cell growth as well as expression of AR target genes leading to a more differentiated and less aggressive phenotype [7–11]. Moreover AI tumours are heterogeneous and comprised of various subpopulations of cells, which respond differently to androgens [12, 13].

Whatever the role of androgens and AR in the different phases of PCa is yet a matter of research and discussion, even if consolidate evidence in the literature demonstrate that the well characterized genomic effects of androgens are integrated with the non-classical ones (also known as non-genomic or non-genotropic) in contributing to PCa development and progression.

In this chapter we will first summarize the main non-classic androgen effects described in PCa cells and then their involvement, together with classic ones, in the main phases of PCa growth.

2 Non-Genomic Effects of AR in PCa Cells

AR non-genomic signalling pathways are characterized by rapid responses and may involve a membrane-localized AR as well as rapid cytoplasmic signalling. Localization in the membrane of the classical AR may occur through both a direct insertion in the lipid bylayer and/or interaction with membrane-associated proteins [14, 15]. It has been demonstrated that post-translational modifications such as palmitoylation are involved in recruitment of AR to the plasma membrane where it interacts with membrane-associated proteins such as caveolins [14], which are the main protein component of lipid raft micro-domains. More recently, it has been shown that localization of AR (as well as of other sex steroid receptors) in membrane lipid raft domains, requires the action of the heat shock protein 27 (Hsp27), which binds steroid receptors promoting their palmitoylation and consequent interaction with caveolar raft domains of the plasma membrane [16]. Interestingly, siRNA of Hsp27 in LNCaP cells inhibits rapid signalling (such as ERK and PI3-K activation) induced by testosterone, indicating that the effect of the hormone requires AR localization to the plasma membrane.

AR localized to a lipid raft sub-cellular compartment in LNCaP cells has been shown to associate with Akt and activate it independently of PI3-K [17, 18]. Moreover, the rapid PI3-K activation by androgens reported in non transformed androgen-sensitive epithelial cells as well as in carcinoma cells was based on the direct interaction between AR and p85alpha regulatory subunit of class I(A) PI3-K [19, 20]. These data indicate that cholesterol-rich membrane micro-domains play an important role in transmitting non-genomic signals involving androgen and the Akt pathway in PCa cells [18, 21]. Moreover, particular cholesterol-rich membrane domains, namely caveolae, harbour caveolin-1 protein that acts as scaffolding protein by controlling many signalling effectors through direct binding [22]. Interaction between AR and caveolin-1 through an androgen-mediated process has been demonstrated in PCa cells, where the NH(2) terminal region of caveolin-1 interacts with both the NH(2)-terminal domain and the ligand binding domain (LBD) of AR [23]. The pathophysiological significance of such interaction, however, is still obscure.

Rapid effects mediated by AR in PCa cells include the release of intracellular calcium [15], activation of protein kinase A (PKA), Akt and protein kinase C (PKC) [24, 25] and a direct association with c-Src leading to the activation of Raf-1/ERK and PI3-K signalling pathways [19, 26]. The association of AR with Src kinase is of particular relevance as it can lead to AR activation both directly (inducing its tyrosine phosphorylation) and indirectly (through activation of other kinase pathways and through src function as scaffold protein leading to direct interaction with other proteins) [27]. In particular, AR has been shown to associate,through c-Src, to MNAR (modulator of non-genomic action of estrogen receptor) forming a complex that leads to Mitogen-Activated Protein Kinase (MAPK) activation both in AD and AI cell lines [28]. However, while in AD cells testosterone is required to activate the complex, in AI cells the complex appears to be constitutively active. The demonstration that disruption of AR/c-Src interaction in AI-PCa cells selectively inhibits AR-mediated cell growth without changing the ability of AR to regulate the transcription of androgen-responsive genes [29] further supports such a complexity.

The characterization in metastatic PCa of a splicing variant of AR, termed AR23, where 23 amino acids inserted between the two zinc fingers determines an exclusive cytoplasmic location inhibiting nuclear entry and activation of target genes has further supported a role for cytoplasmic, non-genomic signalling of androgens in PCa [30]. This receptor variant is indeed able to activate NF-kappa B transcriptional activity contributing to PCa progression [30]. Recently, it has been shown that AR23 increases AR activation when the two isoforms are co-expressed in PCa cells and decreases its sensitivity to anti-androgens [31].

Overall, these studies demonstrate that rapid effects of androgens are integrated with the genomic ones to mediate the complexity of AR signalling in inducing proliferation and cell survival [15, 32]. However evidence exists that both genomic and non-genomic effects of AR are also involved in maintaining a differentiated and less aggressive phenotype [33] of PCa cells. Our and other groups have shown that re-expression of a functional AR in the AR-negative PCa cell line PC3 conferred a more differentiated phenotype characterized by decreased ability of anchorage-independent growth, reduced laminin adhesion and Matrigel invasion in response to epidermal growth factor (EGF) [7, 8, 10, 11]. We have shown that, besides a genomic effect of androgens on alpha6beta4 integrin expression [8], these effects are also mediated by a non-genomic effect of AR on EGF receptor (EGFR) activation [34, 35]. We have demonstrated that AR and EGFR interact at the plasma membrane in PC3-AR cells [34] leading to a decreased EGF-mediated phosphorylation and PI3-K/Akt downstream signalling of the EGFR as well as of receptor internalization [34, 35]. In line with our results, it has been recently shown that EGFR signalling and internalization are reduced in AR positive-PCa cells with respect to AR negative ones [36] and that such effect is mediated by the endocytosis protein REPS2, whose expression is higher in AR-positive PCa cells. Our data also show evidences that in PC3-AR cells a pool of classical ARs and EGFRs are located within cholesterol-rich membrane microdomains (namely as lipid raft), but the interaction between these two proteins, which is increased by androgens, does not co-localize within the same cholesterol-rich lipid rafts domains [37]. Our results have been recently substantiated by a study showing that addition of a functional AR in PC3 cells using a vector whose expression is regulated by a natural AR promoter leads to expression of a functional AR conferring a less invasive phenotype with respect to parental cells, indicating that AR is mostly tumor suppressive in carcinoma cells [38]. However, whether these effects are mediated by non-classical pathways has not been investigated in the study [38]. It must be mentioned that androgens have been shown to induce cell migration and invasion in non prostatic sarcoma cancer cells and normal fibroblasts through a direct association between AR, cytoskeletal elements and integrins inducing the activation of rapid signalling pathways responsible for cell migration [39].

In general, it appears that the non-genomic pathways of AR may contribute to promote or inhibit the migratory behaviours depending on the cell type and/or the signalling pathway involved. In most of the examples described above, a direct involvement of "classic" AR in eliciting non-genomic effects has been demonstrated. However, the fact that some effects can be obtained using membrane impermeable dihydrotestosterone (DHT) analogues, which are not inhibited by anti-androgens, and that Ras/MAPK signalling in response to androgen has been demonstrated also in AR-negative cell lines has supported the hypothesis of the involvement of a membrane AR different from the classic one [33]. Recently, the group of Castanas reported the identification of a membrane AR (mAR) [32], preferentially expressed in tumors rather than benign tissue. Furthermore, they demonstrated that mAR agonists, alone or in combination with anti-mitotic agents, decreased in vitro PCa cell growth and induced apoptosis, whereas in vivo they reduced tumor size [33, 40, 41]. However, the nature of such androgen binding proteins localized on the membrane still remains obscure [42]. In addition, the recent demonstration that the so-called AR-negative PCa cell lines express low levels of AR [43] and that these low levels are sufficient to support androgen-stimulated proliferation [44] through a non-genomic pathway, has raised questions about the existence of such putative non-classic AR isoforms.

3 Role of Androgens and AR in the Pathogenesis and Development of PCa

One important question about PCa concerns the cells of origin of the cancer and the characteristics of stem cells within it. According to Arnold and Isaacs [13], PCa may originate from three distinct cells within the prostate: (1) from an AI stem cell leading to a mixture of androgen-sensitive and AD cells; (2) from an androgen-sensitive amplifying basal cell, giving rise to androgen-sensitive malignant cells that may differentiate into AD cells; iii) from an AD transit glandular cell, leading to a homogenous tumor composed of AD cells. According to this hypothesis PCa may originate also from AI cells, questioning the role of androgens in the very initial phases of the tumor. Recently Hu et al. [45], using adult prostate stem/early progenitor cells, demonstrated that they are negative for AR and highly positive for all known estrogen receptors, including the membrane GPR30 [45]. Interestingly, the exposure of these cells to estradiol for a long time promotes their differentiation towards a basal and luminal epithelial phenotype expressing AR and becoming responsive to androgens. These cells were able to induce the formation of tumors in nude mice, if the animals were exposed to high levels of estradiol and testosterone (but not the two alone) pointing to an important role for estrogens in prostate carcinogenesis. In line with this hypothesis, it has been shown that PCa stem cells, which support self-renewal and continuous growth, appear to be AR negative [13] although it cannot be excluded that AR has not been detected in these cells because of expression at very low levels [46]. How these cells may generate a tumor which expresses high levels of AR is yet unclear, but the three hypothesis postulated by Arnold and Isaacs (see above) indicate that the developing tumour always become androgen-dependent. On the other hand, a role for AR in the development of PCa is suggested by the identification of chromosomal translocations that fuses untraslated sequences of an androgen-regulated gene, TMPRSS2, with the coding sequences of the ETS family transcription factors (in most of cases of ERG). This fusion, which is detected in approximately 50% of PCa [47, 48], renders ERG expression under the control of androgens and, since ETS transcription factors are involved in uncontrolled proliferation of cancer cells, the occurrence of translocation could be involved in the pathogenesis of the disease. It has been recently reported that long-term (up to 5 months) treatment with androgens at high doses may induce the chromosomal rearrangement in non-malignant immortalized prostate epithelial cells, whereas short-term treatment with androgens at physiologic levels is sufficient to induce it in malignant prostatic epithelial cells [49]. This finding suggests that androgen-induced fusion occurs prior to cancer development through a mechanism that induces gene proximity after AR activation by its ligand. Whether non-genotropic signalling is involved in the generation of the rearrangement is presently unknown. It must be mentioned however, that the translocation, per se, is not sufficient to induce complete tumorigenesis in transgenic animals bearing it [48]. Since the frequency of rearrangement doesn't increase with the progression of the tumor, the fusion appears to be an early event although not sufficient to promote the transition from prostatic intraepithelial neoplasia (PIN) to PCa [48]. Probably other (more or less) concomitant events are needed, such as PTEN loss, frequently found in PCa [50], which leads to Akt activation. In conclusion, at present the role of the chromosomal rearrangement in the pathogenesis of PCa needs to be further clarified, but it could be important for an early diagnosis of PCa especially if included in a multiplex model with other biomarkers, such as PCA3, Annexin A3 and Sarcosine, to improve the diagnostic performance [51].

4 Role of Androgens and AR in Progression of PCa

As mentioned above, at least in the initial phases, PCa cells are completely dependent on androgens for growth and survival, the disease is considered 'hormone-dependent' and responds well to ADT, but, after a few months, most tumors become hormone-resistant with a more aggressive phenotype. The process that leads to AI is complex and the molecular mechanisms underlying it are not fully disclosed and are matter of discussion. The complexity is due to the fact that PCa is a very heterogeneous tumor and includes a variety of subpopulations cells which respond differently to androgens. Reflecting these peculiar characteristics, more than one theory has been developed to explain the transition. One of these theories supports the idea that pre-existing subpopulations of AI malignant cells, or developed in consequence of genetic changes, may later support complete AI. According to another theory, called "adaptative," cells may respond differently to ADT: most of them die but others undergo several molecular changes that render them AI with activation of alternative pathways of growth. It has been observed that AR continues to be expressed both in AD and in a large proportion of AI tumors [52]. Indeed, the androgen-regulated gene PSA continues to be expressed in most patients at this stage of the disease, indicating that AR continues to be present and activated. In models of AI cells and xenografts derived from LNCaP cells grown in vivo in castrated nude mice, AR expression increases as a consequence of the pressure of the androgen-deprived environment [53–55]. In addition, in these models, AR becomes responsive to anti-androgens.

The alternative mechanisms that may be responsible for the transition include mutations and amplifications of the AR, alterations of receptor coregulators, ligand-independent activation of AR, and increase of androgen intraprostatic levels. It has been demonstrated that AR mutations are quite rare in patients with clinically localized disease and usually do not play a role in the initial phases of prostatic carcinogenesis, whereas a significant number of AR mutations are found in metastatic disease suggesting that hormonal environment may induce spontaneous mutations that, in turn, promote the metastatic phenotype [56, 57]. Activating AR mutations regards about 25% of AD tumors and may rise, depending on the study, to 50% in metastatic or AI tumors [57].

Evidence also exists that AR may be activated by non-androgenic steroid molecules as well as antiandrogens through a promiscuous way leading to ligand-independent AR activation [58]. AR can be also activated by growth factors (GFs), which induce AR phosphorylation through their tyrosine kinase receptors (TKRs) [52, 58]. Among the growth factors demonstrated to be able to activate AR, insulin-like growth factor (IGF), keratinocyte growth factor (KGF), platelet-derived growth factor (PDGF), EGF, and interleukin-6 (IL-6) are now being targeted in PCa clinical trials using antibodies or inhibitors of their receptor kinase activity [59, 60]. Up-regulation of the anti-apoptotic molecule Bcl-2 and inactivation of the tumor-suppressor gene PTEN, leading to the constitutive activation of PI3-K/AKT/m-TOR pathway, support an AR-bypassed survival of AI cells [61]. Moreover, in AI cells, growth factors have been shown to stimulate the transcription of androgen-responsive genes in ligand-independent manner [62].

The mechanisms that lead to PCa progression could involve also non-genotropic effects of AR. Indeed, Unni et al. [28] demonstrated that in LNCaP-HP, an AI cell line, AR regulates transcription either directly upon ligand binding and nuclear translocation or indirectly through kinase pathways leading to activation of downstream transcription factors. In particular, in this cell line the Src-MEK-1/2-ERK-1/2-CREB pathway was found constitutively active, whereas in the correspondent AD LNCaP cell line, the activation of the pathway was dependent on androgens. In addition, using an in vivo prostate regeneration system, a direct synergy between Akt and AR signalling has been demonstrated to be responsible for PCa progression and development of AI [63]. Indeed, cells infected both with Akt and wild-type AR form larger tumors with respect to cells infected with the two alone. If cells are infected with AR mutated in the proline-rich region which supports its binding with c-Src [64], but allowing genotropic signalling, the synergistic effect is lost. At the same time, the synergy is also lost with AR mutated in domains supporting genotropic signalling. Overall, this study demonstrates that both genotropic and non-genotropic signalling are required for PCa progression [63].

Another mechanism by which prostate epithelial cells could achieve AI is the alteration of AR expression and function in the stroma surrounding the tumor. Indeed, the reciprocal interaction between stroma and epithelium seems to play a crucial role in the initiation and progression of PCa [65]. In a recent study, Niu et al. [66] generated two mouse models in which AR was knocked down in epithelium and stroma (ind-ARKO-TRAMP), or only in epithelium (pes-ARKO-TRAMP), of the prostate. In both cases PCa develops; however, in ind-ARKO-TRAMP mice, tumors were smaller and with lower proliferation rate. In addition, pes-ARKO-TRAMP mice showed lower survival rates, with respect to both wild type and ind-ARKO-TRAMP mice, which showed the better survival rate. These results indicate that stromal AR functions as a stimulator for PCa proliferation and metastasic events, whereas epithelial AR acts as a tumor suppressor and survival factor [66, 67], supporting a differential role of AR in PCa depending on its location and highlighting the importance of crosstalk between stroma and epithelium in carcinogenesis and progression of PCa. Further studies are required to understand the complexity of molecular mechanisms underlying the interaction between stroma and epithelial tissues in PCa, and in particular whether non-genotropic signalling of AR is also involved.

There is a body of evidence about the occurrence of neuroendocrine differentiation (NED) in androgen-deprived conditions. NED is involved in the transition to AI [13, 68] and is related to greater tumor aggressiveness and poorer patient prognosis [69]. In a recent study, we demonstrated that different PCa cell lines do not respond univocally to in vitro treatments inducing NED, in particular to androgen deprivation and EGF supplementation. We observed that growth in androgen-depleted conditions induces NED in AR expressing AD LNCaP cells, whereas EGF induces NED in androgen-irresponsive DU145, but not in androgen-responsive LNCaP and 22Rv1 cell lines [70]. These results indicate that NED may develop in steroid-deprived conditions when a functional AR is present.

5 Conclusions

AR remains a crucial factor in the pathogenesis, development and progression of PCa, either alone or, more likely, in concert with other factors. The goal for researchers is to more clearly elucidate all the signalling pathways that lead to AR activation in response to, and independently of, androgens to define alternative therapeutic targets for new treatments of highly aggressive PCa. In such a scenario, AR signalling effects outside the nucleus should be greatly taken into account, as they have profound implications in all the stages of PCa and may lead to the identification of new potential therapeutic targets that might be otherwise ignored.

References

1. Lippman SM, Hawk ET (2009) Cancer prevention: from 1727 to milestones of the past 100 years. Cancer Res 69:5269–5284
2. Fibbi B, Penna G, Morelli A, Adorini L, Maggi M (2009) Chronic inflammation in the pathogenesis of benign prostatic hyperplasia. Int J Androl 33:475–488
3. Isaacs JT (2004) Testosterone and the prostate. In: Nieschlag E, Behre HM (eds) Testosterone: action, deficiency, substitution, 3rd edn. Cambridge University Press, Cambridge
4. Roehrborn CG (2008) Pathology of benign prostatic hyperplasia. Int J Impot Res 3:S11–S18
5. Tomlins SA, Bjartell A, Chinnaiyan AM, Jenster G, Nam RK, Rubin MA, Schalken JA (2009) ETS gene fusions in prostate cancer: from discovery to daily clinical practice. Eur Urol 56:275–286
6. Bonaccorsi L, Nesi G, Nuti F, Paglierani M, Krausz C, Masieri L, Serni S, Proietti-Pannunzi L, Fang Y, Jhanwar SC, Orlando C, Carini M, Forti G, Baldi E, Luzzatto L (2009) Persistence of expression of the TMPRSS2:ERG fusion gene after pre-surgery androgen ablation may be associated with early prostate specific antigen relapse of prostate cancer: preliminary results. J Endocrinol Invest 32:590–596
7. Cinar B, Koeneman KS, Edlund M, Prins GS, Zhau HE, Chung LW (2001) Androgen receptor mediates the reduced tumor growth, enhanced androgen responsiveness, and selected target gene transactivation in a human prostate cancer cell line. Cancer Res 61:7310–7317
8. Bonaccorsi L, Carloni V, Muratori M, Salvadori A, Giannini A, Carini M, Serio M, Forti G, Baldi E (2000) Androgen receptor expression in prostate carcinoma cells suppresses alpha6beta4 integrin-mediated invasive phenotype. Endocrinology 141:3172–3182
9. Links Chuu CP, Hiipakka RA, Fukuchi J, Kokontis JM, Liao S (2005) Androgen causes growth suppression and reversion of androgen-independent prostate cancer xenografts to an androgen-stimulated phenotype in athymic mice. Cancer Res 65:2082–2084
10. Moehren U, Papaioannou M, Reeb CA, Grasselli A, Nanni S, Asim M, Roell D, Prade I, Farsetti A, Baniahmad A (2008) Wild-type but not mutant androgen receptor inhibits expression of the hTERT telomerase subunit: a novel role of AR mutation for prostate cancer development. FASEB J 22:1258–1267
11. Akashi T, Koizumi K, Nagakawa O, Fuse H, Saiki I (2006) Androgen receptor negatively influences the expression of chemokine receptors (CXCR4, CCR1) and ligand-mediated migration in prostate cancer DU-145. Oncol Rep 16:831–836
12. Goldstein AS, Huang J, Guo C, Garraway IP, Witte ON (2010) Identification of a cell of origin for human prostate cancer. Science 329:568–571
13. Arnold JT, Isaacs JT (2002) Mechanisms involved in the progression of androgen-independent prostate cancers: it is not only the cancer cell's fault. Endocr Relat Cancer 9:61–73
14. Pedram A, Razandi M, Sainson RC, Kim JK, Hughes CC, Levin ER (2007) A conserved mechanism for steroid receptor translocation to the plasma membrane. Biol Chem 31:22278–22288
15. Baron S, Manin M, Beaudoin C, Leotoing L, Communal Y, Veyssiere G, Morel L (2004) Androgen receptor mediates non-genomic activation of phosphatidylinositol 3-OH kinase in androgen-sensitive epithelial cells. J Biol Chem 279:14579–14586

16. Razandi M, Pedram A, Levin ER (2010) Heat shock protein 27 is required for sex steroid receptor trafficking to and functioning at the plasma membrane. Mol Cell Biol 30:3249–3261
17. Freeman MR, Cinar B, Lu ML (2005) Membrane rafts as potential sites of nongenomic hormonal signaling in prostate cancer. Trends Endocrinol Metab 16:273–279
18. Cinar B, Mukhopadhyay NK, Meng G, Freeman MR (2007) Phosphoinositide 3-kinase-independent non-genomic signals transit from the androgen receptor to Akt1 in membrane raft microdomains. Rapid signalling pathway activation by androgens in epithelial and stromal cells. J Biol Chem 282:29584–29593
19. Castoria G, Lombardi M, Barone MV, Bilancio A, Di Domenico M, Bottero D, Vitale F, Migliaccio A, Auricchio F (2003) Androgen-stimulated DNA synthesis and cytoskeletal changes in fibroblasts by a non transcriptional receptor action. J Cell Biol 161:547–556
20. Gatson JW, Kaur P, Singh M (2006) Dihydrotestosterone differentially modulates the mitogen-activated protein kinase and the phosphoinositide 3-kinase/Akt pathways through the nuclear and novel membrane androgen receptor in C6 cells. Endocrinology 147:2028–2034
21. Zhuang L, Lin J, Lu ML, Solomon KR, Freeman MR (2002) Cholesterol-rich lipid rafts mediate Akt-regulated survival in prostate cancer cells. Cancer Res 62:2227–2231
22. Simons K, Toomre D (2000) Lipid rafts and signal transduction. Nat Rev Mol Cell Biol 1:31–39
23. Lu ML, Schneider MC, Zheng Y, Zhang X, Richie JP (2001) Caveolin-1 interacts with androgen receptor. A positive modulator of androgen receptor mediated transactivation. J Biol Chem 276:13442–13451
24. Foradori CD, Weiser MJ, Handa RJ (2008) Non-genomic actions of androgens. Front Neuroendocrinol 29:169–181
25. Li J, Al-Azzawi F (2009) Mechanism of androgen receptor action. Maturitas 63:142–148
26. Migliaccio A, Castoria G, Giovannelli P, Auricchio F (2010) Cross talk between epidermal growth factor (EGF) receptor and extra nuclear steroid receptors in cell lines. Mol Cell Endocrinol 327:19–24
27. Cai H, Babic I, Wei X, Huang J, Witte ON (2011) Invasive prostate carcinoma driven by c-Srcc-Src and androgen receptor synergy. Cancer Res 71:862–872
28. Unni E, Sun S, Nan B, McPhaul MJ, Cheskis B, Mancini MA, Marcelli M (2004) Changes in androgen receptor nongenotropic signaling correlate with transition of LNCaP cells to androgen independence. Cancer Res 64:7156–7168
29. Zhoul J, Hernandez G, Tu SW, Huang CL, Tseng CP, Hsieh JT (2005) The role of DOC-2/DAB2 in modulating androgen receptor-mediated cell growth via the nongenomic c-Srcc-Src-mediated pathway in normal prostatic epithelium and cancer. Cancer Res 65:9906–9913
30. Jagla M, Fève M, Kessler P, Lapouge G, Erdmann E, Serra S, Bergerat JP, Céraline J (2007) A splicing variant of the androgen receptor detected in a metastatic prostate cancer exhibits exclusively cytoplasmic actions. Endocrinology 148:4334–4343
31. Steinkamp MP, O'Mahony OA, Brogley M, Rehman H, Lapensee EW, Dhanasekaran S, Hofer MD, Kuefer R, Chinnaiyan A, Rubin MA, Pienta KJ, Robins DM (2009) Treatment-dependent androgen receptor mutations in prostate cancer exploit multiple mechanisms to evade therapy. Cancer Res 69:4434–4442
32. Hatzoglou A, Kampa M, Kogia C, Charalampopoulos I, Theodoropoulos PA, Anezinis P, Dambaki C, Papakonstanti EA, Stathopoulos EN, Stournaras C, Gravanis A, Castanas E (2005) Membrane androgen receptor activation induces apoptotic regression of human prostate cancer cells in vitro and in vivo. J Clin Endocrinol Metab 90:893–903
33. Papakonstanti EA, Kampa M, Castanas E, Stournaras C (2003) A rapid, nongenomic, signaling pathway regulates the actin reorganization induced by activation of membrane testosterone receptors. Mol Endocrinol 17:870–881
34. Bonaccorsi L, Carloni V, Muratori M, Formigli L, Zecchi S, Forti G, Baldi E (2004) EGF receptor (EGFR) signaling promoting invasion is disrupted in androgen-sensitive prostate cancer cells by an interaction between EGFR and androgen receptor (AR). Int J Cancer 112:78–86

35. Bonaccorsi L, Nosi D, Muratori M, Formigli L, Forti G, Baldi E (2007) Altered endocytosis of epidermal growth factor receptor in androgen receptor positive prostate cancer cell lines. J Mol Endocrinol 38:51–66
36. Oosterhoff JK, Kühne LC, Grootegoed JA, Blok LJ (2005) EGF signalling in prostate cancer cell lines is inhibited by a high expression level of the endocytosis protein REPS2. Int J Cancer 113:561–567
37. Bonaccorsi L, Nosi D, Quercioli F, Formigli L, Zecchi S, Maggi M, Forti G, Baldi E (2008) Prostate cancer: a model of integration of genomic and non-genomic effects of the androgen receptor in cell lines model. Steroids 73:1030–1037
38. Niu Y, Altuwaijri S, Lai KP, Wu CT, Ricke WA, Messing EM, Yao J, Yeh S, Chang C (2008) Androgen receptor is a tumor suppressor and proliferator in prostate cancer. Proc Natl Acad Sci U S A 105:12182–12187
39. Castoria G, D'Amato L, Ciociola A, Giovannelli P, Giraldi T, Sepe L, Paolella G, Barone MV, Migliaccio A, Auricchio F (2011) Androgen-induced cell migration: role of androgen receptor/filamin A association. PLoS One 6:e17218
40. Kampa M, Kogia C, Theodoropoulos PA, Anezinis P, Charalampopoulos I, Papakonstanti EA, Stathopoulos EN, Hatzoglou A, Stournaras C, Gravanis A, Castanas E (2006) Activation of membrane androgen receptors potentiates the antiproliferative effects of paclitaxel on human prostate cancer cells. Mol Cancer Ther 5:1342–1351
41. Kampa M, Theodoropoulou K, Mavromati F, Pelekanou V, Notas G, Lagoudaki ED, Nifli AP, Morel-Salmi C, Stathopoulos EN, Vercauteren J, Castanas E (2011) Novel oligomeric proanthocyanidin derivatives interact with membrane androgen sites and induce regression of hormone-independent prostate cancer. J Pharmacol Exp Ther 337:24–32
42. Lange CA, Gioeli D, Hammes SR, Marker PC (2007) Integration of rapid signaling events with steroid hormone receptor action in breast and prostate cancer. Annu Rev Physiol 69:171–199
43. Alimirah F, Chen J, Basrawala Z, Xin H, Choubey D (2006) DU-145 and PC-3 human prostate cancer cell lines express androgen receptor: implications for the androgen receptor functions and regulation. FEBS Lett 580:2294–2300
44. Martinez HD, Jasavala RJ, Hinkson I, Fitzgerald LD, Trimmer JS, Kung HJ, Wright ME (2008) RNA editing of androgen receptor gene transcripts in prostate cancer cells. J Biol Chem 283:29938–29949
45. Hu WY, Shi GB, Lam HM, Hu DP, Ho SM, Madueke I, Kajdacsy-Balla A, Prins GS (2011) Estrogen-initiated transformation of prostate epithelium derived from normal human prostate stem-progenitor cells. Endocrinology 6:437–451
46. Wang ZA, Shen MM (2011) Revisiting the concept of cancer stem cells in prostate cancer. Oncogene 30:1261–1271
47. Tomlins SA, Rhodes DR, Perner S, Dhanasekaran SM, Mehra R, Sun XW, Varambally S, Cao X, Tchinda J, Kuefer R, Lee C, Montie JE, Shah RB, Pienta KJ, Rubin MA, Chinnaiyan AM (2005) Recurrent fusion of TMPRSS2 and ETS transcription factor genes in prostate cancer. Science 310:644–648
48. Tomlins SA, Laxman B, Dhanasekaran SM, Helgeson BE, Cao X, Morris DS, Menon A, Jing X, Cao Q, Han B, Yu J, Wang L, Montie JE, Rubin MA, Pienta KJ, Roulston D, Shah RB, Varambally S, Mehra R, Chinnaiyan AM (2007) Distinct classes of chromosomal rearrangements create oncogenic ETS gene fusions in prostate cancer. Nature 448:595–599
49. Bastus NC, Boyd LK, Mao X, Stankiewicz E, Kudahetti SC, Oliver RT, Berney DM, Lu YJ (2010) Androgen-induced TMPRSS2:ERG fusion in nonmalignant prostate epithelial cells. Cancer Res 70:9544–9548
50. Chen Z, Trotman LC, Shaffer D, Lin HK, Dotan ZA, Niki M, Koutcher JA, Scher HI, Ludwig T, Gerald W, Cordon-Cardo C, Pandolfi PP (2005) Crucial role of p53-dependent cellular senescence in suppression of Pten-deficient tumorigenesis. Nature 436:725–730
51. Cao DL, Ye DW, Zhang HL, Zhu Y, Wang YX, Yao XD (2011) A multiplex model of combining gene-based, protein-based, and metabolite-based with positive and negative markers in urine for the early diagnosis of prostate cancer. Prostate 71:700–710

52. Lamont KR, Tindall DJ (2011) Minireview: alternative activation pathways for the androgen receptor in prostate cancer. Mol Endocrinol 25:897–907
53. Chen CD, Welsbie DS, Tran C, Baek SH, Chen R, Vessella R, Rosenfeld MG, Sawyers CL (2004) Molecular determinants of resistance to antiandrogen therapy. Nat Med 10:33–39
54. Marques RB, van Weerden WM, Erkens-Schulze S, de Ridder CM, Bangma CH, Trapman J, Jenster G (2006) The human PC346 xenograft and cell line panel: a model system for prostate cancer progression. Eur Urol 49:245–257
55. Zhou JR, Yu L, Zerbini LF, Libermann TA, Blackburn GL (2004) Progression to androgenindependent LNCaP human prostate tumors: cellular and molecular alterations. Int J Cancer 110:800–806
56. Marcelli M, Ittmann M, Mariani S, Sutherland R, Nigam R, Murthy L, Zhao Y, Di Concini D, Puxeddu E, Esen A, Eastham J, Weigel NL, Lamb DJ (2000) Androgen receptor mutations in prostate cancer. Cancer Res 60:944–949
57. Koochekpour S (2010) Androgen receptor signaling and mutations in prostate cancer. Asian J Androl 12:639–657
58. Taichman RS, Loberg RD, Mehra R, Pienta KJ (2007) The evolving biology and treatment of prostate cancer. J Clin Invest 117:2351–2361
59. Singh P, Uzgare A, Litvinov I, Denmeade SR, Isaacs JT (2006) Combinatorial androgen receptor targeted therapy for prostate cancer. Endocr Relat Cancer 13:653–666
60. Karkera J, Steiner H, Li W, Skradski V, Moser PL, Riethdorf S, Reddy M, Puchalski T, Safer K, Prabhakar U, Pantel K, Qi M, Culig Z (2011) The anti-interleukin-6 antibody siltuximab down-regulates genes implicated in tumorigenesis in prostate cancer patients from a phase I study. Prostate (Epub ahead of print)
61. Pienta KJ, Smith DC (2005) Advances in prostate cancer chemotherapy: a new era begins. CA Cancer J Clin 55:300–318
62. Culig Z, Hobisch A, Cronauer MV, Radmayr C, Trapman J, Hittmair A, Bartsch G, Klocker H (1994) Androgen receptor activation in prostatic tumor cell lines by insulin-like growth factor-I, keratinocyte growth factor, and epidermal growth factor. Cancer Res 54:5474–5478
63. Xin L, Teitell MA, Lawson DA, Kwon A, Mellinghoff IK, Witte ON (2006) Progression of prostate cancer by synergy of AKT with genotropic and nongenotropic actions of the androgen receptor. Proc Natl Acad Sci U S A 103:7789–7794
64. Migliaccio A, Castoria G, Di Domenico M, de Falco A, Bilancio A, Lombardi M, Barone MV, Ametrano D, Zannini MS, Abbondanza C, Auricchio F (2000) Steroid-induced androgen receptor-oestradiol receptor beta-Src complex triggers prostate cancer cell proliferation. EMBO J 19:5406–5417
65. Niu YN, Xia SJ (2009) Stroma-epitheliumepithelium crosstalk in prostate cancer. Asian J Androl 11:28–35
66. Niu Y, Altuwaijri S, Yeh S, Lai KP, Yu S, Chuang KH, Huang SP, Lardy H, Chang C (2008) Targeting the stromal androgen receptor in primary prostate tumors at earlier stages. Proc Natl Acad Sci U S A 105:12188–12193
67. Niu Y, Chang TM, Yeh S, Ma WL, Wang YZ, Chang C (2010) Differential androgen receptor signals in different cells explain why androgen-deprivation therapy of prostate cancer fails. Oncogene 29:3593–3604
68. Yuan TC, Veeramani S, Lin MF (2007) Neuroendocrine-like prostate cancer cells: neuroendocrine transdifferentiation of prostate adenocarcinoma cells. Endocr Relat Cancer 14:531–547
69. Amorino GP, Parsons SJ (2004) Neuroendocrine cells in prostate cancer. Crit Rev Eukaryot Gene Expr 14:287–300
70. Marchiani S, Tamburrino L, Nesi G, Paglierani M, Gelmini S, Orlando C, Maggi M, Forti G, Baldi E (2010) Androgen-responsive and -unresponsive prostate cancer cell lines respond differently to stimuli inducing neuroendocrine differentiation. Int J Androl 33:784–793

Mechanisms of Signal Transduction in Prostate Cancer: The Role of PI3-Kinase Pathway in Androgen Action

Laurent Morel and Silvère Baron

Abstract The androgen receptor deregulation is described as one of the key initiator event leading to a carcinogenetic process in the prostate gland. Canonical molecular mechanism of AR activation by its cognate ligands, testosterone and dihydrotestosterone (DHT), leads to the receptor translocation in the nucleus and to subsequent transcription of Androgen Response Element (ARE)-containing target genes that control cell cycle progression (e.g. p21) and cell survival (e.g. Bcl-2, IL6). Accumulating data suggests that intracellular signaling pathways are also the mediators of androgen action. Current knowledge indicates that connection between androgen receptor and Phosphatidylinositol 3-kinase (PI3K) both contributes to modulate genomic and non genomic activity of this nuclear receptor. Here we describe the modalities and discuss the consequences of such a connection on the prostate epithelium homeostasis. PI3K activation by AR occurs rapidly and in a transient fashion and represent a flexible and adaptive mechanism that may help to override apoptotic signals and to strengthen survival in normal prostatic epithelium. A dysregulation in this crosstalk may represent an oncogenic signal for cell maintenance and consequently promote prostate cancer development.

Keywords Prostate cancer · Phosphatidylinositol 3-kinase · Androgen receptor · Cell survival · Epithelial cell

---

L. Morel · S. Baron (✉)
Laboratoire Génétique, Reproduction et Développement (GRe D),
UMR CNRS 6247—Clermont Université—INSERM U931, 24,
Avenue des Landais, 80026 63171 Aubiere Cedex, France
e-mail: silvere.baron@univ-bpclermont.fr

L. Morel
e-mail: laurent.morel@univ-bpclermont.fr

G. Castoria and A. Migliaccio (eds.), *Advances in Rapid Sex-Steroid Action*,
DOI: 10.1007/978-1-4614-1764-4_11,

Abbreviations

AR	Androgen receptor
BAD	Bcl-2-associated death promoter
DHT	Dihydrotestosterone
EGF	Epidermal growth factor
EGFR	Epidermal growth factor receptor
Elk-1	Ets like gene1
ER	Estrogen receptor
ERK	Extracellular signal-regulated kinase
Fox	Forkhead box O transcription factors
GSK-3β	Glycogen synthase kinase-3 β
HER2	Human Epidermal growth factor Receptor 2
IGF	Insulin like growth factor
MAPK	Mitogen activated protein kinase
MDM2	Mouse double minute 2
MEK-1	Mitogen-activated protein (MAP) Kinase-1
mTOR	Mammalian target of rapamycin
mTORC1 and 2	mTOR Complex 1 and 2
PDK1	3-phosphoinositide-dependent protein kinase 1
PI3K	Phosphatidylinositol 3-kinase
PIN	Prostatic intraepithelial neoplasia
PTEN	Phosphatase and tensin homologue deleted on chromosome 10 gene
SH2	Src homology 2
SH3	Src homology 3
TSC1 and 2	Tuberous sclerosis complex 1 and 2

Contents

1 PI3Kinase/AKT Pathway and Prostate Cancer

1.1 The PI3K Family

Phosphatidylinositol 3-kinase (PI3K) enzymes are lipid kinases involved in diverse cellular processes including cell growth, migration, apoptosis, proliferation and differentiation. The PI3K signaling pathway is then considered as a driver of cell homeostasis, most notably in cells that are responding to growth-factor–receptor engagement. Although the PI3K pathway is considered as a single entity, there are multiple isoforms of PI3K. They can be divided in three classes according to their structure and substrate specificity in vitro [1–3]. Unlike class I PI3Ks, class II and class III enzymes are not yet linked to oncogenesis [4]. Class I are divided further into Class IA and IB subclasses. Class IA PI3Ks are heterodimeric proteins which consist of a regulatory subunit and a catalytic subunit. In mammals, three different genes encode the regulatory subunits. The PI3KR1 gene encodes p85α and the alternatively spliced variants p55α and p50α while the PI3KR2 and PI3KR3 genes encode p85β and p55γ subunits respectively. Associated to these regulatory subunits are three types of catalytic subunits, p110α, p110β and p110δ, which are encoded respectively by the PI3KCAα, PIK3CAβ and PIK3CAδ genes. Class IB is made of only one complex that associates the p110γ catalytic subunit, encoded by the PIK3CAγ gene to the p101 regulatory subunit. Such a dimer is activated by G protein-coupled receptors (GPCR) and Ras.

Considering class IA PI3Ks, the p85 regulatory subunit contains two Src homology domain (SH2), that recognizes phosphorylated tyrosine (T) residues, an inter-SH2 (iSH2) domain which constitutes a rigid tether for p110, a BCR domain (conserved domain related to sequences present in the break point cluster region—BCR-gene) and a SH3 domain able to bind to proline-rich motifs and mediate protein–protein interactions [5]. This subunit is activated by tyrosine-kinase coupled receptors such as EGF receptor or IGF-I receptor [6]. Firstly, p85 is recruited to the phosphorylated tyrosine residues of receptors via its SH2 domain. Secondly, the regulatory subunit associates to the p110 catalytic domain. This localizes the class IA p110 subunits in the membranes where their lipid substrates reside. The enzyme then catalyzes the phosphorylation of the PI[4,5]P2 phosphoinositides (PIP2) on the carbon at the D3 position of the inositol ring to generate PI[3,4,5]P3 (PIP3) [7]. The PIP3 target both the phosphoinositide-dependent kinase-1 (PDK-1) and its substrate, the protein kinase B (PKB/AKT), at the plasma membrane. The phosphorylation of AKT on the threonine (Thr)-308 residue by PDK1 leads to the subsequent phosphorylation of serine (Ser)-473 by the mTORC2 complex [8] and full activation of AKT.

1.2 AKT: The Main Transducer of the PI3K Signaling Pathway

AKT is a master kinase for a large panel of non redundant substrates [9]. In all cases AKT stimulates cell survival, cell proliferation and cell growth by favoring either the inhibition or the activation of downstream substrates. On one hand, AKT inhibits pro-apoptotic proteins (e.g. Bad, caspase 9) [10, 11], inhibitors of metabolic and cell growth signaling (e.g. GSK-3α/β and the mTOR pathway regulator TSC1/2) [12], cell cycle controllers and DNA damage response proteins (e.g. p27, Chk1) [13, 14], or transcription factors that promote apoptosis, cell-cycle arrest, and metabolic processes (e.g. the forkhead box O (FOXO) transcription factors −1, −3, and −4) [15–17]. On the other hand, AKT activates MDM2/HDM2 [18, 19], a negative regulator of p53, and the NFκB pathway following an activating phosphorylation of the IκB kinase IKKα [20, 21].

2 Deregulation of the PI3K Pathway and Prostate Cancer

The tight control of the PI3K/AKT pathway is dependent on the activity of two specific phosphatases. PTEN/MMAC1 (phosphatase and tensin homolog deleted on chromosome 10, mutated in multiple advanced cancers 1) was characterized to dephosphorylate PIP3 at the D3 position while SHIP1/2 (SH2-domain-containing inositol phosphatase 1/2) targets PIP3 dephosphorylation at the D5 position. In the absence of a fully active PTEN, activation of the PI3K dependent signaling can occur constitutively, in the absence of any exogenous stimulus [22]. The PI3K–PTEN signalling network thus functions as a crucial regulator of cell survival decisions and plays a central role in tumorigenesis. The importance of loss of function of PTEN was investigated in both localized and metastatic prostate cancers. Although frequency of PTEN inactivation consecutive to missense mutations, to loss of heterozygoty or to homozygous deletion vary considerably depending on the stage of the pathology and on the study considered, about 40% of primary and 70% of metastatic prostate cancers have genomic alterations involving the PTEN gene [23–29]. Transgenic mouse models that recapitulate features of the disease have also advanced understanding of this pathway. Mice with conditional, prostate-specific PTEN deletion have revealed the presence of prostate intraepithelial neoplasia (PIN) foci, invasive adenocarcinoma progressing to metastatic disease [30]. In accordance, a specific over-expression of AKT in mice prostate epithelium induces a similar development of PIN [31].

Prostate cancer progression is also dependent on androgens, given that prostate carcinoma dramatically regresses after androgen deprivation by castration or anti-hormonal therapy [32]. Most of androgens effects, but not all, are mediated by the androgen receptor (AR) that belongs to the nuclear receptor superfamily. Current knowledge indicates that connection between androgen receptor and PI3K both contributes to modulate genomic and non genomic activity of this nuclear receptor.

Various studies demonstrated that many posttranslational modifications of AR are PI3K and/or AKT-dependent, thus resulting in changes in AR trancriptional activity in normal and tumoral cells [16, 33–35].

In the present review, we report part of the connections that associate "androgen signaling" to PI3K/AKT pathway by focusing on the non genomic and genomic activation of the PI3K by the androgen receptor in prostate cancer.

3 Rapid Androgen Response and PI3K Crosstalk in Prostate Cancer

3.1 Genomic vs Non-genomic: the Two "Janus Faces" of Androgens Action

The androgen receptor is defined as a ligand-dependent transcription factor belonging to the "nuclear" receptor superfamily. Canonical molecular mechanism of AR activation by testosterone and dihydrotestosterone (DHT) leads to AR translocation in the nucleus and to subsequent transcription of Androgen Response Element (ARE)-containing target genes. Accumulating data suggests that intracellular signaling pathways, such as the PI3K/AKT pathway, can also be the target of the androgen receptor through both its classical transcriptional activity and a non-genomic mechanism. We and others have shown that upon R1881 binding, AR is able to contact the regulatory subunit p85α of the PI3K complex by direct interaction in normal epithelial cells [33]. This interaction leads to the activation of the p110α catalytic subunit. It results in an increase of PIP3 levels in the plasma membrane, subsequent AKT activation and phosphorylation of its downstream targets such as GSK3β, FKHRL1 and Bad. Interestingly, this system could be re-activated in PC3 prostatic cell line following AR re-expression. This was strengthened by experiments using AR inhibitor, bicalutamide and siRNA targeting AR [27, 33] indicating that this nuclear receptor, and not only a membrane receptor such as already suggested [36, 37], is able to trigger a non genomic signaling pathway. Kang et al. described a similar activation of the PI3K/AKT pathway by AR in an osteoblastic cell line [27] indicating that this mechanism is not restraint to prostate cells.

The association between AR and p85α is the basis of a larger complex that also involves the Src kinase [38]. Dominant negative Src completely abolished PI3K activation by AR indicating that this kinase plays a central role to integrate androgens non-genomic signal. Moreover, the presence of Src together with p85α and AR indicate that other signaling pathway could be activated, especially the MAPK pathway [39, 40]. Further evidences demonstrate that the level of activated AKT is directly correlated to androgens stimulation of cells and that it participates to the inhibition of TNFα and TRAIL induced apoptosis [41]. However, as AKT phosphorylation status was monitored 48 h following androgens treatment, it cannot be excluded that the PI3K pathway's stimulation result from AR genomic activities.

At the opposite, in some specific conditions, PI3K/AKT signaling may be down-regulated by androgens. Re-expression of AR in PC-3 cells was shown to interfere with EGFR signaling and to lead to changes in the cell proliferation and invasion properties. Stimulation of these cells with R1881 decreases the EGF-dependent activity of PI3K compared to native PC-3 cells. This demonstrates that liganded AR may negatively regulate the PI3K/AKT pathway by targeting upstream regulators of the kinase. This down-regulation originates from a direct interaction between EGFR and AR and then drives a decrease in the autophosphorylation of EGFR [42]. Such mechanism targets the interaction between EGFR and integrin $\alpha6\beta4$, and could explain the low malignant potential of PC3-AR cells [43].

Repression of PI3K activity may also be dependent on genomic action of AR. Recent study demonstrated a reciprocal feedback regulation of PI3K and androgen receptor signaling in prostate PTEN-deficient mice and in human prostate tumors [44]. High PI3K activity is here correlated with a down-regulation of numerous AR-target genes such as FKBP5. FKBP5 acts as a chaperone for the PHLPP, a phosphatase targeting phospho-AKT. Consequently, an increase in FKBP5 expression leads to PHLPP accumulation and to AKT inhibition. Further evidences for a negative regulation of PI3K/AKT pathway by AR nuclear activity were given by N-methyl-N-nitroso-urea (MNU) prostate tumor induced rat models. In these animals, the percentage of positive AR nuclei decreased during carcinogenesis while phospho-AKT staining increased [45]. This could result from acquisition of androgen independency since androgen deprivation of LNCaP cells results in a similar increase of PI3K activity associated with neuro-endocrine differentiation [46]. These data support the idea that AR can antagonize the PI3K/AKT pathway through a transcriptional process in the nucleus.

Altogether, these results demonstrate that AR and PI3K are connected at different levels that could modulate each other through mechanisms involved genomic and non-genomic action.

3.2 Androgen Receptor Subcellular Localisation: Reconcile Transcription and Transduction

As described above, binding of androgens to AR leads to the receptor translocation into the nucleus. However, most of studies showed that, depending on the ligand or the antagonist, AR exhibits different features of nuclear translocation [47] suggesting that AR cellular sub-localisation is a tightly regulated process. Paradoxically, the existence of AR non-genomic activities implies that a fraction of the liganded-receptor remains outside the nucleus and is targeted to the plasma membrane. We can assume that protein, such as HSPs [48] and the actin-binding protein FlnA [49], known to affect AR localisation in the sub-cellular compartment, play an important role in non-genomic androgen receptor action.

The cross-talk between AR and PI3K/AKT pathway takes place at the plasma membrane and was particularly analysed in LNCaP cells. AKT activity in membrane microdomains have been described to sustain most of the oncogenic properties of LNCaP cells [50]. Androgen receptor associated with lipid raft microdomain is able to interact directly with AKT in a PI3K independent mechanism since this crosstalk is insensitive to LY294002 [51]. Moreover, androgens promoted AKT activity in lipid rafts and myristoylated anchoring form of AR enhanced its localization in microdomains and limit the cell dependency from the PI3K in term of cell survival.

Finally, the existence of a membrane associated activity of the androgen receptor is consistent with a decisive role of the mechanisms controlling its subcellular localization in response to androgens. The challenge is now to better understand the relevance and the precise role of these mechanisms and of AR membrane activity in vivo during prostate carcinogenesis.

3.3 Features of Activation and Interaction Between Androgen Receptor and PI3K

The rapid response to androgens is characterized by its insensitivity to transcription and translation inhibitors and by the activation of downstream transduction pathways on the scale of a second or a minute. Although AR was shown to stimulate the PI3K/AKT pathway independently of its transcription activities, it cannot be ruled out whether a membrane receptor can also transduce the androgenic signal. Like for other steroids, rapid effects of androgens were first described to modulate (Ca^{2+}) in the cytoplasm [52–56] and this can be achieved by a testosterone-BSA conjugate suggesting that this effect is mediated by a cell surface receptor. This clearly raises the question of the nature of the complex that integrates the androgenic signal at the plasma membrane. Current knowledge indicates that at least three proteins are present in such a complex and are required to mediate the androgens signal: p85α, AR and Src (Fig. 1).

Convergent investigations demonstrated that AR interacts with the C-SH2 domain of p85α [33, 38]. More precisely, in vitro binding experiments demonstrated that the binding motif on AR, probably a phospho-tyrosine residue, is located between amino acids 1-537 [33] or 1-371 [38] even though the exact position of the interaction remains to be established. Baron et al. additionally identified an interaction between AR and the SH3 motif of p85α that probably engages the proline-rich motif located in the N-term region of AR (372–382). Unexpected results showed that AR deleted for the ligand binding domain is still able to mediate PI3K activation [38] suggesting that AR is necessary for building a functional protein complex but that it is not the receptor that integrates the

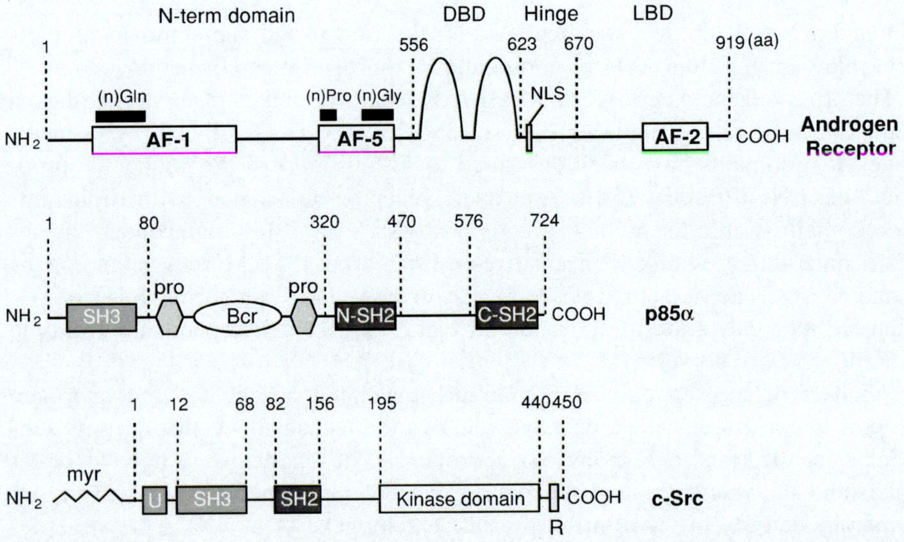

Fig. 1 Structural domains of Androgen Receptor (AR), p85α regulatory subunit of PI3-kinase and c-Src kinase *Androgen receptor* - AF-1 (Activating Factor), AF-2, AF-5: transactivation domains; Glu(n), Pro(n), Gly(n): Glutamine, Proline, Glycine strech respectively; DBD: DNA binding domain; Hinge: flexible domain; NLS: nuclear localisation signal; LBD: Ligand Binding Domain. *p85α* - SH3: protein interacting domain; pro: proline rich domain; Bcr: Breakpoint Cluster Region; N-SH2, C-SH2: Src-homology-2 located in N-term and in C-term, respectively. *c-Src* – myr, myristoylated sequence; U; unique region; SH3, protein interacting domain; SH2: Src-homology-2; R: regulatory domain

androgens signal. The authors then postulate the involvement of a putative androgen membrane receptor in the complex but this still needs to be demonstrated. Surprisingly, AR interaction with p85α is enhanced by R1881 treatment in vivo. This result is questioning since bicalutamide, an anti-androgen that specifically inhibits AR, also antagonizes androgen-dependent PI3K stimulation [33]. However, it still remains possible that a membrane receptor sensitive to anti-androgens mediates androgens signal. Further investigation should clarify how androgens signal is integrated in order to activate the PI3K.

Another important player present in the transducing complex is the Src kinase. Src represents an important transduction crossroad since it is able to connect PI3K to MAPK pathways. Other steroids receptor such ERα and PR have been described to interact with Src [40, 57, 58]. In order to propose a model of the complex associating AR, p85α and Src, we need to give an overview of already identified interactions. Sun et al. [38] proposed that p85α interacts with the N-terminal domain of AR (1-371) via its SH2 carboxy-terminal motif (624-718) (Fig. 2). But they did not identify precisely the motif of Src involved. Migliaccio et al. [40] demonstrated that, in LNCaP as well as MCF-7 and T47D cells, ERβ and ERα are involved in the complex and that they interact through the phosphorylated tyrosine

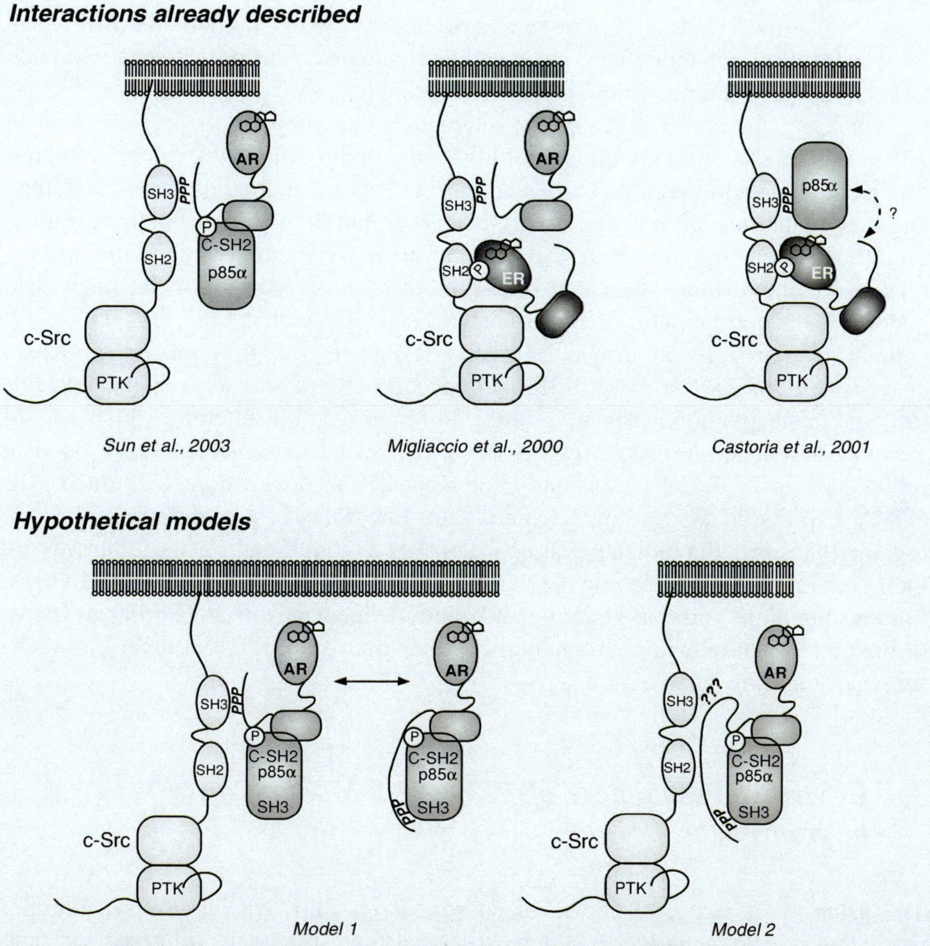

Fig. 2 Interactions already described and hypothetical models for AR/c-Src/p85α complex. AR: Androgen receptor; ER: Estrogen receptor; P: phosphorylation; SH3: protein interacting domain; PPP: proline rich domain; SH2: Src-homology-2; PTK: kinase domain

residue 537 with the SH2 domain of Src. In these experiments, in presence of R1881, AR is able to interact with the SH3 motif of Src via its proline-rich motif, providing evidence that this domain of AR is competent for the interaction with other proteins exhibiting SH3 domain, such as p85α. Finally, p85α association with AR engages both its SH3 and carboxyterminal SH2 domain [33]. These observations could be confusing since Proline-rich domain of AR cannot be engaged in the same time in an interaction with the SH3 motif of p85α and the SH3 motif of Src. Thus, we propose two different models that integrate this restricting parameter (Fig. 2). In a first model, we can consider the interaction between AR, p85α and Src as a dynamic process in which AR binding to the SH3 motif of the p85α and Src proteins is dependent of the kinetics and/or the presence of chaperone. The second model assumes that the SH3 motifs of p85α and Src interact with a domain of AR distinct from the proline-rich motif. This point will be elucidated by using AR construct with targeted domain deletion in the proline rich-domain.

Well characterized features of the interaction that supports the engagement of AR in this transduction complex could offer the opportunity to develop strategies for uncoupling non-genomic from genomic effects of androgens. It is clear that targeted mutations in AR could be an answer but it would need to carefully investigate their impact on AR transcription activity and co-regulators trans-repression. Interesting data came out from the use of NIH-3T3 cells, in which genomic and non-genomic activities have been dissociated [59]. In fact, small amount of androgens, as low as 0.001 nM R1881, is able to stimulate the association between AR, Src and PI3K without any AR translocation in the nucleus [60] and this activation is sensitive to the anti-androgen bicalutamide. Such a non-genomic mobilisation of AR triggers DNA synthesis in these cells. This was also reproduced in COS cells transiently transfected with low amont of human AR cDNA expression vector and treated with low R1881 concentrations. Taken together, these results indicate that non-genomic action of androgens, contrarily to their genomic activities, can be mediated by a small fraction of cellular AR. These findings highlight that non-genomic and genomic mechanisms are similar in terms of binding to natural and pharmacological ligand but very different regarding their sensitivity and mode of action.

3.4 *In vivo* Consequences of PI3K/AKT Modulation by Androgens

The *prima facie* opposite effects of androgens on PI3K/AKT pathway, alternatively positive or negative, could be disconcerting. The main difference is that positive regulation is mediated through AR non-genomic action and negative one through AR transcriptional activity. PI3K activation by AR occurs rapidly and in a transient fashion. This could be necessary in normal epithelial cell to override apoptotic signals and strengthen survival. Such a mechanism presents the advantage to be flexible and to support rapid adaptation for the maintenance of prostatic epithelium. On the contrary, genomic effects of AR mediate long term action of androgens since they mobilize the gene expression machinery [61]. We could assume that this process is dedicated to a long term cell regulation phenomenon such as cell differentiation and cell metabolism. The importance of each effect, genomic and non-genomic, in the field of prostate cancer needs to be deciphered. It is now clear that the crosstalk between AR and PI3K is involved in carcinogenesis, but the relevance of activation or inhibition process needs to be clarified. Using grafted mesenchyme of embryonic urogenital sinus under the kidney capsule, Xin et al. demonstrated that AKT synergizes with genotropic and nongenotropic actions of AR [62]. Unlike previous findings, Carver et al. [44] observed a reciprocal feedback regulation between AR signaling and PI3K/AKT pathway suggesting that AR activation results in a negative control of AKT activity [44]. Altogether, in vivo studies need to be extended in order to reconcile and decipher the "janus" effects of AR in prostate cancer.

References

1. Hawkins PT, Anderson KE, Davidson K, Stephens LR (2006) Signalling through class I PI3Ks in mammalian cells. Biochem Soc Trans 34:647–662
2. Leevers SJ, Vanhaesebroeck B, Waterfield MD (1999) Signalling through phosphoinositide 3-kinases: the lipids take centre stage. Curr Opin Cell Biol 11:219–225
3. Vanhaesebroeck B, Waterfield MD (1999) Signaling by distinct classes of phosphoinositide 3-kinases. Exp Cell Res 253:239–254
4. Zhao L, Vogt PK (2008) Class I PI3K in oncogenic cellular transformation. Oncogene 27:5486–5496
5. Vanhaesebroeck B, Leevers SJ, Panayotou G, Waterfield MD (1997) Phosphoinositide 3-kinases: a conserved family of signal transducers. Trends Biochem Sci 22:267–272
6. Inukai K, Funaki M, Anai M, Ogihara T, Katagiri H, Fukushima Y, Sakoda H, Onishi Y, Ono H, Fujishiro M, Abe M, Oka Y, Kikuchi M, Asano T (2001) Five isoforms of the phosphatidylinositol 3-kinase regulatory subunit exhibit different associations with receptor tyrosine kinases and their tyrosine phosphorylations. FEBS Lett 490:32–38
7. Rameh LE, Cantley LC (1999) The role of phosphoinositide 3-kinase lipid products in cell function. J Biol Chem 274:8347–8350
8. Sarbassov DD, Guertin DA, Ali SM, Sabatini DM (2005) Phosphorylation and regulation of Akt/PKB by the rictor-mTOR complex. Science 307:098–1101
9. Manning BD, Cantley LC (2007) AKT/PKB signaling: navigating downstream. Cell 129:1261–1274
10. Cardone MH, Roy N, Stennicke HR, Salvesen GS, Franke TF, Stanbridge E, Frisch S, Reed JC (1998) Regulation of cell death protease caspase-9 by phosphorylation. Science 282:1318–1321
11. Datta SR, Dudek H, Tao X, Masters S, Fu H, Gotoh Y, Greenberg ME (1997) Akt phosphorylation of BAD couples survival signals to the cell-intrinsic death machinery. Cell 91:231–241
12. Cross DA, Alessi DR, Cohen P, Andjelkovich M, Hemmings BA (1995) Inhibition of glycogen synthase kinase-3 by insulin mediated by protein kinase B. Nature 378:85–789
13. Fujita N, Sato S, Katayama K, Tsuruo T (2002) Akt-dependent phosphorylation of p27Kip1 promotes binding to 14–3-3 and cytoplasmic localization. J Biol Chem 277:28706–28713
14. Shtivelman E, Sussman J, Stokoe D (2002) A role for PI 3-kinase and PKB activity in the G2/M phase of the cell cycle. Curr Biol 12:919–924
15. Biggs WH 3rd, Meisenhelder J, Hunter T, Cavenee WK, Arden KC (1999) Protein kinase B/Akt-mediated phosphorylation promotes nuclear exclusion of the winged helix transcription factor FKHR1. Proc Natl Acad Sci USA 96:7421–7426
16. Brunet A, Bonni A, Zigmond MJ, Lin MZ, Juo P, Hu LS, Anderson MJ, Arden KC, Blenis J, Greenberg ME (1999) Akt promotes cell survival by phosphorylating and inhibiting a forkhead transcription factor. Cell 96:857–868
17. Rena G, Guo S, Cichy SC, Unterman TG, Cohen P (1999) Phosphorylation of the transcription factor forkhead family member FKHR by protein kinase B. J Biol Chem 274:17179–17183
18. Ashcroft M, Ludwig RL, Woods DB, Copeland TD, Weber HO, MacRae EJ, Vousden KH (2002) Phosphorylation of HDM2 by Akt. Oncogene 21:1955–1962

19. Mayo LD, Donner DB (2001) A phosphatidylinositol 3-kinase/Akt pathway promotes translocation of Mdm2 from the cytoplasm to the nucleus. Proc Natl Acad Sci USA 98:11598–11603
20. Beraud C, Henzel WJ, Baeuerle PA (1999) Involvement of regulatory and catalytic subunits of phosphoinositide 3-kinase in NF-kappa B activation. Proc Natl Acad Sci USA 96:429–434
21. Thomas KW, Monick MM, Staber JM, Yarovinsky T, Carter AB, Hunninghake GW (2002) Respiratory syncytial virus inhibits apoptosis and induces NF-kappa B activity through a phosphatidylinositol 3-kinase-dependent pathway. J Biol Chem 277:492–501
22. Stambolic V, Suzuki A, de la Pompa JL, Brothers GM, Mirtsos C, Sasaki T, Ruland J, Penninger JM, Siderovski DP, Mak TW (1998) Negative regulation of PKB/Akt-dependent cell survival by the tumor suppressor PTEN. Cell 95:29–39
23. Carracedo A, Pandolfi PP (2008) The PTEN-PI3K pathway: of feedbacks and cross-talks. Oncogene 27:5527–5541
24. Hollander MC, Blumenthal GM, Dennis PA (2011) PTEN loss in the continuum of common cancers, rare syndromes and mouse models. Nat Rev Cancer 11:289–301
25. Lee JT, Lehmann BD, Terrian DM, Chappell WH, Stivala F, Libra M, Martelli AM, Steelman LS, McCubrey JA (2008) Targeting prostate cancer based on signal transduction and cell cycle pathways. Cell Cycle 7:1745–1762
26. McMenamin ME, Soung P, Perera S, Kaplan I, Loda M, Sellers WR (1999) Loss of PTEN expression in paraffin-embedded primary prostate cancer correlates with high gleason score and advanced stage. Cancer Res 59:4291–4296
27. Rhei E, Kang L, Bogomolniy F, Federici MG, Borgen PI, Boyd J (1997) Mutation analysis of the putative tumor suppressor gene PTEN/MMAC1 in primary breast carcinomas. Cancer Res 57:3657–3659
28. Singh B, Ittmann MM, Krolewski JJ (1998) Sporadic breast cancerbreast cancers exhibit loss of heterozygosity on chromosome segment 10q23 close to the cowden disease locus. Genes Chromosom Cancer 21:166–171
29. Steelman LS, Stadelman KM, Chappell WH, Horn S, Basecke J, Cervello M, Nicoletti F, Libra M, Stivala F, Martelli AM, McCubrey JA (2008) Akt as a therapeutic target in cancer. Expert Opin Ther Targets 12:1139–1165
30. Ma X, Ziel-van der Made AC, Autar B, van der Korput HA, Vermeij M, van Duijn P, Cleutjens KB, de Krijger R, Krimpenfort P, Berns A, van der Kwast TH, Trapman J (2005) Targeted biallelic inactivation of P ten in the mouse prostate leads to prostate cancer accompanied by increased epithelial cell proliferation but not by reduced apoptosis. Cancer Res 65:5730–5739
31. Majumder PK, Yeh JJ, George DJ, Febbo PG, Kum J, Xue Q, Bikoff R, Ma H, Kantoff PW, Golub TR, Loda M, Sellers WR (2003) Prostate intraepithelial neoplasia induced by prostate restricted Akt activation: the MPAKT model. Proc Natl Acad Sci USA 100:7841–7846
32. Huggins C, Hodges CV (1941) The effect of castration, of estrogen and of androgen injection on serum phosphatases in metastatic carcinoma of the prostate. Cancer Res 1:293–297
33. Baron S, Manin M, Beaudoin C, Leotoing L, Communal Y, Veyssiere G, Morel L (2004) Androgen receptor mediates non-genomic activation of phosphatidylinositol 3-OH kinase in androgen-sensitive epithelial cells. J Biol Chem 279:14579–14586
34. Sharma M, Chuang WW, Sun Z (2002) Phosphatidylinositol 3-kinasePhosphatidylinositol 3-kinase/Akt stimulates androgen pathway through GSK3beta inhibition and nuclear beta-catenin accumulation. J Biol Chem 277:30935–30941
35. Wen Y, Hu MC, Makino K, Spohn B, Bartholomeusz G, Yan DH, Hung MC (2000) HER-2/neu promotes androgen-independent survival and growth of prostate cancer cells through the Akt pathway. Cancer Res 60:6841–6845
36. Hatzoglou A, Kampa M, Kogia C, Charalampopoulos I, Theodoropoulos PA, Anezinis P, Dambaki C, Papakonstanti EA, Stathopoulos EN, Stournaras C, Gravanis A, Castanas E (2005) Membrane androgen receptor activation induces apoptotic regression of human prostate cancer cells in vitro and in vivo. J Clin Endocrinol Metab 90:893–903

37. Papadopoulou N, Charalampopoulos I, Anagnostopoulou V, Konstantinidis G, Foller M, Gravanis A, Alevizopoulos K, Lang F, Stournaras C (2008) Membrane androgen receptor activation triggers down-regulation of PI-3K/Akt/NF-kappa B activity and induces apoptotic responses via Bad, FasL and caspase-3 in DU145 prostate cancer cells. Mol Cancer 7:88
38. Sun M, Yang L, Feldman RI, Sun XM, Bhalla KN, Jove R, Nicosia SV, Cheng JQ (2003) Activation of phosphatidylinositol 3-kinase/Akt pathway by androgen through interaction of p85alpha, androgen receptor, and Src. J Biol Chem 278:42992–43000
39. Kousteni S, Bellido T, Plotkin LI, O'Brien CA, Bodenner DL, Han L, Han K, DiGregorio GB, Katzenellenbogen JA, Katzenellenbogen BS, Roberson PK, Weinstein RS, Jilka RL, Manolagas SC (2001) Nongenotropic, sex-nonspecific signaling through the estrogen or androgen receptors: dissociation from transcriptional activity. Cell 104:719–730
40. Migliaccio A, Castoria G, Di Domenico M, de Falco A, Bilancio A, Lombardi M, Barone MV, Ametrano D, Zannini MS, Abbondanza C, Auricchio F (2000) Steroid-induced androgen receptor-oestradiol receptor beta-Src complex triggers prostate cancer cell proliferation. EMBO J 19:5406–5417
41. Rokhlin OW, Taghiyev AF, Guseva NV, Glover RA, Chumakov PM, Kravchenko JE, Cohen MB (2005) Androgen regulates apoptosis induced by TNFR family ligands via multiple signaling pathways in LNCaP. Oncogene 24:6773–6784
42. Bonaccorsi L, Marchiani S, Muratori M, Carloni V, Forti G, Baldi E (2004) Signaling mechanisms that mediate invasion in prostate cancer cells. Ann N Y Acad Sci 1028:283–288
43. Bonaccorsi L, Muratori M, Carloni V, Zecchi S, Formigli L, Forti G, Baldi E (2003) Androgen receptor and prostate cancer invasion. Int J Androl 26:21–25
44. Carver BS, Chapinski C, Wongvipat J, Hieronymus H, Chen Y, Chandarlapaty S, Arora VK, Le C, Koutcher J, Scher H, Scardino PT, Rosen N, Sawyers CL (2011) Reciprocal feedback regulation of PI3K and androgen receptor signaling in PTEN-deficient prostate cancer. Cancer Cell 19:575–586
45. Liao Z, Wang S, Boileau TW, Erdman JW Jr, Clinton SK (2005) Increased phospho-AKT is associated with loss of the androgen receptor during the progression of N-methyl-N-nitrosourea-induced prostate carcinogenesis in rats. Prostate 64:186–199
46. Murillo H, Huang H, Schmidt LJ, Smith DI, Tindall DJ (2001) Role of PI3K signaling in survival and progression of LNCaP prostate cancer cells to the androgen refractory state. Endocrinology 14:4795–4805
47. Georget V, Terouanne B, Lumbroso S, Nicolas JC, Sultan C (1998) Trafficking of androgen receptor mutants fused to green fluorescent protein: a new investigation of partial androgen insensitivity syndrome. J Clin Endocrinol Metab 83:3597–3603
48. Zoubeidi A, Zardan A, Beraldi E, Fazli L, Sowery R, Rennie P, Nelson C, Gleave M (2007) Cooperative interactions between androgen receptor (AR) and heat-shock protein 27 facilitate AR transcriptional activity. Cancer Res 67:10455–10465
49. Ozanne DM, Brady ME, Cook S, Gaughan L, Neal DE, Robson CN (2000) Androgen receptor nuclear translocation is facilitated by the f-actin cross-linking protein filamin. Mol Endocrinol 14:1618–1626
50. Adam RM, Mukhopadhyay NK, Kim J, Di Vizio D, Cinar B, Boucher K, Solomon KR, Freeman MR (2007) Cholesterol sensitivity of endogenous and myristoylated Akt. Cancer Res 67:6238–6246
51. Cinar B, Mukhopadhyay NK, Meng G, Freeman MR (2007) Phosphoinositide 3-kinase-independent non-genomic signals transit from the androgen receptor to Akt1 in membrane raft microdomains. J Biol Chem 282:29584–29593
52. Benten WP, Lieberherr M, Sekeris CE, Wunderlich F (1997) Testosterone induces Ca^{2+} influx via non-genomic surface receptors in activated T cells. FEBS Lett 407:211–214
53. Falkenstein E, Tillmann HC, Christ M, Feuring M, Wehling M (2000) Multiple actions of steroid hormones–a focus on rapid, nongenomic effects. Pharmacol Rev 52:513–556
54. Gorczynska E, Handelsman DJ (1995) Androgens rapidly increase the cytosolic calcium concentration in sertoli cells. Endocrinology 136:2052–2059

55. Kampa M, Papakonstanti EA, Alexaki VI, Hatzoglou A, Stournaras C, Castanas E (2004) The opioid agonist ethylketocyclazocine reverts the rapid, non-genomic effects of membrane testosterone receptors in the human prostate LNCaP cell line. Exp Cell Res 294:434–445
56. Lyng FM, Jones GR, Rommerts FF (2000) Rapid androgen actions on calcium signaling in rat sertoli cells and two human prostatic cell lines: similar biphasic responses between 1 picomolar and 100 nanomolar concentrations. Biol Reprod 63:736–747
57. Ballare C, Uhrig M, Bechtold T, Sancho E, Di Domenico M, Migliaccio A, Auricchio F, Beato M (2003) Two domains of the progesterone receptor interact with the estrogen receptor and are required for progesterone activation of the c-Src/Erk pathway in mammalian cells. Mol Cell Biol 23:1994–2008
58. Boonyaratanakornkit V, Scott MP, Ribon V, Sherman L, Anderson SM, Maller JL, Miller WT, Edwards DP (2001) Progesterone receptor contains a proline-rich motif that directly interacts with SH3 domains and activates c-Src family tyrosine kinases. Mol Cell 8:269–280
59. Castoria G, Lombardi M, Barone MV, Bilancio A, Di Domenico M, De Falco A, Varricchio L, Bottero D, Nanayakkara M, Migliaccio A, Auricchio F (2004) Rapid signalling pathway activation by androgens in epithelial and stromal cells. Steroids 69:517–522
60. Castoria G, Lombardi M, Barone MV, Bilancio A, Di Domenico M, Bottero D, Vitale F, Migliaccio A, Auricchio F (2003) Androgen-stimulated DNA synthesis and cytoskeletal changes in fibroblasts by a nontranscriptional receptor action. J Cell Biol 161:547–556
61. Wang Y, Kreisberg JI, Ghosh PM (2007) Cross-talk between the androgen receptor and the phosphatidylinositol 3-kinase/Akt pathway in prostate cancer. Curr Cancer Drug Targets 7:591–604
62. Xin L, Teitell MA, Lawson DA, Kwon A, Mellinghoff IK, Witte ON (2006) Progression of prostate cancer by synergy of AKT with genotropic and nongenotropic actions of the androgen receptor. Proc Natl Acad Sci USA 103:7789–7794

The IGF-I Axis in Prostate Cancer: The Role of Rapid Steroid Actions

Antonino Belfiore

Abstract Dysregulation of the IGF-I axis involving increased IGF-I receptor (IGF-IR) expression and/or increased/aberrant production of cognate ligands insulin-like growth factors (IGF) I and II plays a role in the development and progression of a variety of malignancies, including prostate cancer. Recent studies indicate that membrane-initiated effects of both androgens and estrogens provide a non-mutational mechanism for marked IGF-IR upregulation in prostate cancer cells. This mechanism is specific and does not affect the homologous insulin receptor. IGF-IR upregulation by sex steroids requires steroid receptor location at the membrane level and the activation of the Src/ERK pathway. This pathway eventually activates the transcription factor CREB by phosphorylating it at Ser133. Activated CREB binds to a newly identified region located at the 5′UTR fragment of the IGF-IR promoter and stimulates IGF-IR gene transcription. IGF-IR upregulation sensitizes prostate cancer cells to the proliferative and protumor effects of IGFs. As IGF-IR activation by IGFs contributes to CREB activation, this mechanism may be involved in a positive feed-back loop implicated in IGF-IR overexpression in prostate cancer cells. These data suggest that current anti-hormone therapies should be complemented with inhibitors of this Src/ERK/CREB/IGF-IR pathway.

Keywords Prostate cancer · Rapid steroid effects · Androgens · Estrogens · Nongenomic · IGF-I receptor · Insulin receptor · IGF-I · IGF-II · IGF axis

A. Belfiore (✉)
Department of Clinical and Experimental Medicine,
University of Catanzaro, 88100 Catanzaro, Italy
e-mail: belfiore@unicz.it

G. Castoria and A. Migliaccio (eds.), *Advances in Rapid Sex-Steroid Action*,
DOI: 10.1007/978-1-4614-1764-4_12,

Abbreviations

AR	Androgen receptor
ATF	Activating transcription factor
BAD	Bcl-2-associated death promoter
BMax	Bound maximum
CaMKII	Calcium/Calmodulin-Dependent Protein Kinase II
Cav-1	Caveolin-1
CBP	CREB-binding protein
C/EBPb	CCAAT enhancer binding protein-b
ChIP	Chromatin Immunoprecipitation
CRE	cAMP response elements
CREB	cAMP response element-binding
CREM	cAMP-responsive element modulator
DHT	Diidrotestosterone
4EBP1	eukaryotic initiation factor 4E binding protein
EGFR	Epidermal growth factor receptor
Elk-1	Ets LiKe gene1
ER	Estrogen receptor
ERK	Extracellular signal-regulated kinase
EREs	Estrogen response elements
E2	Estradiol
Fox	Forkhead box O transcription factors
GH	Growth hormone
GHRH	Growth-hormone-releasing hormone
GSK-3β	Glycogen synthase kinase-3β
GTPase	Guanosine triphosphate hydrolase
HB-EGF	Heparin-binding EGF-like growth factor
HER2	Human Epidermal growth factor Receptor 2
HR	Hybrid receptor
HB-EGF	Heparin-binding EGF
IGF	Insulin growth factor
IGF-IR	IGF-I receptor
IGFBP	IGF-binding protein
IR	Insulin receptor
IRS-1 and-2	Insulin receptor substrates 1 and-2
MAPK	Mitogen activated protein kinase
MEK-1	Mitogen-activated protein (MAP) Kinase Kinase
MISS	Membrane initiated steroid effects
MMP-2 and MMP-9	Matrix metalloproteinases 2 and 9
mTOR	Mammalian target of rapamycin
mTORC1 and 2	mTOR Complex 1 and 2
M6P/IGF-IIR	Mannose-6-phosphate/IGF-II receptor
NEFA	Non-esterificated fatty acids
PDK1	3-phosphoinositide-dependent protein kinase 1
PKC	Protein kinase C

PI3-K	Phosphatidylinositol 3-kinase
PIP3	Phosphatidylinositol 3,4,5-trisphosphate
PTEN	Phosphatase and tensin homologue deleted on chromosome 10 gene
p38-MAPK	p38 mitogen-activated protein kinase
p70S6K	ribosomal S6 Kinase
Ras	RAt Sarcoma
SH2	Src homology 2
SV40	Simian virus-40
TRAMP	Transgenic adenocarcinoma of the mouse prostate
TSC1 and 2	Tuberous sclerosis complex 1 and 2
UTR	UnTraslated Region
WT-1	Wilms tumor protein 1

Contents

1 Introduction

The insulin-like growth factor I (IGF-I) axis plays a key role in regulating growth, resistance to apoptosis, and invasion in a variety of malignancies, including prostate cancer [1, 2]. The IGF-I axis comprises three closely related growth factors (IGF-I, IGF-II, and insulin), which bind and activate two homologous but distinct receptors of the tyrosine kinase superfamily, the IGF-I receptor (IGF-IR) and the insulin receptor (IR). The activity of the IGF-I axis is also regulated by a third, unrelated receptor, the mannose-6-phosphate receptor/IGF-II receptor (M6P/IGF-IIR), which has no enzymatic activity and binds only IGF-II, targeting it to lysosomal degradation, and by six IGF binding proteins (IGFBP-1 to -6) that control the bioavailability of both IGF-I and IGF-II [3].

Prostate cancer is commonly responsive to androgens at its early stages and may regress with androgen deprivation therapy. However, at later stages it is resistant to androgen deprivation as well as to other available therapies [4]. Many factors account for prostate cancer progression to androgen independence, including the activation of androgen receptor (AR) signaling pathway in androgen-independent ways [5]. Moreover, abnormal activation of the IGF-I axis should be considered a candidate factor implicated in prostate cancer progression to androgen independence [6–10]. IGF-IR overexpression and autocrine/paracrine expression of cognate ligands are common mechanisms underlying dysregulation of the IGF-I axis during cancer progression [2]. IGF-IR overexpression is only rarely caused by gene amplification whereas it is often associated to mutations or functional activation of anti-oncogenes [11]. Moreover, there is evidence of extensive cross-talk between the IGF-IR and sex steroid signaling in various model systems, especially in breast cancer, where the two pathways synergize for tumor growth promotion [12].

In prostate cancer we recently described a new, non-mutational mechanism for IGF-IR overexpression induced by membrane initiated steroid effects (MISS). Through this mechanism, both androgens and estrogens may sensitize cancer cells to the biological effects of IGFs and contribute, therefore, to cancer progression to androgen independence.

2 Dysregulation of the IGF Axis and Prostate Cancer

2.1 Experimental Studies

Transgenic mice overexpressing IGF-I usually develop organomegaly [13]. However, transgenic mice expressing human IGF-I in basal epithelial cells of prostate and undergoing selective IGF-IR activation develop stepwise prostate oncogenesis, including hyperplasia, intraepithelial neoplasia, and adenocarcinoma [14]. Other studies have found that IGF-I overexpression induces spontaneous preneoplastic changes in the prostate in a genetically engineered mouse model but that the development of aggressive metastatic tumors requires selection against IGF-I signals [15]. An explanation of these findings was provided in a further study where abrogation of IGF-IR expression in the prostate induced p53-regulated apoptosis while conditional abrogation of IGF-IR expression in young animals was associated with cell proliferation and the emergence of aggressive prostate cancer in mice with compromised p53 activity [16]. These data suggest that IGF-IR has a dual role in the prostate epithelium. On one hand it suppresses cellular senescence and apoptosis allowing deregulated cell survival and transformation, while, on the other hand, it induces a p53-dependent differentiation block. Aggressive cancers ensue when this block become inefficient.

The transgenic adenocarcinoma of the mouse prostate (TRAMP) model obtained by transgenic expression of SV40 T antigen is often used to study the pathogenesis of prostate cancer, as male TRAMP mice spontaneously develop prostate tumors following the onset of puberty. In the TRAMP mouse, when circulating levels of both GH and IGF-I are reduced by a germ-line mutation that inactivates the GHRH receptor, the risk to develop prostate cancer is reduced and cancer progression is slowed [17].

Collectively, these data in the animal model support a complex role for IGF-IR signaling in prostate tumorigenesis and are in good agreement with data obtained in human prostate cancer cell cultures where IGF-I increases cell proliferation and survival [10, 18]. In addition, IGF-IR is often overexpressed in human prostate cancer as compared to matched normal prostate tissues [19].

Conflicting data are available for the role of IGF-IR in progression of human prostate cancer. Some studies have found either a direct correlation between IGF-IR expression and metastatic behavior [17, 20] while others have found no such correlation [21], or even an inverse correlation [22]. In a model where human primary prostate epithelial cells were immortalized with SV40 T antigen (P69 line) or rendered malignant and metastatic by further selection in nude mice (M12 line), IGF-IR was transcriptionally repressed in malignant and metastatic cells as a result of increased expression of the WT-1 tumor suppressor [23]. However, in human prostate cancer xenografts, progression to androgen independence is associated with increased expression of both IGF-IR and IGF-I [24, 25] and increased responsiveness to IGF-I [26]. A recent study found a positive immunostaining for both IRs and IGF-IR in prostate carcinomas, implying the presence of IR/IGF-IR hybrids [27]. According to this study, IGF-IR were similarly expressed in cancer tissues and in benign prostate hyperplasia whereas IRs were more intensely expressed in cancer tissues and increased with Gleason score [27] suggesting that, in advanced prostate cancers IGF-I binding sites increase as a result of increased IR/IGF-IR hybrids.

As far as blocking therapies targeting the IGF axis are concerned, IGF-IR downregulation obtained by an antisense RNA strategy resulted in significant suppression of human prostate cancer cell invasion and proliferation in vitro [19]. Human monoclonal antibodies, which specifically recognize IGF-II, have been used to specifically inhibit IGF-IR phosphorylation and downstream kinases Akt and MAPK [28]. One of these antibodies, at nanomolar concentrations, was shown to inhibit growth of human prostate cancer cells. A similar antibody inhibited the growth of human prostate cancer cells transplanted in the context of human bone in immunodeficient mice [29]. In a recent study it was found that suppression of IGF-IR expression by a 2′-MOE-modified antisense oligonucleotide was associated with decreased proliferation and survival of cultured prostate cancer cells and suppressed or delayed prostate tumor growth in xenografts [30].

Enhanced IGF-IR signaling also correlates with resistance to therapies that target other kinases, including the EGFR [31], HER2, mTOR and others [32].

2.2 Epidemiology

Several studies have reported an association between abdominal obesity and increased risk for various malignancies, including carcinomas of the breast, colon-rectus, endometrium, stomach and prostate [33–35] while weight control is associated with a decreased cancer risk [36, 37]. With regard to prostate cancer, obesity is especially associated with an increased risk of cancer aggressiveness and mortality [38].

Although several factors may contribute to the increased cancer risk of obese patients, hyperinsulinemia and increased free levels of IGFs are considered major factors underlying the increased cancer risk associated with obesity. Various studies have directly correlated the level of circulating IGFs and the occurrence of prostate cancer [6, 39]. Forty-two studies published worldwide and correlating levels of IGFs or IGFBPs with prostate cancer occurrence have been recently examined and subjected to meta-analysis [40]. Results have shown a 21% increased risk per standard deviation increase in IGF-I, while a modestly reduced risk was associated to IGFBP-3 increase. Both IGF-I and IGFBP-3 were more strongly associated with advanced disease. Similar results have been reached by a previous analysis of 12 prospective studies, which found a 38% increased risk of prostate cancer when considering the highest quintiles vs. lowest quintiles of IGF-I [41].

The degree of this increased risk of prostate cancer in relationship to IGF-I is in the same range as the increase of ischemic heart disease in relationship to increased diastolic blood pressure or increased total cholesterol [40, 42].

Taken together, these data indicate that the IGF axis is an important role in prostate cancer initiation and progression.

3 Cross-Talk Between Sex Steroids and the IGF Axis

3.1 The IGF-I Receptor and Its Signaling Pathways

The IGF-IR is a transmembrane receptor with intrinsic tyrosine kinase activity. Upon ligand binding IGF-IR becomes phosphorylated on several tyrosine residues [43] located in the juxta-membrane region, in the catalytic domain, and in the carboxy-terminal [44]. These phosphotyrosine residues are docking sites for Src homology 2 (SH2)-containing domain substrates. Major substrates that bind to IGF-IR include Insulin Receptor Substrates (IRS) and Shc proteins [45, 46]. These proteins bind the juxtamembrane domain and are phosphorylated on several tyrosine residues that act as docking sites for other kinases or adaptors, such as Phosphatidyl-inositol-3-kinase (PI3-kinase) [47], Grb2 [48] and others. These reactions activate two major signaling pathways: the ERK1/2 cascade, which is mainly implicated in the stimulation of cell proliferation and the PI3-K pathway, which is mainly implicated in the regulation of cell growth and survival.

Activation of the ERK1/2 cascade requires the recruitment of Grb/Sos complex to IRS or Shc proteins, which triggers the activation of GTPase Ras and downstream signaling effectors RAF kinase, MEK1/2 and ERK1/2; Activated ERK1/2 phosphorylate proteins in the cytosol and also translocate into the nucleus, where they regulate important cellular processes [49, 50]. The activation of the PI3-K cascade involves the activation of the PI3-K catalytic subunit (p110) following the binding of the regulatory domain (p85) to IRS or Shc proteins and PI3-K recruitment to the plasma membrane where it induces the production of the phosphatidylinositol-3, 4, 5-triphosphate (PIP3). PIP3 activates the 3-phosphoinositide-dependent protein kinase 1 (PDK1) and AKT, which are negatively regulated by the lipid phosphatase PTEN, which dephosphorylates PIP3.

AKT activates several targets involved in various cell processes, including cell survival (BAD), gene transcription (FoxO) and ribosome biogenesis (TSC1/TSC2 and mTOR) [51, 52]. mTOR exists in two distinct complexes: mTORC1 (mTOR-raptor) and mTORC2 (mTOR-rictor). IGF-I modulates mTORC1 complex activity through the activation of both the ERK1/2 and the PI3-K cascades. Activated mTORC1 enhances protein synthesis by the phosphorylation of two major targets: ribosomal S6 Kinase (p70S6K) and eukaryotic initiation factor 4E binding protein (4EBP1), both of which positively regulate cell growth [53]. AKT also inhibits GSK-3β function allowing β-catenin to translocate into the nucleus, where it regulates the transcription of genes involved in proliferation, such as cyclin D1 [54].

3.2 IGF-I May Affect AR Transcriptional Activity

Various studies have shown cross-talk between the IGF axis and sex steroids in cancer. IGF-I may affect AR signaling in prostate cancer by various mechanisms. Whether IGF-I may transactivate the AR in human prostate cancer cells in the absence of androgens is controversial. While some studies have obtained positive results [55], others have been unable to confirm these findings [56]. More recently, the possibility has been raised that the IGF-I effect on AR transcriptional activity is complex [57]. IGF-I could enhance androgen-stimulated AR transcriptional activity in non-metastatic prostate cancer cells while suppressing it in metastatic cells. In LNCaP prostate cancer cells, IGF-I, via Ras/MAPK pathway, may sensitize the AR transcriptional complex to sub-physiological androgens concentrations [58]. Moreover, the activation of the PI3-K/Akt pathway by IGF-I may phosphorylate the AR at Ser-210 and Ser-790 and inhibit the interaction between AR and co-regulators [59].

3.3 IGF-IR and Membrane-Initiated Effects of Sex Steroids

Little is known about the possible interrelationship between the IGF-IR and membrane-initiated actions of sex steroids. Membrane ER and AR appear to be located in specialized membrane domains named lipid rafts, which are privileged locations for the assembly of multiprotein signal some complexes. These complexes may include nonreceptor tyrosine kinases, such as Src and PI3-K [60], G proteins, but also receptor tyrosine kinase such as IGF-IR [61].

For the human ER-α the mechanism of transport to the membrane has been recently characterized. It requires receptor palmitoylation at cystine 447 [62] and subsequent binding to caveolin-1 (Cav-1), which facilitates ER transport to and localization at the membrane [63]. ER-α palmitoylation as well as the integrity of the E domain (ligand-binding domain) are required for ER-dependent ERK1/2 and PI3-K activation and consequent cell proliferation [64]. Recently, a lipid raft association has been reported also for ARs in LNCap prostate cancer cells [65]. A conserved mechanism for translocation to the plasma membrane seems, therefore, to be common to ER-α and AR [65].

IGF-IR is also present in lipid rafts and interacts directly with Cav-1 in caveolae [66]. Cav-1 is tyrosine phosphorylated after IGF-I stimulation and Cav-1 silencing greatly reduces IGF-IR activation and downstream signaling [66].

It has been suggested that ERK1/2 activation by E2 occurs as the consequence of the activation of a cascade which involves Src-mediated activation of MMP2, and MMP9, followed by proteolytic release of HB-EGF and consequent EGFR activation and ERK1/2 phosphorylation [63].

However, it has recently been shown that the activation of this cascade by E2 in MCF-7 breast cancer cells is initiated by the activation of IGF-IR [67]. Blockade of EGFR was not sufficient to abrogate IGF-I-induced ERK1/2 activation, suggesting that IGF-IR has EGFR independent ways to activate ERK1/2. In contrast, other authors have shown that IGF-IR may activate EGFR by physical binding and not by activating the IGF-IR-MMP-EGFR cascade [68]. In any case, the involvement of IGF-IR in the activation of the ERK pathway in breast cancer cells exposed to estrogens seems very likely while it is unclear whether a similar mechanism operates for androgen-dependent ERK1/2 activation in prostate cancer.

4 Sex Steroids Induce IGF-IR Up-Regulation via Membrane-Initiated Effects

4.1 Effects of Androgens

Using LNCaP AR positive human prostate cells, we found that androgens induced a marked increase (approximately 7 folds) in IGF-IR expression [69]. This effect was relatively rapid, starting 6–12 h after androgen exposure, and dose-dependent through a concentration range of 0.01–10.0 nM. IGF-I binding sites concomitantly increased with a BMax of 36.0 pM in androgen-exposed cells vs. 5.6 pM in untreated cells while IGF-I binding affinity was not significantly affected [69]. Androgens were able to activate ERK1/2 by c-Src-dependent mechanism, as previously described by others [60] and inhibition of either MEK-1 or c-Src completely blocked IGF-IR upregulation. Classical antiandrogens, instead, were only marginally effective.

In AR negative PC-3 cells, IGF-IR expression did not change in response to androgens. AR-transfected PC-3 cell clones, however, responded to androgens with IGF-IR upregulation proportional to the level of AR expression [69]. While these findings suggested the involvement of a rapid, membrane-initiated effect of androgens, the use of AR variants lacking the ability to bind DNA, provided proof-of-concept that the classical genomic pathway was not involved. We used two different AR mutants (AR-C619Y and AR-881), both lacking DNA binding capacity and transcriptional activity, although able to elicit rapid membrane-initiated effects. The AR-C619Y mutant, previously identified in prostate cancer cells, carries a substitution of a tyrosine for a cysteine at amino acid 619, near the cysteine that coordinates zinc in the AR DNA-binding domain [70]. The AR-881 mutant was found in a male affected by a phenotype of complete androgen insensitivity and is characterized by the inability to translocate into the nucleus [71, 72]. Both AR mutants enhanced IGF-IR promoter activity and induced IGF-IR up-regulation similarly to the AR wt. This activity was inhibited by co-transfection with Src or MEK dominant-negative constructs [69].

LNCaP cells, which have low basal IGF-IR expression and are unresponsive to IGF-I, responded to IGF-I with increased mitogenesis, migration and protection from apoptosis only after pre-incubation with androgens (Fig. 1). Others have also reported increased responsiveness to IGF-I in LNCaP cells exposed to androgens [73] although they have not explained the mechanism of this finding.

4.2 *Effects of Estrogens*

Various evidences suggest that, besides androgens, estrogens may also play a role in prostate cancer. Most primary prostate cancers express the beta subtype of the estrogen receptor (ER-β) [74] while the classical alpha subtype (ER-α) is mostly silenced by DNA hyper-methylation. ER-β is commonly expressed in prostate cancer metastases, suggesting a role of this receptor in late-stage cancer [75]. Moreover, ER antagonists may inhibit growth and/or induce apoptosis in prostate cancer cell lines that express either only ER-β or both ER subtypes [74, 76].

A number of studies, mostly carried out in breast cancer cells, have shown that estrogens and the IGF system may functionally interact, resulting in reciprocal potentiation of their signaling pathways [12, 77, 78]. By binding to the ER-α estrogens are able to increase IGF-I actions with a variety of mechanisms. Estrogens increase IGF-I binding and IGF-IR mRNA expression [79] and are also

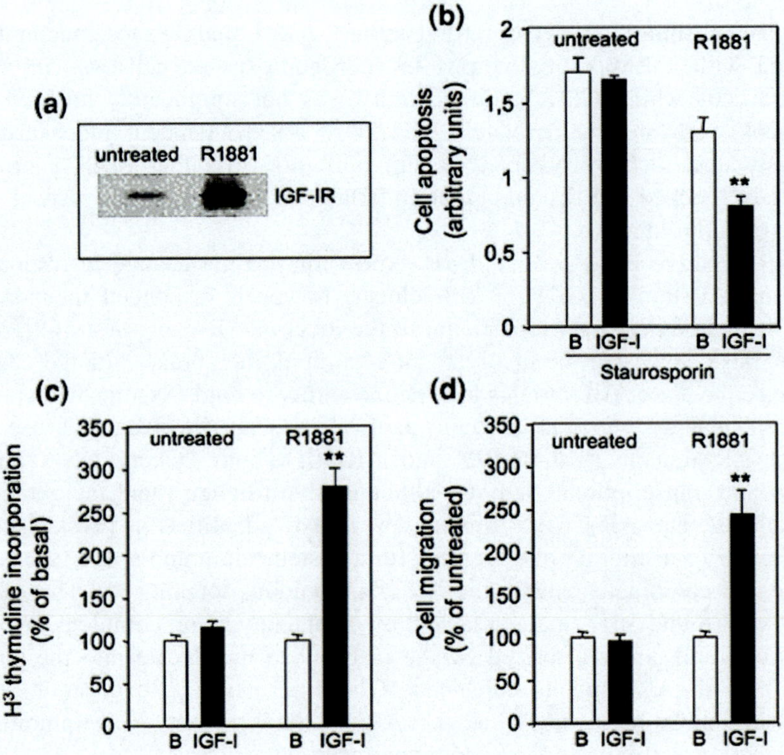

Fig. 1 Enhanced biological responses to IGF-I in LNCaP cells exposed to androgen R1881. **a** R1881-pretreated LNCaP cells show up-regulated IGF-IR levels. **b** IGF-I (10 nM) exposure induces significant protection from staurosporin-induced apoptosis, **c** increase of [3H]thymidine incorporation, **d** or migration, only after pretreatment of LNCaP cells with the synthetic androgen R1881 (10 nM for 48 h). $^{**}P = 0.001$, IGF-I versus basal, two-tailed Student's t test for paired values ([69] and our unpublished data)

able to up-regulate IRS-1 expression [80, 81] and to down-regulate IGFBPs [82]. This synergy between IGF and estrogens can explain cancer resistance to antiestrogen therapies. The two ER subtypes, however, often behave in a different way. For instance, only ER-α, but not ER-β, transactivates the IGF-I promoter [83]. However, very limited data are available regarding prostate cancer.

We hypothesized that estrogens could also contribute to upregulate IGF-IR in prostate cancer. Indeed, exposure to 17β-estradiol (E2) caused a 4-5-fold IGF-IR increase. Similarly to androgens, E2 effects did not require ER binding to specific DNA sequences (EREs) but involved membrane-initiated effects with the activation of cytosolic kinases such as c-Src, ERK1/2 and PI3-K [84]. Various lines of evidences supported this conclusion. First, Src and MEK1 inhibitors were able to completely block the IGF-IR up-regulation induced by E2 exposure, both in LNCaP cells and in HEK293 transfected with either ER-α or ER-β. Second, estren, a synthetic ER ligand that induces ERK1/2 and Elk-1 activation without affecting

ER binding to DNA [85], reproduced this E2 effect, while pyrazole, a compound that activates only membran-initiated effects of E2, was ineffective. Third, E2 activated the IGF-IR promoter in cells transfected with a mutant ER that localizes at the membrane level while it was without effect in cells expressing a mutant ER that localizes only in the nucleus [84]. Since LNCaP cells express a mutated AR (AR-T877A) we evaluated the possibility that E2 could cross-react with AR-T877A. Experiments in transfected HEK293 cells, however, indicated that E2 induces IGF-IR upregulation via both ER-α and ER-β but not via AR-T877A [84]. The individual role of the two ER subtypes in prostate cancer is unclear. However, these findings show that, as far as IGF-IR upregulation is concerned, both receptor subtypes behave similarly.

The present results showing a major role of c-Src in mediating E2 effects are supported by previous studies indicating that E2 activates a Src-dependent pathway by inducing an interaction between the ER phosphotyrosine 537 and the SH2 domain of Src [60]. Other studies have also demonstrated that ER, Src and p85 form a ternary complex, whose assembly is stimulated by E2 and that induces the activation of both c-Src and the PI3-K/AKT pathway [86]. The PI3-K inhibitor LY294002 partially blocked the E2 effect in LNCaP cells, suggesting an involvement of PI3-K. Moreover, E2 exposure stimulates the association of both ER-α and ER-β with c-Src and with p85, the regulatory subunit of PI3-K [84].

In summary, these data demonstrate that E2 specifically up-regulates IGF-IR in prostate cancer cells and sensitizes cancer cells to the biologic effects of IGF-I. This E2 effect can occur through both ER-α and ER-β and does not involve ER binding to DNA but rather the activation of kinase cascades initiated by the association between ER- Src and PI3-K and followed by ERK1/2 phosphorylation. AR expression is not required, although it may potentiate E2 effect by forming a complex with ER.

These data raise several potential implications in prostate cancer development and treatment. First, estrogens may enhance the biological effects of IGFs by up-regulating IGF-IR both in AR positive and AR negative prostate cancers. Second, since ER-β is expressed in both normal and pre-cancerous prostate epithelium, it is possible that environmental xenoestrogens may mimic rapid effects of E2 and represent a risk factor for prostate cancer.

4.3 Transcription Factors Involved

MISS may eventually regulate gene transcription by various mechanisms that may include regulation of coactivators or corepressors involved in the classical genomic pathway, but may also involve different transcription factors [87]. One mechanism reported for androgens (DHT) involves ERK-dependent activation of Elk-1, which in turn activates c-fos expression thus eliciting gene transcription independently of AR binding to DNA response elements [88]. Noteworthy, the activation of this pathway is insensitive to anti-androgens [88]. Gene transcription elicited by membrane-initiated actions of androgens may also involve other mechanisms, as reported by various studies [60, 88–91]. Similar studies have regarded the rapid effects of estrogens [87, 92].

In prostate cancer cells, we found that rapid effects of both androgens and estrogens converge into phosphorylation and activation of CREB, a member of the CREB/CREM/ATF family of transcription factors [93]. Both sex steroids, at nanomolar concentrations (0.1–1.0 nmol/L) were able to induce CREB phosphorylation at Ser133 residue, with an early peak after 30–60 min exposure followed by a late peak at 18 h [93]. CREB-Ser133 is a phosphosite required for CREB-binding protein (CBP) recruitment and formation of the CREB transcriptional complex, which binds to a conserved CREB responsive element (CRE), a palindromic 8-bp sequence (TGACGTCA) found in the enhancer regions of various genes [94].

In LNCaP cells, transfection with a dominant negative construct for CREB abrogated the increase of CRE activity and IGF-IR promoter activity in response to sex steroids. CREB activation was clearly downstream the c-Src/ERK pathway, in agreement with the notion that CREB is a substrate of p90Rsk, a kinase downstream ERK-1/2 [95–97] (Fig. 2). Various other kinases, such as PKA, PKC and CaMKII that may be involved in CREB activation do not have a role in our model. The PI3-K pathway has a role after exposure to estrogens but seems to be dispensable for androgen action [84].

The concept that the AR or ER response element are not involved in IGF-IR upregulation is reinforced by the finding that AR or ER mutants that do not bind to DNA are able to induce CREB phosphorylation as well as the wild type receptors. Furthermore, transfection of AR or ER, as well as of their mutants lacking genomic activity, in either PC-3 or HEK293 cells, was equally able to induce CREB phosphorylation after sex steroid stimulation. As expected, untransfected AR/ER negative cells were unresponsive to sex steroids.

CREB binding elements had not been previously described in the IGF-IR promoter. The human IGF-IR promoter consists in a sequence of 1557 bp, including a 5′-flanking region (−518/−1 fragment) and a 5′-UTR region (+1/+1038 fragment). Both regions are highly GC-rich, and show a very high homology to the corresponding regions of the rat IGF-IR gene [98], with 75% homology in the 5′-flanking region and 85% homology in the 5′-UTR region. Major regulators of the IGF-IR gene include Sp1 transcription factor [99], WT-1 [100] and p53 [101, 102].

We identified sex steroid responsive CREB elements in the 5′UTR promoter region. In cells transfected with either ER or AR (or their mutants lacking genomic activity), the response of the 5′UTR fragment to sex steroids was similar to that of the full-length promoter. Mutation of one CREB site at the 5′UTR markedly reduced both basal and sex steroid stimulated promoter activity while deletion of this region completely abolished the response to sex steroids. The role of this sequence was further confirmed by DNA affinity precipitation assay and by ChIP analysis [93]. In addition to CREB, CCAAT enhancer binding protein-β (C/EBPβ) seems also involved in mediating E2 effects, as C/EBPβ inhibition actually

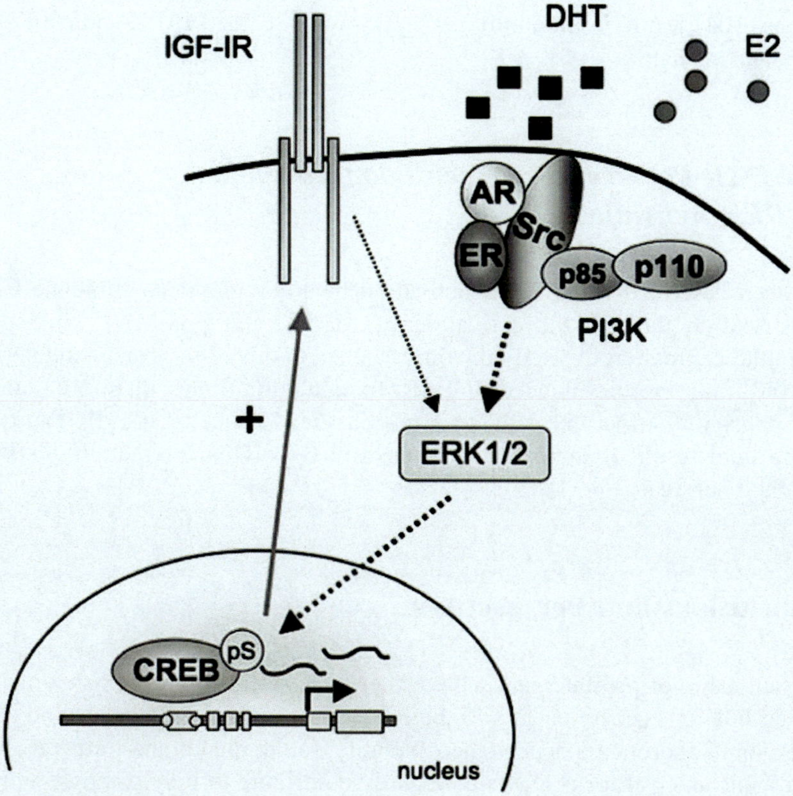

Fig. 2 Schematic representation of IGF-IR upregulation by membrane-initiated sex steroid signals in prostate cancer cells. Exposure to either androgens or estrogens induces the formation of multiprotein complexes involving c-Src and AR and/or ER with the possible participation of PI3-K, and subsequent activation of ERK1/2. CREB is then phosphorylated at Ser133 and activated. Activated CREB directly binds to the IGF-IR promoter and induces IGF-IR gene transcription and protein overexpression. In turn, ligand-activated IGF-IR increases ERK1/2 and CREB activation, promoting a positive feed-back loop, which induces IGF-IR overexpression

blocked E2-induced IGF-IR promoter activity. Further work is needed to elucidate the precise role of this transcription factor.

While CREB activation by MISS is a novel mechanism of IGF-IR upregulation, limited data have been reported by others regarding CREB activation by sex steroids As far as androgens are concerned, DHT has been found to induce c-fos promoter activity in LNCaP cells through a c-Src/MEK/ERK/CREB pathway [72]. In Sertoli cells androgens may also induce CREB phosphorylation downstream ERK1/2, although at much higher concentrations (10-25-folds higher) than those required for IGF-IR upregulation in LNCaP cells [103].

With regard to estrogens, CREB activation has been studied in brain, where it is involved in plasticity and resistance to apoptosis. In hippocampal primary cell cultures, both MAPK and CaMKII activities have a role in CREB activation by estrogens [104], while in immortalized hippocampal cells, MAPK and p90Rsk are the primary mediators [105].

4.4 IGF-IR Positive Feed-Back Loop Through CREB Activation

It has been described that IGF-IR activation by IGFs may also stimulate CREB phosphorylation through the activation of MAPK and p38-MAP kinases and regulate the expression of CRE-containing genes involved in growth and survival [106–108]. Sex steroid-induced IGF-IR upregulation may, therefore, amplify CREB phosphorylation and activate a positive feed-back for IGF-IR expression with the final result of increased cell sensitivity to IGFs for the stimulation of growth and survival (Fig. 1).

5 Conclusions and Perspectives

The relationship of prostate cancer with the IGF axis is well established, as dysregulated IGF axis is associated with both increased cancer occurrence and cancer progression to androgen independence. Notably, rapid, membrane-initiated actions of androgens and estrogens may significantly contribute to IGF axis dysregulation by stimulating IGF-IR promoter activity and IGF-IR upregulation through the c-Src/ERK/CREB pathway. There is evidence that the proportion of classical sex steroid receptors located at the membrane level, and therefore their relevance, increases in aggressive prostate cancers. In turn, the upregulated IGF-IR may be involved in a positive feed-back loop involving further stimulation of CREB phosphorylation and increased IGF-IR expression. IGF-IR upregulation sensitizes prostate cancer cells to the biological effects of IGFs, thus contributing to tumor progression and resistance to therapy. It might also increase AR classical genomic effects by inducing AR phosphorylation.

This sequence of events may occur not only in AR positive but also in AR negative/ER positive prostate cancer cells and in malignant cells that express AR and/or ER mutants unable to bind DNA and are only partially inhibited by currently available anti-androgens and anti-estrogens. This mechanism may synergize with classical genomic effects of sex steroids and contribute to prostate cancer progression to androgen-independence. These novel findings strongly suggest that inhibitors of the c-Src/ERK/PI3-K/CREB pathway and/or IGF-IR inhibitors should be used to complement the classical anti-hormone therapy in prostate cancer patients.

Acknowledgments This work was partially supported by grants from the AIRC (Associazione Italiana per la Ricerca sul Cancro) and PRIN-MIUR 2008 (Ministero Italiano Università e Ricerca).

Conflict of interest The Author declares that he has no conflict of interest.

References

1. Baserga R (1995) The insulin-like growth factor I receptor: a key to tumor growth? Cancer Res 55:249–252
2. Samani AA, Yakar S, LeRoith D et al (2007) The role of the IGF system in cancer growth and metastasis: overview and recent insights. Endocr Rev 28:20–47
3. Clemmons DR, Busby WH, Arai T et al (1995) Role of insulin-like growth factor binding proteins in the control of IGF actions. Prog Growth Factor Res 6:357–366
4. Trapman J, Brinkmann AO (1996) The androgen receptor in prostate cancer. Pathol Res Pract 192:752–760
5. Marcelli M, Ittmann M, Mariani S et al (2000) Androgen receptor mutations in prostate cancer. Cancer Res 60:944–949
6. Pollak M, Beamer W, Zhang JC (1998) Insulin-like growth factors and prostate cancer. Cancer Metastasis Rev 17:383–390
7. Baserga R (2000) Insulin-like growth factor I receptor signalling in prostate cancer cells. Growth Horm IGF Res 10 Suppl A:S43–S44
8. Roberts CT Jr (2000) Insulin-like growth factor I receptor regulation in prostate carcinoma. Growth Horm IGF Res 10 Suppl A:S20–S21
9. Djavan B, Waldert M, Seitz C et al (2001) Insulin-like growth factors and prostate cancer. World J Urol 19:225–233
10. LeRoith D, Roberts CT Jr (2003) The insulin-like growth factor system and cancer. Cancer Lett 195:127–137
11. Werner H, Bruchim I (2009) The insulin-like growth factor-I receptor as an oncogene. Arch Physiol Biochem 115:58–71
12. Sisci D, Surmacz E (2007) Crosstalk between IGF signaling and steroid hormone receptors in breast cancer. Curr Pharm Des 13:705–717
13. Mathews LS, Hammer RE, Behringer RR et al (1988) Growth enhancement of transgenic mice expressing human insulin-like growth factor I. Endocrinology 123:2827–2833
14. Di Giovanni J, Kiguchi K, Frijhoff A et al (2000) Deregulated expression of insulin-like growth factor 1 in prostate epithelium leads to neoplasia in transgenic mice. Proc Natl Acad Sci U S A 97:3455–3460
15. Kaplan-Lefko PJ, Sutherland BW, Evangelou AI et al (2008) Enforced epithelial expression of IGF-1 causes hyperplastic prostate growth while negative selection is requisite for spontaneous metastogenesis. Oncogene 27:2868–2876
16. Sutherland BW, Knoblaugh SE, Kaplan-Lefko PJ et al (2008) Conditional deletion of insulin-like growth factor-I receptor in prostate epithelium. Cancer Res 68:3495–3504
17. Majeed N, Blouin MJ, Kaplan-Lefko PJ et al (2005) A germ line mutation that delays prostate cancer progression and prolongs survival in a murine prostate cancer model. Oncogene 24:4736–4740
18. Cohen P, Peehl DM, Lamson G et al (1991) Insulin-like growth factors (IGFs), IGF receptors, and IGF-binding proteins in primary cultures of prostate epithelial cells. J Clin Endocrinol Metab 73:401–407

19. Burfeind P, Chernicky CL, Rininsland F et al (1996) Antisense RNA to the type I insulin-like growth factor receptor suppresses tumor growth and prevents invasion by rat prostate cancer cells in vivo. Proc Natl Acad Sci U S A 93:7263–7268
20. Hellawell GO, Turner GD, Davies DR et al (2002) Expression of the type 1 insulin-like growth factor receptor is up-regulated in primary prostate cancer and commonly persists in metastatic disease. Cancer Res 62:2942–2950
21. Figueroa JA, De Raad S, Speights VO et al (2001) Gene expression of insulin-like growth factors and receptors in neoplastic prostate tissues: correlation with clinico-pathological parameters. Cancer Invest 19:28–34
22. Tennant MK, Thrasher JB, Twomey PA et al (1996) Protein and messenger ribonucleic acid (mRNA) for the type 1 insulin-like growth factor (IGF) receptor is decreased and IGF-IIIGF-II mRNA is increased in human prostate carcinoma compared to benign prostate epithelium. J Clin Endocrinol Metab 81:3774–3782
23. Damon SE, Plymate SR, Carroll JM et al (2001) Transcriptional regulation of insulin-like growth factor-I receptor gene expression in prostate cancer cells. Endocrinology 142:21–27
24. Nickerson T, Chang F, Lorimer D et al (2001) In vivo progression of LAPC-9 and LNCaP prostate cancer models to androgen independence is associated with increased expression of insulin-like growth factor I (IGF-I) and IGF-I receptor (IGF-IR). Cancer Res 61:6276–6286
25. Hellawell GO, Brewster SF (2002) Growth factors and their receptors in prostate cancer. BJU Int 89:230–240
26. Krueckl SL, Sikes RA, Edlund NM et al (2004) Increased insulin-like growth factor I receptor expression and signaling are components of androgen-independent progression in a lineage-derived prostate cancer progression model. Cancer Res 64:8620–8629
27. Cox ME, Gleave ME, Zakikhani M et al (2009) Insulin receptor expression by human prostate cancers. Prostate 69:33–40
28. Feng Y, Zhu Z, Xiao X et al (2006) Novel human monoclonal antibodies to insulin-like growth factor (IGF)-II that potently inhibit the IGF receptor type I signal transduction function. Mol Cancer Ther 5:114–120
29. Goya M, Miyamoto S, Nagai K et al (2004) Growth inhibition of human prostate cancer cells in human adult bone implanted into nonobese diabetic/severe combined immunodeficient mice by a ligand-specific antibody to human insulin-like growth factors. Cancer Res 64:6252–6258
30. Furukawa J, Wraight CJ, Freier SM et al (2010) Antisense oligonucleotide targeting of insulin-like growth factor-1 receptor (IGF-1R) in prostate cancer. Prostate 70:206–218
31. Jones HE, Goddard L, Gee JM et al (2004) Insulin-like growth factor-I receptor signalling and acquired resistance to gefitinib (ZD1839; Iressa) in human breast and prostate cancer cells. Endocr Relat Cancer 11:793–814
32. Belfiore A, Frasca F, Pandini G et al (2009) Insulin receptor isoforms and insulin receptor/insulin-like growth factor receptor hybrids in physiology and disease. Endocr Rev 30:586–623
33. Schapira DV (1991) Diet, obesity, fat distribution and cancer in women. J Am Med Womens Assoc 46:126–130
34. Bray GA (2002) The underlying basis for obesity: relationship to cancer. J Nutr 132:3451S–3455S
35. Calle EE, Thun MJ (2004) Obesity and cancer. Oncogene 23:6365–6378
36. Kaaks R, Lukanova A (2002) Effects of weight control and physical activity in cancer prevention: role of endogenous hormone metabolism. Ann N Y Acad Sci 963:268–281
37. Vainio H, Kaaks R, Bianchini F (2002) Weight control and physical activity in cancer prevention: international evaluation of the evidence. Eur J Cancer Prev 11 Suppl 2:S94–S100
38. Hsing AW, Sakoda LC, Chua S Jr (2007) Obesity, metabolic syndrome, and prostate cancer. Am J Clin Nutr 86:S843–S857
39. Wolk A, Mantzoros CS, Andersson SO et al (1998) Insulin-like growth factor 1 and prostate cancer risk: a population-based, case-control study. J Natl Cancer Inst 90:911–915

40. Rowlands MA, Gunnell D, Harris R et al (2009) Circulating insulin-like growth factor peptides and prostate cancer risk: a systematic review and meta-analysis. Int J Cancer 124:2416–2429
41. Roddam AW, Allen NE, Appleby P et al (2008) Insulin-like growth factors, their binding proteins, and prostate cancer risk: analysis of individual patient data from 12 prospective studies. Ann Intern Med 149(461–471):W468–W483
42. Juul A, Scheike T, Davidsen M et al (2002) Low serum insulin-like growth factor I is associated with increased risk of ischemic heart disease: a population-based case-control study. Circulation 106:939–944
43. Hubbard SR, Wei L, Ellis L et al (1994) Crystal structure of the tyrosine kinase domain of the human insulin receptor. Nature 372:746–754
44. Pawson T (1994) Signal transduction. Look at a tyrosine kinase. Nature 372:726–727
45. White MF (1998) The IRS-signalling system: a network of docking proteins that mediate insulin action. Mol Cell Biochem 182:3–11
46. Chiang SH, Baumann CA, Kanzaki M et al (2001) Insulin-stimulated GLUT4 translocation requires the CAP-dependent activation of TC10. Nature 410:944–948
47. Backer JM, Myers MG Jr, Shoelson SE et al (1992) Phosphatidylinositol 3′-kinase is activated by association with IRS-1 during insulin stimulation. EMBO J 11:3469–3479
48. Skolnik EY, Lee CH, Batzer A et al (1993) The SH2/SH3 domain-containing protein GRB2 interacts with tyrosine-phosphorylated IRS1 and Shc: implications for insulin control of ras signalling. EMBO J 12:1929–1936
49. Sebolt-Leopold JS, Herrera R (2004) Targeting the mitogen-activated protein kinase cascade to treat cancer. Nat Rev Cancer 4:937–947
50. Dhillon AS, Hagan S, Rath O et al (2007) MAP kinase signalling pathways in cancer. Oncogene 26:3279–3290
51. Foster FM, Traer CJ, Abraham SM et al (2003) The phosphoinositide (PI) 3-kinase family. J Cell Sci 116:3037–3040
52. Harrington LS, Findlay GM, Lamb RF (2005) Restraining PI3K: mTOR signalling goes back to the membrane. Trends Biochem Sci 30:35–42
53. Holland EC, Sonenberg N, Pandolfi PP et al (2004) Signaling control of mRNA translation in cancer pathogenesis. Oncogene 23:3138–3144
54. Liang J, Slingerland JM (2003) Multiple roles of the PI3K/PKB (Akt) pathway in cell cycle progression. Cell Cycle 2:339–345
55. Culig Z, Hobisch A, Cronauer MV et al (1994) Androgen receptor activation in prostatic tumor cell lines by insulin-like growth factor-I, keratinocyte growth factor, and epidermal growth factor. Cancer Res 54:5474–5478
56. Orio F Jr, Terouanne B, Georget V et al (2002) Potential action of IGF-1 and EGF on androgen receptor nuclear transfer and transactivation in normal and cancer human prostate cell lines. Mol Cell Endocrinol 198:105–114
57. Plymate SR, Tennant MK, Culp SH et al (2004) Androgen receptor (AR) expression in AR-negative prostate cancer cells results in differential effects of DHT and IGF-I on proliferation and AR activity between localized and metastatic tumors. Prostate 61:276–290
58. Bakin RE, Gioeli D, Sikes RA et al (2003) Constitutive activation of the Ras/mitogen-activated protein kinase signaling pathway promotes androgen hypersensitivity in LNCaP prostate cancer cells. Cancer Res 63:1981–1989
59. Lin HK, Yeh S, Kang HY et al (2001) Akt suppresses androgen-induced apoptosis by phosphorylating and inhibiting androgen receptor. Proc Natl Acad Sci U S A 98:7200–7205
60. Migliaccio A, Castoria G, Di Domenico M et al (2000) Steroid-induced androgen receptor-oestradiol receptor beta-Src complex triggers prostate cancer cell proliferation. EMBO J 19:5406–5417
61. Song RX, Barnes CJ, Zhang Z et al (2004) The role of Shc and insulin-like growth factor 1 receptor in mediating the translocation of estrogen receptor alpha to the plasma membrane. Proc Natl Acad Sci U S A 101:2076–2081

62. Acconcia F, Ascenzi P, Fabozzi G et al (2004) S-palmitoylation modulates human estrogen receptor-alpha functions. Biochem Biophys Res Commun 316:878–883
63. Razandi M, Alton G, Pedram A et al (2003) Identification of a structural determinant necessary for the localization and function of estrogen receptor alpha at the plasma membrane. Mol Cell Biol 23:1633–1646
64. Acconcia F, Ascenzi P, Bocedi A et al (2005) Palmitoylation-dependent estrogen receptor alpha membrane localization: regulation by 17β-estradiol. Mol Biol Cell 16:231–237
65. Freeman MR, Cinar B, Lu ML (2005) Membrane rafts as potential sites of nongenomic hormonal signaling in prostate cancer. Trends Endocrinol Metab 16:273–279
66. Salani B, Briatore L, Garibaldi S et al (2008) Caveolin-1 down-regulation inhibits insulin-like growth factor-I receptor signal transduction in H9C2 rat cardiomyoblasts. Endocrinology 149:461–465
67. Song RX, Zhang Z, Chen Y et al (2007) Estrogen signaling via a linear pathway involving insulin-like growth factor I receptor, matrix metalloproteinases, and epidermal growth factor receptor to activate mitogen-activated protein kinase in MCF-7 breast cancer cells. Endocrinology 148:4091–4101
68. Ahmad T, Farnie G, Bundred NJ et al (2004) The mitogenic action of insulin-like growth factor I in normal human mammary epithelial cells requires the epidermal growth factor receptor tyrosine kinase. J Biol Chem 279:1713–1719
69. Pandini G, Mineo R, Frasca F et al (2005) Androgens up-regulate the insulin-like growth factor-I receptor in prostate cancer cells. Cancer Res 65:1849–1857
70. Nazareth LV, Stenoien DL, Bingman WE 3rd et al (1999) A C619Y mutation in the human androgen receptor causes inactivation and mislocalization of the receptor with concomitant sequestration of SRC-1 (steroid receptor coactivator 1). Mol Endocrinol 13:2065–2075
71. Zoppi S, Marcelli M, Deslypere JP et al (1992) Amino acid substitutions in the DNA-binding domain of the human androgen receptor are a frequent cause of receptor-binding positive androgen resistance. Mol Endocrinol 6:409–415
72. Unni E, Sun S, Nan B et al (2004) Changes in androgen receptor nongenotropic signaling correlate with transition of LNCaP cells to androgen independence. Cancer Res 64:7156–7168
73. Iwamura M, Sluss PM, Casamento JB et al (1993) Insulin-like growth factor I: action and receptor characterization in human prostate cancer cell lines. Prostate 22:243–252
74. Lau KM, LaSpina M, Long J et al (2000) Expression of estrogen receptor (ER)-alpha and ER-beta in normal and malignant prostatic epithelial cells: regulation by methylation and involvement in growth regulation. Cancer Res 60:3175–3182
75. Lai JS, Brown LG, True LD et al (2004) Metastases of prostate cancer express estrogen receptor-beta. Urology 64:814–820
76. Kim IY, Kim BC, Seong DH et al (2002) Raloxifene, a mixed estrogen agonist/antagonist, induces apoptosis in androgen-independent human prostate cancer cell lines. Cancer Res 62:5365–5369
77. Umayahara Y, Kawamori R, Watada H et al (1994) Estrogen regulation of the insulin-like growth factor I gene transcription involves an AP-1 enhancer. J Biol Chem 269:16433–16442
78. Dupont J, Karas M, LeRoith D (2000) The potentiation of estrogen on insulin-like growth f actor I action in MCF-7 human breast cancer cells includes cell cycle components. J Biol Chem 275:35893–35901
79. Stewart AJ, Johnson MD, May FE et al (1990) Role of insulin-like growth factors and the type I insulin-like growth factor receptor in the estrogen-stimulated proliferation of human breast cancer cells. J Biol Chem 265:21172–21178
80. Lee AV, Jackson JG, Gooch JL et al (1999) Enhancement of insulin-like growth factor signaling in human breast cancer: estrogen regulation of insulin receptor substrate-1 expression in vitro and in vivo. Mol Endocrinol 13:787–796
81. Mauro L, Salerno M, Panno ML et al (2001) Estradiol increases IRS-1 gene expression and insulin signaling in breast cancer cells. Biochem Biophys Res Commun 288:685–689

82. Huynh H, Yang X, Pollak M (1996) Estradiol and antiestrogens regulate a growth inhibitory insulin-like growth factor binding protein 3 autocrine loop in human breast cancer cells. J Biol Chem 271:1016–1021
83. Fournier B, Gutzwiller S, Dittmar T et al (2001) Estrogen receptor (ER)-alpha, but not ER-beta, mediates regulation of the insulin-like growth factor I gene by antiestrogens. J Biol Chem 276:35444–35449
84. Pandini G, Genua M, Frasca F et al (2007) 17β-estradiol up-regulates the insulin-like growth factor receptor through a nongenotropic pathway in prostate cancer cells. Cancer Res 67:8932–8941
85. Kousteni S, Chen JR, Bellido T et al (2002) Reversal of bone loss in mice by nongenotropic signaling of sex steroids. Science 298:843–846
86. Castoria G, Migliaccio A, Bilancio A et al (2001) PI3-kinase in concert with Src promotes the S-phase entry of oestradiol-stimulated MCF-7 cells. EMBO J 20:6050–6059
87. Hammes SR, Levin ER (2007) Extranuclear steroid receptors: nature and actions. Endocr Rev 28:726–741
88. Peterziel H, Mink S, Schonert A et al (1999) Rapid signalling by androgen receptor in prostate cancer cells. Oncogene 18:6322–6329
89. Abreu-Martin MT, Chari A, Palladino AA et al (1999) Mitogen-activated protein kinase kinase kinase 1 activates androgen receptor-dependent transcription and apoptosis in prostate cancer. Mol Cell Biol 19:5143–5154
90. Price DT, Rocca GD, Guo C et al (1999) Activation of extracellular signal-regulated kinase in human prostate cancer. J Urol 162:1537–1542
91. Castoria G, Lombardi M, Barone MV et al (2003) Androgen-stimulated DNA synthesis and cytoskeletal changes in fibroblasts by a nontranscriptional receptor action. J Cell Biol 161:547–556
92. Kousteni S, Han L, Chen JR et al (2003) Kinase-mediated regulation of common transcription factors accounts for the bone-protective effects of sex steroids. J Clin Invest 111:1651–1664
93. Genua M, Pandini G, Sisci D et al (2009) Role of cyclic AMP response element-binding protein in insulin-like growth factor-i receptor up-regulation by sex steroids in prostate cancer cells. Cancer Res 69:7270–7277
94. Benbrook DM, Jones NC (1990) Heterodimer formation between CREB and JUN proteins. Oncogene 5:295–302
95. Sturgill TW, Ray LB, Erikson E et al (1988) Insulin-stimulated MAP-2 kinase phosphorylates and activates ribosomal protein S6 kinase II. Nature 334:715–718
96. Xing J, Ginty DD, Greenberg ME (1996) Coupling of the RAS-MAPK pathway to gene activation by RSK2, a growth factor-regulated CREB kinase. Science 273:959–963
97. Frodin M, Gammeltoft S (1999) Role and regulation of 90 kDa ribosomal S6 kinase (RSK) in signal transduction. Mol Cell Endocrinol 151:65–77
98. Cooke DW, Bankert LA, Roberts CT Jr et al (1991) Analysis of the human type I insulin-like growth factor receptor promoter region. Biochem Biophys Res Commun 177:1113–1120
99. Werner H, Bach MA, Stannard B et al (1992) Structural and functional analysis of the insulin-like growth factor I receptor gene promoter. Mol Endocrinol 6:1545–1558
100. Werner H, Re GG, Drummond IA et al (1993) Increased expression of the insulin-like growth factor I receptor gene, IGF1R, in Wilms tumor is correlated with modulation of IGF1R promoter activity by the WT1 Wilms tumor gene product. Proc Natl Acad Sci U S A 90:5828–5832
101. Werner H, Shalita-Chesner M, Abramovitch S et al (2000) Regulation of the insulin-like growth factor-I receptor gene by oncogenes and antioncogenes: implications in human cancer. Mol Genet Metab 71:315–320
102. Idelman G, Glaser T, Roberts CT Jr et al (2003) WT1–p53 interactions in insulin-like growth factor-I receptor gene regulation. J Biol Chem 278:3474–3482

103. Cheng J, Watkins SC, Walker WH (2007) Testosterone activates mitogen-activated protein kinase via Src kinase and the epidermal growth factor receptor in Sertoli cells. Endocrinology 148:2066–2074
104. Lee SJ, Campomanes CR, Sikat PT et al (2004) Estrogen induces phosphorylation of cyclic AMP response element binding (pCREB) in primary hippocampal cells in a time-dependent manner. Neuroscience 124:549–560
105. Wade CB, Dorsa DM (2003) Estrogen activation of cyclic adenosine 5′-monophosphate response element-mediated transcription requires the extracellularly regulated kinase/mitogen-activated protein kinase pathway. Endocrinology 144:832–838
106. Ginty DD, Bonni A, Greenberg ME (1994) Nerve growth factor activates a Ras-dependent protein kinase that stimulates c-fos transcription via phosphorylation of CREB. Cell 77:713–725
107. Monnier D, Boutillier AL, Giraud P et al (1994) Insulin-like growth factor-I stimulates c- fos and c-jun transcription in PC12 cells. Mol Cell Endocrinol 104:139–145
108. Linnerth NM, Baldwin M, Campbell C et al (2005) IGF-IIIGF-II induces CREB phosphorylation and cell survival in human lung cancer cells. Oncogene 24:7310–7319

Androgen Receptor Pathway in Prostate Cancer: Old Target and New Drugs

Christophe Massard and Karim Fizazi

Abstract Prostate cancer is the most common cancer, and the second leading cause of death from cancer, in males in most Western countries. Prostate cancer has an exquisite sensitivity to androgen deprivation therapy and is the most endocrine-sensitive solid neoplasm, although the disease may eventually progress to the castration-resistant status (CRPC). However, recent evidence was provided that the cancer progression at the CRPC stage is often mediated by androgen receptor signaling, so that subsequent androgen receptor targeting may further contribute to disease control and eventually survival improvement. Several novel agents targeting the androgen receptor signaling are currently being evaluated including Abiraterone, MDV-3100, orteronel (TAK-700), and other compounds currently in early development.

Keywords CRPC · Androgen receptor · Abiraterone · MDV-3100

Contents

C. Massard (✉) · K. Fizazi
Department of Medicine, Institut Gustave Roussy,
39 rue Camille Desmoulins, 94805 Villejuif, France
e-mail: christophe.massard@igr.fr

K. Fizazi
e-mail: fizazi@igr.fr

G. Castoria and A. Migliaccio (eds.), *Advances in Rapid Sex-Steroid Action*,
DOI: 10.1007/978-1-4614-1764-4_13, © Springer Science+Business Media, LLC 2012

1 Introduction

Prostate cancer is the commonest malignancy in Western countries and the second leading cause of cancer-related deaths in males [1–3]. Although advanced disease is initially sensitive to androgen deprivation therapy (ADT) most deaths occur following progression towards castration resistant prostate cancer (CRPC), which is currently incurable, and metastatic dissemination and resistance to ADT [4–6]. Until recently, only docetaxel-based chemotherapy had been shown to modestly improve survival since the identification of therapeutic castration by Charles Huggins in 1941 [7–10] (Fig. 1).

The recent discovery of molecular alterations in prostate cancer led to the development of various agents targeting these alterations [11]. This includes drugs targeting angiogenesis (bevacizumab, VEGF-Trap), agents targeting molecules involved in the onset of bone metastases such as endothelin-1 receptor A (zibotentan), RANK ligand (denosumab) [12], bone-targeting radiopharmaceutical agents [13], immunotherapy [14], and also new generation hormonal manipulations.

During the last decade, the androgen receptor (AR) axis has been demonstrated to be active in both early and late metastatic prostate cancer [15], which justifies the development of drugs that directly or indirectly target this receptor such as abiraterone [16], MDV-3100 [17]. This review aims at describing the rationale of AR pathway inhibition and the main drugs under development (Table 1).

2 AR Signaling in Prostate Cancer

The AR belongs to the steroid hormone receptor family of ligand-activated nuclear transcription factors. It contains four functional regions: an amino terminal regulatory domain (AF-1 site), a DNA- binding domain, a hinge region containing a nuclear localization signal, and a carboxy-terminal ligand-binding domain (AF-2 site). Unligated AR are bound to heat shock proteins (HSP) in the cytoplasm; androgen binding leads to dissociation from HSPs, dimerization, phosphorylation, translocation in the nucleus, DNA binding, co-activator recruitment, and transcription of androgen-regulated genes.

Since androgens and AR signaling pathways are regarded as the main oncogene drivers in prostate carcinogenesis, they represent a logical target for prostate cancer treatment. The clinical activity of ADT (castration) was first reported more

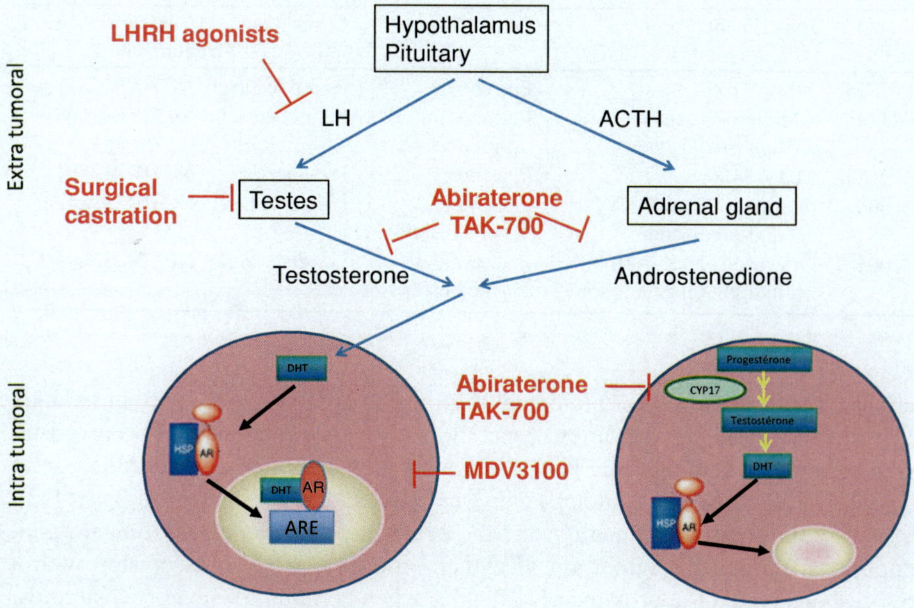

Fig. 1 AR signaling in prostate cancer

than 70 years ago by Huggins and Hodges [18], and remains the mainstay of systemic therapy. Since then, the treatment of patients with advanced or high-risk disease has been based on ADT (orchidectomy or pharmacological strategies), which improves survival in high-risk localized disease, and results in at least a 80% response rate when initiated in patients with newly diagnosed metastatic disease. Nonetheless, despite continuous ADT, the disease eventually progresses, usually after a delay of several years [5].

There are several known mechanisms of resistance to ADT, including AR amplification, hyper-activation without any androgen-binding, mutations in the AF-2 site, possible activation by steroids or other ligands, and co-activation by tyrosine kinases or other molecules. More recently, several studies showed that intracrine androgen synthesis is able to activate the AR pathway and maintain cancer survival [19]. Moreover, recent reports showed that CRPC cells can also express AR splicing variants without the AF-2 site [20, 21], which could represent a novel mechanism of resistance to castration.

The traditional and empiric use of second-line hormonal therapy in patients with CRPC was retrospectively supported by the demonstration of sustained AR expression and intact AR signaling as the disease evolves from androgen-sensitive to castration resistance [4]. Withdrawing anti-androgens may result in a biological response in 15–20% of cases (as a likely consequence of AR mutations making the receptor sensitive to inappropriate anti-androgen stimulation) and adding an anti-androgen or using an estrogen in patient progressing while on castration alone

Table 1 AR targeting agents in advanced phase III trials for advanced metastatic CRPC

Clinical trials	Experimental arm	Control arm	Clinical setting	Clinicaltrials.gov number
AFFIRM	MDV-3100	Placebo	Post-docetaxel	NCT00974311
COU-302	Abiraterone acetate and prednisone	Placebo and prednisone	Pre-docetaxel	NCT00887198
PREVAIL	MDV-3100	Placebo	Pre-docetaxel	NCT01212991
C21005	Orteronel (TAK-700) and prednisone	Placebo and prednisone	Post-docetaxel	NCT01193257
C21004	Orteronel (TAK-700) and prednisone	Placebo and prednisone	Pre-docetaxel	NCT01193244

may also result in clinical or biological response in approximately 25% of patients [22]. Finally, targeting the adrenal secretion of testosterone can be achieved by using steroids or ketoconazole [23]. Prednisone demonstrated a similar biological response rate compared to an anti-androgen (flutamide), but increased benefits in terms of pain control and quality of life [24]. Ketoconazole, an antifungal agent which acts through the inhibition of cytochrome P450, is also associated with a PSA response rate of approximately 20–40% when combined with corticosteroids. Unfortunately a phase III trial testing anti-androgen withdrawal with or without ketoconazole was closed early and therefore, the contribution of this compound on overall survival remains unknown [25]. The potential importance of subsequent hormonal manipulation in patients with CRPC was strengthened by data showing that combining chemotherapy with estramustine, a nitrogen mustard-estradiol conjugate, can improve overall survival compared with chemotherapy alone (HR = 0.77 [95% CI, 0.63–0.93], $p = 0.02$) [9]. A significant benefit was also reported in PSA response rate, and time to PSA progression. The routine use of estramustine, however, is limited by its toxicity, including a risk of thromboembolism.

3 Targeting the AR Axis with New Molecules in CRPC

3.1 Inhibition of Steroidogenic Pathways: Abiraterone and Other Compounds

Several enzymes, such as CYP17, can be targeted to inhibit adrenal and intracrine steroid synthesis. Abiraterone acetate (CB 7630), is an irreversible inhibitor of cytochrome P450-17 (CYP17), with 17α–hydroxylase and C17,20-lyase properties [26]. Since CYP17 is a key enzyme in the production of androgens and estrogens in the adrenal glands and tumor tissue [27–29], abiraterone inhibits both adrenal androgen and intratumoral androgen synthesis. However, due to the upstream inhibition of the C-21 steroid, the levels of serum cortisol decrease, which can result in a positive feed-back on ACTH and a risk of hypokalemia and hypertension, which was circumvented by the concomitant administration of dexamethasone or prednisone in the clinic.

A Phase I study (COU-AA-001) evaluated the safety of continuous daily administration of abiraterone (250–2,000 mg) without steroid adjunction in chemotherapy-naive men [16]. No dose-limiting toxicity was observed; the most frequent side effects were related to the mineralocorticoid excess, including hypertension, hypokaliemia and lower-limb edema. Antitumor activity was reported at all dose levels; in total, 66% of the patients exhibited a PSA decrease above 30 and 38% had a partial response by RECIST criteria. A second Phase I study (COU-AA-002) [30] evaluated the safety and tolerability of abiraterone acetate at doses ranging from 250 to 1,000 mg with steroids and confirmed the acceptable safety profile for further development. The 1,000 mg dose that offered consistent and well tolerated pharmacological target inhibition was selected for subsequent evaluation.

Several Phase II studies were conducted [31–33] in both chemotherapy-naïve and taxane pre-treated CRPC patients. In docetaxel-naive patients, the PSA response rate was 60–80% [30, 32]. Two Phase II studies (COU-AA-003 and COU-AA-004) were conducted in post-docetaxel CRPC patients. In the first, 47 patients were treated with abiraterone acetate 1,000 mg/day alone ($n = 10$), or combined with prednisone ($n = 37$). Declines in PSA $\geq 30 \geq 50$ and $\geq 90\%$ were observed in 32 (69), 24 (51) and 7 (15%) patients respectively. Among 35 patients evaluable by RECIST, 6 (17%) had a partial response [33]. The drug was well tolerated in the post-docetaxel setting with similar toxicities to pre-docetaxel patients.

An international, multicentre randomized Phase III double-blind placebo-controlled was performed on 1,195 patients with metastatic CRPC who had failed docetaxel-based chemotherapy to compare the efficacy and safety of abiraterone acetate plus prednisone (AP) with those of placebo plus prednisone (PP) [34]. The results of the intermediate analysis were recently released and the median overall survival in the AP group was 450 versus 332 days in the PP group ($P < 0.0001$; $HR = 0.65$). Time to PSA progression, radiographic progression-free survival and PSA response rate were also significantly improved in the AR arm. Mineralo-corticoid-related AEs were more common in the AP arm: fluid retention 30.5 versus 22.3%, and hypokaliemia 17.1 versus 8.4%. However, Grade 3/4 hypokaliemia (3.8 versus 0.8%), and Grade 3/4 hypertension (1.3 versus 0.3%) were infrequent. This trial showed for the first time that targeting the AR pathway can prolong overall survival in patients with metastatic CRPC. Another placebo-controlled randomized Phase III study in the pre-docetaxel setting is closed to accrual after more than 1,000 patients have been randomized 1:1 for abiraterone acetate plus prednisolone versus prednisolone plus placebo. The results of this second trial are awaited.

Different other compounds inhibiting the androgen synthesis are also evaluating in clinical trials: TAK-700, a selective, non-steroidal inhibitor of 17, 20-lyase [35–37] (ClinicalTrials.gov-NCT01084655); HE3235 (17a-ethynyl-5a-androstane-3a, 17b-diol) a synthetic androstenediol (ClinicalTrials.gov-NCT00716794) [38].

3.2 Androgen Receptor Antagonists: MDV-3100 and Other Compounds

MDV-3100 is a novel AR antagonist that binds to the AR more avidly than bicalutamide. Unlike bicalutamide, MDV-3100 also inhibits AR function by blocking nuclear translocation and DNA binding, and has no agonist activity [38].

In a large multi-center, open-label, dose-escalation phase I/II study performed in 140 CRPC patients treated with doses ranging from 30 to 600 mg/day, the authors reported antitumor activity including PSA declines of >50% or more in 78 patients (56%), response in soft tissue in 13 out of 59 patients (22%), and bone disease stabilization in 61 out of 109 patients (56%) [39] (ClinicalTrials.gov-NCT00510718). Circulating tumor cells (CTC) count was performed prospectively: 92% of patients with favorable pretreatment counts (i.e. <5 cells/7.5 mL of blood) maintained favorable post-treatment counts, while 49% of patients converted from unfavorable pretreatment (i.e. >5 cells/7.5 mL of blood) to favorable post-treatment counts. At the 600 mg/day doses, two of three subjects had dose-limiting toxicities (seizure and rash, respectively). Fatigue was the most frequently reported adverse event with Grade 3 fatigue occurring in 9, 15 and 20% of patients in the 240, 360 and 480 mg/day groups, respectively. The dose of 240 mg/day was defined as the maximum tolerated dose.

A large phase III randomized, double-blind, placebo-controlled study was performed to determine the benefit in overall survival of MDV-3100 as compared to placebo in patients with progressive CRPC previously treated with docetaxel-based chemotherapy. More than 1,100 patients were enrolled and randomized 2:1 (MDV-3100 versus placebo); the accrual was completed in 2010 and the results are awaited. Another phase III study performed in chemotherapy naïve patients with the same design and methodology has started recently. This study will enroll patients with progressive metastatic cancer that have progressed despite ADT, but who have not been previously treated with cytotoxic chemotherapy (ClinicalTrials.gov Identifier NCT01212991).

Other potent antagonists of human AR with affinity to AR superior to that of bicalutamide are in development in phase I/II trials in CRPC patients: ARN-509, (ClinicalTrials.gov Identifier NCT01171898); BMS-641988 (ClinicalTrials.gov Identifier NCT00326586); EPI-001 which targets the AF-1 region and inhibits transactivation of the amino-terminal domain of the AR, without interacting with the ligand-binding domain with a potential activity against AR splicing variant in CRPC [40–42].

Finally, many other drugs targeting the AR pathway are currently in early clinical development, including CYP17 inhibitors (TOK-001), AR antagonists (ODM-201), drugs aiming to annihilate AR production (*SARA or ZD* 3514), 17βHSD5 inhibitor (ASP9521), and steroid sulphatase inhibitors (irosustat).

4 Perspectives: From AR Inhibition to Personalized Medicine

Several issues have significantly limited the development of new active treatments (including atrasentan, satraplatin, DN 101, oblimersen, GVAX) in metastatic prostate cancer, therefore leading to a series of negative randomized trials [11]. First of all, the response to treatment is notoriously difficult to assess: metastatic prostate cancer does not usually generate radiologically measurable lesions and measuring changes in existing lesions on bone scans is highly unreliable. Secondly, European and American agencies have requested a demonstrated benefit in overall survival for drug approval and there is a lack of reliable surrogates for long-term outcome and clinical benefit. Thirdly, the correlation between PSA changes and long-term outcome is controversial, and PSA progression does not qualify as a surrogate for overall survival [5]. In the absence of any other potential outcome measures, these issues have led to the development of a consensus guideline for the restricted use of PSA as an endpoint in clinical trials [17]. Finally, and probably most importantly, metastatic prostate cancer is currently still treated as a "single disease", in contrast to the other frequent cancers, although there is evidence of considerable heterogeneity in outcome and sensitivity to anti-prostate cancer therapies. In contrast, the other three most frequent cancers in Western countries have all been sub-classified based on molecular features (e.g. ER, PR, HER2/neu, and BRCA-1 in breast cancer, EGF-R in non-small cell lung cancer, and K-ras in colo-rectal cancer), leading to successful drug development in specific subgroups [43]. However, increased knowledge in prostate cancer biology has led to the identification of a number of molecular alterations, some of which are promising potential targets [44].

Prostate cancer demonstrates great molecular heterogeneity in which several pathways are simultaneously active, leading to tumourigenesis. Several molecular alterations have recently been discovered that affect cell proliferation and homeostasis, such as alterations in angiogenesis, signal transduction, apoptosis, immortalisation and invasion. The discovery of recurrent gene fusions in prostate cancers has important clinical and biological implications [45]. The fusion of TMPRSS2 and ETS genes was reported by Tomlins et al. [26, 46] as the first recurrent genomic alteration in prostate cancer and has now been confirmed by multiple independent groups. The genes involved are the androgen-regulated gene TMPRSS2 and ETS transcription factor family members, ERG, ETV1, or ETV4. TMPRSS2-ERG fusions are the most predominant molecular subtype, since they have been identified in approximately 40–80% of prostate cancers. The detection of the translocation of TMPRSS2 to the ERG gene in prostate cancer tissue could be used as a biomarker in clinical drug development. Moreover, various molecular abnormalities in the AR pathway lead to resistance to castration. AR gene amplification has been reported in 25–30% of patients with CRPC but is present at very low rates (1–2%) in those with primary prostate cancer, indicating that AR amplification is involved in the development of CRPC. AR gene amplification is associated with increased mRNA expression and augmented levels of AR protein. Point mutations in the AR can result in altered ligand specificity such that mutated ARs can be activated by non-androgenic ligands such as anti-androgens [47]. Another pathway with a prominent role in prostate cancer is the PI3 K/Akt/mTOR pathway, with upregulated signaling found in 30–50% of prostate cancers, often through loss of PTEN. Molecular changes in the PI3 K/Akt/mTOR signaling pathway have been demonstrated to differentiate benign from malignant prostatic epithelium and are associated with a higher tumour stage, grade, and risk of biochemical recurrence [48]. Other important pathways have also been identified in prostate cancer progression to the castration-resistant stage including but not exclusively the endothelin-1 axis, clusterin expression and activation, and the implication of tumour angiogenesis.

Ultimately, molecular characterization of prostate cancer shall lead to the identification of different molecular alterations (such as TMPRSS2-ERG, loss of PTEN, activation of AR signaling pathway) and probably subsets of prostate cancer disease with a different natural history, sensitivity and resistance to treatment. In the future, clinical trials will likely need to consider the stratification of patients by molecular subtypes.

5 Conclusion

In conclusion, recent evidence has demonstrated that progression in prostate cancer is often mediated by androgen receptor signaling, so that subsequent androgen receptor targeting may further contribute to disease control and eventually survival improvement. Abiraterone acetate, an androgen biosynthesis inhibitor, was tested in patients with CRPC pre-treated with docetaxel in a phase III trial with demonstration of an overall survival benefit, confirming that CRPC remains hormone-driven, even in advanced stages of the disease. Several novel agents also targeting the androgen receptor signaling are currently being evaluated including MDV-3100, orteronel (TAK-700), and other agents are currently in earlier development phases. Several studies are ongoing to identify potential predictors of response or resistance to AR signaling pathway targeting agents. In the future, tumor samples (initial prostate cancer, biopsy of a metastatic lesion, molecular characterization of CTC), should allow the identification of various molecular alterations predictive for sensitivity to subsequent hormone manipulations (abiraterone, MDV-3100, already approved anti-hormonal agents), to taxane-based chemotherapy (docetaxel or cabazitaxel), and non-endocrine, non-chemotherapy agents including immunotherapy.

References

1. Jemal A, Siegel R, Xu J, Ward E (2010) Cancer statistics. CA Cancer J Clin 60:277–300
2. La Vecchia C, Bosetti C, Lucchini F et al (2010) Cancer mortality in Europe, 2000–2004, and an overview of trends since 1975. Ann Oncol 21:1323–1360

3. Guerin S, Hill C (2010) Cancer epidemiology in France in 2010, comparison with the USA. Bull Cancer 97:47–54
4. Nelson WG, De Marzo AM, Isaacs WB (2003) Prostate cancer. N Engl J Med 349:366–381
5. Fitzpatrick JM, Anderson J, Sternberg CN et al (2008) Optimizing treatment for men with advanced prostate cancer: expert recommendations and the multidisciplinary approach. Crit Rev Oncol Hematol 68 Suppl 1:S9–S22
6. Attard G, Sarker D, Reid A, Molife R, Parker C, de Bono JS (2006) Improving the outcome of patients with castration-resistant prostate cancer through rational drug development. Br J Cancer 95:767–774
7. Tannock IF, de Wit R, Berry WR et al (2004) Docetaxel plus prednisone or mitoxantrone plus prednisone for advanced prostate cancer. N Engl J Med 351:1502–1512
8. Petrylak DP, Tangen CM, Hussain MH et al (2004) Docetaxel and estramustine compared with mitoxantrone and prednisone for advanced refractory prostate cancer. N Engl J Med 351:1513–1520
9. Fizazi K, Le Maitre A, Hudes G et al (2007) Addition of estramustine to chemotherapy and survival of patients with castration-refractory prostate cancer: a meta-analysis of individual patient data. Lancet Oncol 8:994–1000
10. Madan RA, Pal SK, Sartor O, Dahut WL (2011) Overcoming chemotherapy resistance in prostate cancer. Clin Cancer Res 17(12):3892–3902
11. Fizazi K, Massard C (2009) New agents in metastatic prostate cancer. Eur J Cancer 45 Suppl 1:379–380
12. Fizazi K, Lipton A, Mariette X et al (2009) Randomized phase II trial of denosumab in patients with bone metastases from prostate cancer, breast cancer, or other neoplasms after intravenous bisphosphonates. J Clin Oncol 27:1564–1571
13. Fizazi K, Beuzeboc P, Lumbroso J et al (2009) Phase II trial of consolidation docetaxel and samarium-153 in patients with bone metastases from castration-resistant prostate cancer. J Clin Oncol 27:2429–2435
14. Gulley JL, Drake CG (2011) Immunotherapy for prostate cancer: recent advances, lessons learned, and areas for further research. Clin Cancer Res 17(12):3884–3891
15. Chen Y, Clegg NJ, Scher HI (2009) Anti-androgens and androgen-depleting therapies in prostate cancer: new agents for an established target. Lancet Oncol 10:981–991
16. Attard G, Reid AH, Yap TA et al (2008) Phase I clinical trial of a selective inhibitor of CYP17, abiraterone acetate, confirms that castration-resistant prostate cancer commonly remains hormone driven. J Clin Oncol; 26:4563–4571
17. Scher HI, Halabi S, Tannock I et al (2008) Design and end points of clinical trials for patients with progressive prostate cancer and castrate levels of testosterone: recommendations of the prostate Cancer clinical trials working group. J Clin Oncol 26:1148–1159
18. Huggins C, Hodges CV (1941) Studies on prostatic cancer. I. The effect of castration, of estrogen and of androgen injection on serum phosphatases in metastatic carcinoma of the prostate. Cancer Res 1:293
19. Montgomery RB, Mostaghel EA, Vessella R et al (2008) Maintenance of intratumoral androgens in metastatic prostate cancer: a mechanism for castration-resistant tumor growth. Cancer Res 68:4447–4454
20. Nacusi LP, Tindall DJ (2009) Androgen receptor abnormalities in castration-recurrent prostate cancer. Expert Rev Endocrinol Metab 4:417–422
21. Vis AN, Schroder FH (2009) Key targets of hormonal treatment of prostate cancer. Part 1: the androgen receptor and steroidogenic pathways. BJU Int 104:438–448
22. Oh WK (2002) The evolving role of estrogen therapy in prostate cancer. Clin Prostate Cancer 1:81–89
23. Ryan CJ, Lin A, Valiente J, Kim J, Small EJ (2007) Phase I evaluation of abiraterone acetate (CB7630), a 17 alpha hydroxylase C17, 20-Lyase inhibitor in androgen-independent prostate cancer (AiPC). J Clin Oncol 25:18S Abstract 5064
24. Fossa SD, Slee PH, Brausi M et al (2001) Flutamide versus prednisone in patients with prostate cancer symptomatically progressing after androgen-ablative therapy: a phase III

study of the European organization for research and treatment of cancer genitourinary group. J Clin Oncol 19:62–71
25. Small EJ, Halabi S, Dawson NA et al (2004) Antiandrogen withdrawal alone or in combination with ketoconazole in androgen-independent prostate cancer patients: a phase III trial (CALGB 9583). J Clin Oncol 22:1025–1033
26. Reid AH, Attard G, Barrie E, de Bono JS (2008) CYP17 inhibition as a hormonal strategy for prostate cancer. Nat Clin Pract Urol 5:610–620
27. Barrie SE, Potter GA, Goddard PM, Haynes BP, Dowsett M, Jarman M (1994) Pharmacology of novel steroidal inhibitors of cytochrome P450(17) alpha (17 alpha-hydroxylase/C17–20 lyase). J Steroid Biochem Mol Biol 50:267–273
28. Potter GA, Barrie SE, Jarman M, Rowlands MG (1995) Novel steroidal inhibitors of human cytochrome P45017 alpha (17 alpha-hydroxylase-C17, 20-lyase): potential agents for the treatment of prostatic cancer. J Med Chem 38:2463–2471
29. Rowlands MG, Barrie SE, Chan F et al (1995) Esters of 3-pyridylacetic acid that combine potent inhibition of 17 alpha-hydroxylase/C17, 20-lyase (cytochrome P45017 alpha) with resistance to esterase hydrolysis. J Med Chem 38:4191–4197
30. Ryan CJ, Smith MR, Fong L et al (2010) Phase I clinical trial of the CYP17 inhibitor abiraterone acetate demonstrating clinical activity in patients with castration-resistant prostate cancer who received prior ketoconazole therapy. J Clin Oncol 28:1481–1488
31. Danila DC, Morris MJ, de Bono JS et al (2010) Phase II multicenter study of abiraterone acetate plus prednisone therapy in patients with docetaxel-treated castration-resistant prostate cancer. J Clin Oncol 28:1496–1501
32. Attard G, Reid AH, A'Hern R et al (2009) Selective inhibition of CYP17 with abiraterone acetate is highly active in the treatment of castration-resistant prostate cancer. J Clin Oncol 27:3742–3748
33. Reid AH, Attard G, Danila DC et al (2010) Significant and sustained antitumor activity in post-docetaxel, castration-resistant prostate cancer with the CYP17 inhibitor abiraterone acetate. J Clin Oncol 28:1489–1495
34. de Bono JL, Logothetis CJ, Fizazi K, North S, Chu L, Chi KN, Kheoh T, Haqq C, Molina A, Scher HI (2010) Abiraterone acetate (AA) plus low dose prednisone or prednisone improves overall survival (OS) in patients with metastatic castration resistant prostate cancer who have progressed after docetaxel-based chemotherapy: results of COU-AA-301, a randomized double-blind placebo-controlled phase III study. ESMO meeting Lba5
35. Dreicer RA, Agus DB, MacVicar GR, Wang J, MacLean D, Stadler WM (2010) Safety, pharmacokinetics, and efficacy of TAK-700 in metastatic castration-resistant prostrate cancer: a phase I/II, open-label study. J Clin Oncol 28 (15S) Suppl Abstract 3084
36. Dreicer RA, Agus DB, MacVicar GR, MacLean D, Zhang T, Stadler WM (2010) Safety, pharmacokinetics, and efficacy of TAK-700 in castration-resistant, metastatic prostate cancer: a phase I/II, open-label study. Genitourinary cancers symposium Abstract 103
37. Montgomery RB, Morris MJ, Ryan CJ, Stickney DR, Frincke JM, Reading CL, Scher, HI (2010).HE3235, a synthetic adrenal hormone, in patients with castration-resistant prostate cancer (CRPC): clinical phase I/II trial results. Genitourinary cancers symposium Abstract 235
38. Tran C, Ouk S, Clegg NJ et al (2009) Development of a second-generation antiandrogen for treatment of advanced prostate cancer. Science 324:787–790
39. Scher HI, Beer TM, Higano CS et al (2010) Antitumour activity of MDV-3100 in castration-resistant prostate cancer: a phase 1–2 study. Lancet 375:1437–1446
40. Attar RM, Jure-Kunkel M, Balog A et al (2009) Discovery of BMS-641988, a novel and potent inhibitor of androgen receptor signaling for the treatment of prostate cancer. Cancer Res 69:6522–6530
41. Rathkopf D, Liu G, Carducci MA et al (2011) Phase I dose-escalation study of the novel antiandrogen BMS-641988 in patients with castration-resistant prostate cancer. Clin Cancer Res 17:880–887

42. Andersen RJ, Mawji NR, Wang J et al (2010) Regression of castrate-recurrent prostate cancer by a small-molecule inhibitor of the amino-terminus domain of the androgen receptor. Cancer Cell 17:535–546
43. Ferte C, Andre F, Soria JC (2010) Molecular circuits of solid tumors: prognostic and predictive tools for bedside use. Nat Rev Clin Oncol 7:367–380
44. Attard G, de Bono JS (2011) Translating scientific advancement into clinical benefit for castration-resistant prostate cancer patients. Clin Cancer Res 17(12):3867–3875
45. Kumar-Sinha C, Tomlins SA, Chinnaiyan AM (2008) Recurrent gene fusions in prostate cancer. Nat Rev Cancer 8:497–511
46. Tomlins SA, Rhodes DR, Perner S et al (2005) Recurrent fusion of TMPRSS2 and ETS transcription factor genes in prostate cancer. Science 310:644–648
47. Taplin ME (2007) Drug insight: role of the androgen receptor in the development and progression of prostate cancer. Nat Clin Pract Oncol 4:236–244
48. Reid AH, Attard G, Ambroisine L et al (2010) Molecular characterisation of ERG, ETV1 and PTEN gene loci identifies patients at low and high risk of death from prostate cancer. Br J Cancer 102:678–684

Part III
New Tools for Steroid Receptor Analysis and Regulatory Networks

Quantitative Visualization of Sex Steroid Receptor Functions: AR and ERα

Michael J. Bolt, Sean M. Hartig, Adam T. Szafran, Sanjay N. Mediwala, Marco Marcelli and Michael A. Mancini

Abstract The nuclear receptors (NR) are a critical superfamily of gene regulatory proteins involved in all of human physiology. Classic biochemical techniques have provided deep insights into NR function but, due to their nature as single endpoint assays derived from pooled cell populations and tissues, these approaches are intrinsically unable to address important mechanistic considerations linked to cellular heterogeneity. Androgen receptor (AR) and estrogen receptor-α (ER) are members of the Type 1 steroid receptor subfamily of NRs that contribute to sex determination. Numerous recent advances have permitted direct, quantitative visualization of AR and ER functions within a cellular context that can be combined with conventional molecular and biochemical approaches. This new approach, essentially single cell-based systems biology, now enables researchers to follow NR shuttling through subcellular compartments in response to physiologic, pathologic or pharmacologic stimuli, to quantify transcriptional activity, and to identify interacting molecules leading to induction, or repression, of transcription. Here, we discuss recent reports that have applied advanced imaging systems [high throughput microscopy (HTM), high content analysis (HCA), FRET, FRAP] to dissect the biology of ER and AR at the single cell level.

M. J. Bolt · S. M. Hartig · A. T. Szafran · M. Marcelli · M. A. Mancini (✉)
Department of Molecular and Cellular Biology, Baylor College of Medicine,
Houston, TX, USA
e-mail: mancini@bcm.edu

M. J. Bolt
e-mail: bolt@bcm.edu

S. M. Hartig
e-mail: hartig@bcm.edu

S. N. Mediwala · M. Marcelli
The Michael E. DeBakey VA Medical Center, Baylor College of Medicine,
Houston, TX, USA
e-mail: mediwala@bcm.edu

G. Castoria and A. Migliaccio (eds.), *Advances in Rapid Sex-Steroid Action*,
DOI: 10.1007/978-1-4614-1764-4_14,

First, we discuss the use of HCA to examine AR functions in genital skin fibroblasts derived from normally virilized individuals and patients with androgen insensitivity syndrome (AIS), and in prostate cancer cell lines. Second, we highlight how these imaging techniques have been applied to define compound-specific mechanisms of ER gene regulation and coregulator interactions. These methods reveal new findings about the actions of AR and ER that are overlooked by conventional methods.

Keywords Gene regulation · Estrogen receptor · Androgen receptor · Nuclear receptor · High throughput microscopy · High content analysis

Contents

1 Introduction

1.1 Gene Regulation

Regulation of the genome is a critical step in the process of creating and maintaining life. In normal tissue, transcription factors are activated (through expression and/or signaling), bind to specific sites throughout the genome along with interacting factors (chromatin remodeling complexes, coregulators), and facilitate the recruitment of RNA polymerase II to regulate genes. This process is highly controlled through ligand-activation, kinase signaling [1], feedback loops [2], and proteolysis [3]. Not surprisingly, gene regulation must be tightly controlled for homeostasis. Alterations in the gene regulatory environment can lead to aberrant gene expression and initiate disease progression, as in endocrine disorders and cancer.

Traditional biochemical approaches for studying gene expression (ChIP, qPCR, luciferase assays) are remarkably useful single endpoint assays. However, there is an increasing need to develop multi-level, integrated views based upon more complex assays that enhance our understanding of the intrinsic complexities in gene regulation.

Cell–cell heterogeneity is an important factor that is not addressed in biochemical assays. While there have been outstanding advances in our understanding of the molecular mechanisms involved in NR/CoR (coregulator) biology, these achievements have been largely based upon three different experimental approaches. First, cell free systems [4] that allow a penultimate, reductionist dissection of key functional molecules. Second, animal models [5] have provided great insights into organismic-scale responses to genetic manipulation. Third, and closely tied to our rationale for much of the work presented in this review, tremendous efforts have been applied to the study the biologic responses of large cell populations either in tissue, or cultured cells. While generally not well appreciated, data that are derived from thousands or millions of cells in a dish are best described as "population averages". Such approaches provide *no* ability to appreciate the variation of biological responses within the population, regardless of the clonal nature of the cells, or attempts to chemically synchronize them.

Towards the goal of understanding cell–cell variability, multiplex high-throughput, multi-endpoint analyses (e.g., high-content analysis, HCA) are becoming increasingly utilized. With reference to AR and ER studies as a focal point, this chapter will discuss the utility and benefit of combining modern molecular cell biology and high throughput microscopy (HTM), other fluorescence imaging techniques, and high content analysis (HCA) to study gene regulation at the single cell level.

1.2 Quantitative Imaging of Cell–Cell Heterogeneity

Cellular responsiveness, on a population scale, has largely been thought to function as a linear process in which cells gradually respond to an experimental or environmental perturbation. This concept arises when a specific population-level response marker (e.g., target gene expression, post translational modification (PTM) gradually changes as a function of time and/or stimulus dose. Further, it has been assumed that the average output from the entire cell population is typically regulated in a reproducible manner, yielding deterministic models that can be applied to better understand mechanisms of gene expression. These models predict, validated by the classic, bulk biochemical methods such as RT-PCR, Western blotting, luciferase assays, coIPs, that increasing levels of stimuli-responsive transcription factors interact with gene regulator regions causing the expected transcription output in each cell. Recent work has challenged this model and suggests that gene expression and cellular responsiveness are highly variable amongst isogenic cell variants; this heterogeneity has been observed in lower eukaryotes to mammalian cells derived from human tissue, suggesting that cell-to-cell variation is critical to the process of gene activation and an organized cellular response [6–8]. These results have led to the development of stochastic models where multiple responsive regulatory events (receptor localization, chromatin remodeling, gene expression, etc.) are necessary to produce the population-level deterministic response and adaptation to variable environments [9]. Further, it is now increasingly accepted that cellular functions are not necessarily determined by the ensemble average of a nominally homogeneous population, and that outliers in a heterogeneous cell population do not simply represent irrelevant, short-lived phenotypic states [10]. Because variation in cell-to-cell activities influence genetic selection and evolution [11, 12], the ability to understand and visualize single cell function is absolutely critical to reveal the machinery underlying alterations in promoter regulation, in chromatin structure necessary for epigenetic changes, haploinsufficiency, clonal emergence, and cancer metastasis [13, 14–15]. However, the mechanistic detail of how cell-to-cell variation in gene regulation delivers deterministic behavior has been largely unstudied due to system complexity and unavailability of experimental platforms that can distinguish individual responses from cells.

While cellular heterogeneity is not easy to study, there have been recent advances in exploring cellular heterogeneity in model systems. Slack et al. [16] measured fluorescent markers labeling either DNA/phospho-p30/phospho-ERK or DNA/actin/α-tubulin across a time- and dose-response of 25 different drugs. The 25 drugs were selected from 5 functional categories including effectors of DNA replication and microtubule disruptors. The authors used image analysis to identify cell regions, and then quantified colocalization of the marker set (stated above). Due to the large amount of data, the authors implemented data reduction algorithms (principle component analysis) to reveal distinct phenotypic populations. Based on their analysis of drug perturbation in HeLa cells, the authors argued that heterogeneity within populations represents a redistribution of a limited repertoire of underlying states, i.e. all states are present before treatment, but there are changes to the percentage of cells in a state upon drug treatment. Their system demonstrated the power of using HTM across time- and dose-responses to characterize shifts in the status of a population of cells, ultimately demonstrating that all cell states are present, it is only the distribution that changes.

In 2009, Loo et al. [17] also investigated heterogeneity using an image-based approach to classify phenotypic properties of distinct subpopulations. This manuscript addressed an issue that affects all fluorescent-based experiments: there is a limit to the number of markers that can be used for any given experiment (3–5 depending on the detection equipment in use). The authors used HCA to examine different cell subpopulations based upon expression of known differentiation markers. In 3T3L1 preadipocytes, the population of cells was split into 4 subgroups based on expression of adiponectin and total cellular levels of lipid. The authors trained a classifier to learn the patterns of features that best describe the four subpopulations. This allowed the system to decide for itself what population a specific cell was in according to the features extracted during the imaging process. Next, the authors removed (deleted from the record) all of the features from one marker. The classifiers were recreated from the list of features that still remained that best separated the four classes without relying on features from the removed marker. In this manner, it was iteratively possible to add new markers to further study the subpopulations, without compromising available fluorescent channels or further stressing data collection/management workflows. Ultimately, this approach defined subpopulations of leukemic and lung cancer cells, using a different panel of markers for each cell type. Taken together, the effort clearly highlighted the need and value to apply HCA to studying cell subpopulations.

In another excellent example illustrating the utility of image-based screening in determining drug responses at the single cell level, Loo et al., [18] used a support vector machine (SVM) algorithm to define classifiers for separation of treated versus untreated cells. First, changes in sets of fluorescent markers were evaluated against 100 different compounds in HeLa cells. With the ability to capture thousands of cells per treatment combined with cell cycle determination based upon DNA staining, measurement of broad and specific effects within each cell cycle phase were possible. The study showed how high content analysis and data reduction techniques can be used to contrast feature types (texture- versus intensity-based) for collections of marker sets. These examples of high throughput microscopy and high content analysis highlight the innate ability of these methods to characterize subpopulations of cells under different perturbations and can also be used to study the biology of nuclear receptors.

While Altschuler's lab [17] developed a framework for analysis of subpopulations in 3T3-L1, an additional study used HCA to determine the mechanisms of cell–cell variability in peroxisome proliferator-activated receptor (PPARγ and lipid accumulation during human adipocyte differentiation [19]. To identify potential coactivator interplay and redundancy during human adipogenesis, Hartig et al. used HCA to quantify new links between the nuclear receptor PPARγ, proadipogenic steroid receptor coactivators (SRCs), and lipogenesis in human subcutaneous adipocytes. As expected during the first 96 h of differentiation, there were robust and concomitant increases in PPARγ protein levels and lipid content within the bulk population. When examined on a cell-to-cell basis, marked cell-to-cell heterogeneity was apparent, with PPARγ and lipid levels varying up to a 1,000-fold. Experimentally, they perturbed PPARγ heterogeneity by down-regulating SRC-2 and SRC-3 while, simultaneously, quantifying PPARγ. Knockdowns of SRC-2 and SRC-3, individually or jointly, equally inhibited lipid accumulation by preventing lipogenic gene engagement, without affecting PPARγ protein levels. When this result was analyzed further, SRC-2 and SRC-3 knockdown increased the proportion of cells in a PPARγ^{hi}/Lipid^{lo} state, likely reflecting PPARγ with reduced transcriptional activity. This effect on PPARγ was corroborated when increased levels of phospho- PPAR$\tilde{\gamma}$S114 was detected, which is a post-translational modification that reduces PPARγ transcriptional activity and blocks adipogenesis. This study represents an innovative application of HCA to describe a putative mechanism driving non-genetic, mutation-independent population variability. But also, novel to coregulator biology, SRC-2 and SRC-3 not only 'coactivate' PPARγ biochemically, as established extensively in the literature, but also promote PPARγ population variation and attenuate an anti-adipogenic PPARγ phosphorylation event in a previously undiscovered way. These findings and methodology establish a framework for future studies of molecular heterogeneity and gene regulatory mechanisms overlooked by classic, homogenized, biochemical methods.

1.3 High-Throughput Techniques for Studying Nuclear Receptor Biology

As nuclear receptors are regulated by many inputs and feedback outputs, it is necessary to study a wide range of NR-associated endpoints. Quantitative, image-based, high throughput systems allow the collection of large datasets that, combined with HCA, produce a set of quantitative endpoints on a cell-by-cell basis. This section will introduce and discuss HCA and high throughput screening (HCS) as a means to study mechanisms governing NR activity.

A key, early event in transcription is alteration of the chromatin environment. Activating histone marks such as acetylated Histone 3 Lysine 27 are requirements for transcription [20]. To discover regulators of chromatin modification, a recent study [21] used quantitative high throughput screening (qHTS) to screen 60,000 compounds for reagents that de-repress a repressed GFP locus. Over 400 hits were identified that relieved repression and/or activated transcription of the GFP reporter. Common chemical substructures were extracted from the hits, yielding six varieties of compounds. Analysis of false-positives (fluorescent compounds) identified a series containing quinoline and thisdiazinane cores. Importantly, the hit compounds were not histone deacetylase (HDAC) or DNA methyltransferase inhibitors, but were effective in the slowing cancer cell growth, similar to other epigenetic modulators. Extending qHTS methodology to identify epigenetic modulators highlights the ability of microscopy-based screening to discover new classes of compounds that act through novel biological candidate proteins.

The combination of NR biology with high throughput, multiplexed screening has been applied to identify selective nuclear receptor modulators (SNRMs). Glucocorticoids, acting through the glucocorticoid receptor (GR), are used as anti-inflammatory agents and immunotherapeutics. However, likely linked to the widespread physiological role of GR in numerous organ systems, these drugs can result in hazardous side effects [22]. In order to screen for drugs that exhibit tissue-specific activity without side effects, 1,040 compounds were screened in A549 cells in parallel for transcriptional activity at four different promoters [23]. These promoters each controlled expression of a different fluorescent protein (cerulean fluorescent protein, yellow fluorescent protein, or mOrange fluorescent protein) and were transfected into a GR positive, glucocorticoid-responsive cell type (A549). The fourth promoter controlled a non-dexamethasone (Dex, a GR agonist) responsive mCherry fluorescent protein. The compounds were screened for both agonist and antagonistic activity with a fluorescent plate reader. With this screen, compounds were classified based upon their ability to affect one or more promoters. One class affected all three dex-regulated promoters (for example, Mitoantrone), another class only two promoters (for example rosolic acid), or a class affecting only 1 promoter (forskolin). A new class of GR inhibitors, anthracyclines, was discovered with confirmatory experiments performed in U2OS cells line stably transfected with GR. These findings emphasize the advantage of using fluorescent multiplexing methods to identify compounds that uniquely affect nuclear receptor biology. By standard luciferase assays, these experiments would have to be run in parallel, requiring four times as much source material while being unable to study multiple promoters during the same treatment. However, this multiplexed XFP assay was a plate-based assay that can only assess the bulk average response. Improvements in HTM and HCA are now in place to allow the measurement of cell–cell contributions to GR-mediated reporter activity.

The above systems provided an intellectual framework to study the complex biology of the sex steroid receptors ERα and AR. The ability to separate and classify subpopulations of cells are very important for identifying antagonists against these receptors while also determine the properties of cell populations that predispose disease. It is also known that cells expressing AR and ERα exhibit cellular heterogeneity in the levels of these receptors and receptor-associated coregulators. The next sections will discuss the advances made in the field of AR and ERα biology obtained through the use advanced fluorescence microscopy techniques, including FRAP, FRET, and high throughput microscopy. We will highlight the opportunities that state-of-the-art imaging approaches bring to the study of gene regulation by focusing upon model systems for AR and ER. First, relevant molecular and clinical information will be presented, then followed by examples of imaging based efforts to better understand mechanisms of action and screening.

2 Androgen Receptor

2.1 Basic AR Biology

The androgen receptor (AR) is a member of the nuclear receptor super-family, functions as a ligand-inducible transcription factor, and is involved in the differentiation and development of the male genital apparatus [24]. There are a number of prerequisites leading to wild-type AR activation under physiologic circumstances. Especially in the context of cellular analyses, it is important to note that in the absence of agonist, up to 80% of AR is localized in the cytoplasm where it is complexed to molecular chaperones. Addition of agonist sheds chaperones and allows receptor translocation to the nucleus. Once within the nucleoplasmic compartment, agonist-activated AR forms a hyperspeckled fluorescent pattern that is generally linked to an active transcriptional status [25–27]. These agonist-induced speckles likely represent transient interactions (see below) between AR, nuclear proteins and/or DNA [28]. AR nuclear speckles are not visualized when AR-mediated transcription is repressed by antagonists, for instance in the presence of Casodex [25]. In the nucleus, agonist-bound AR associates with the chromatin of AR-responsive genes and recruits coregulators (CoR) and the transcriptional machinery to induce (or inhibit) target gene transcription. The biological effects of AR are modified by a set of post-translational modifications (PTMs, e.g., phosphorylation, acetylation, sumoylation [29] that can change its function, localization, and protein–protein interaction profile. Briefly summarized below, human diseases associated with hypo or hyperfunction of AR have been described in at least 3 different clinical entities.

More than 400 inactivating mutations of AR have been found in patients affected by androgen insensitivity syndrome (AIS) (http://androgendb.mcgill.ca/). AIS presentation depends on the site of the mutations, the degree of inactivation, and falls within one of the following phenotypes: complete (CAIS complete androgen insensitivity syndrome), partial (PAIS partial androgen insensitivity syndrome) and minimal (MAIS minimal androgen insensitivity syndrome) [24].

A second clinical entity associated with AR is the expansion of a CAG/glutamine (Q) tract in exon 1 of AR, known as Kennedys Disease (also known as Spinal Bulbar Muscular Atrophy) [30], that represents one of nine neurodegenerative disorders associated with the expansion of CAG repeats in the coding region of an otherwise unrelated gene. The clinical picture associated with Kennedys Disease consists of lower motor neuron degeneration in males [31] and signs of partial androgen insensitivity, testicular atrophy, gynecomastia and/or reduced fertility [32]. As with other polyglutamine expanded proteins (e.g., Huntingtin, Spinal Cerebellar Ataxia-1, etc.), AR with an expanded poly Q tract undergoes misfolding and cellular aggregation and it is thought to exert toxic effects in the nervous system through several mechanisms [33]. These include disruption of AR transcriptional activity and sequestration of coregulators [30, 34], interference with the ubiquitin-proteasome pathway followed by induction of a stress response, and possibly interruption of axonal transport and synaptic function [35]. In keeping with cell culture experiments showing a partial reduction of AR function mediated by the expanded CAG tract, it is also possible that reduced transcription function of the mutated protein contributes to the pathogenesis of SBMA disease [36].

The third and most prevalent clinical entity associated with AR dysfunction is prostate cancer. Interestingly, the classic, physiologic model of AR activation has underscored that nuclear translocation, subnuclear organization and PTMs are critically important in prostate cancer. Not only is AR involved in primary tumor development, it is also required for disease progression to androgen-independent disease. Since AR is involved in prostate cancer (PC) growth, most patients affected by this disease undergo androgen depletion therapy (ADT) when surgery is not an option. Although this therapy is initially effective, invariably treatment-resistance occurs after a median of two years leading to castration resistant prostate cancer (CRPC) [37]. Once prostate cancer has transitioned to CRPC, the disease invariably progresses to a fatal outcome, and was expected to kill 27,360 Americans in 2009 [38]. However, ligand-dependent, activation does not apply to CRPC, where AR is active in a ligand-independent way. In CRPC, AR is constitutively found in the nucleus. The fact that AR is active in patients who have undergone ADT creates the paradox that AR agonists, depleted after chemical castration, are not necessary for AR activation under castration resistant conditions. Many reviews over the years [39, 40] have summarized and proposed hypotheses that describe putative mechanisms of ligand-independent AR activity. This section will discuss the advances in fluorescent imaging techniques that have expanded our knowledge of AR action.

2.2 *Microscopy-Based AR Assays for Mechanistic Inquiry of AR Function*

Monitoring reporter gene activity as the functional readout has classically identified AR inhibitors. However, these assays are vulnerable to non-AR effects such as inhibitors of mRNA stability and RNA polymerase II that often yield antagonistic results similar to bona fide inhibition of AR. While extensive biochemical controls are used to minimize problems with enzymatic assays, imaging approaches have been developed to screen for AR inhibitors that specifically examine changes in AR conformation within a cellular context [41]. Here, Fluorescence Resonance Energy Transfer (FRET) can be performed using a dual-tagged AR fusion protein with CFP at the N-terminus and YFP at the C-terminus (C-AR-Y). The well-studied agonist-induced increase in N–C terminal contact results in increased FRET signals [42]. As FRET signals are intrinsically distance-dependent (<60 angstroms), visualization of changes to FRET signals have been considered a form of 'nanoscopy'. For screening purposes, C-AR-Y was stably expressed in both LAPC4 and HEK293 cell lines as an assay to identify new AR inhibitors. In the initial report, this assay was used to screen >1,000 compounds along with a traditional luciferase reporter assays. The imaging approach identified 34 compounds that decrease N–C terminal interactions in the presence of androgen. Hits were also validated in an MMTV-luciferase reporter assay. Tritiated DHT competition assays showed that most of the hits were non-competitive inhibitors. Ultimately, a diverse set of compounds affecting AR were identified, including coumarin derivatives, antimicrobial agents such as sulfaquinoxaline, and interestingly GABA receptor inhibitors, such as Clonazepam. This assay not only showed the power of using a cell-based, conformation assay in screening compounds for AR activity but also provided evidence of new pathways that affect AR signaling.

In a follow-up study, [43] the FRET assay was combined with HTM to quantify both N–C interactions *and* changes in subcellular localization, creating a multiplexed approach that encompasses multiple stages of AR activation (Fig. 1). This screen comprised >4,400 bioactive molecules of which 7% decreased the FRET signal, 0.5% inhibited nuclear translocation, and 0.3% inhibited both measurements. Hits were validated through dose response assays and DHT binding. The screen identified compounds such as Sanguinarine and Ketoconazole as known compounds that inhibit AR by interfering with ligand binding. The authors also identified noncompetitive inhibitors such as radicicol and 17-AAG, two Hsp90 inhibitors that blocked AR activation without affecting DHT binding. Interestingly, the authors found a novel inhibitory compound, oxindole I, that actually increased the FRET signal signifying a more tightly folded receptor. Taken together, these imaging-based assays display the power of immunofluorescence in screening compound libraries while simultaneously looking for distinct outcomes and detecting novel mechanisms.

2.3 *FRAP/FRET Assays for Studying the Mechanisms of AR Activation*

While fluorescence-based assays are useful screening tools, they can also be used to determine basic mechanistic information on AR function in normal tissues or in various disease states. In 2005, Schaufele et al. [42] compared ligand-dependent activation, intramolecular contact, and intermolecular interactions for AR, ER, and PPARγ using CFP-NR-YFP, CFP-NR, and NR-YFP constructs. After validating the ligand-dependent, biological activity of the constructs (in some cases more active than wild-type AR), it was shown that an increase in the inter-molecular FRET ratio was observed between CFP-AR and AR-YFP only in the nucleus. Interestingly, when the same experiment was performed on cells expressing CFP-AR-YFP, an increase in the intra-molecular FRET ratio occurred in both the cytoplasm and the nucleus of the cells. This data provided a cell-based validation for the classic model of ligand binding to AR where agonists act by inducing a conformational change in the receptor. After liganded AR translocates to the nucleus, it then dimerizes with another liganded AR. In contrast to AR, the CFP-ER-YFP did show high levels of FRET without ligand. PPARγ, which only heterodimerizes with RXR [44], showed only intramolecular FRET occurring that was not increased with addition of ligand, suggesting conformational change is not a key step in PPARγ activation. They further showed that O-hydroxyflutamide (OHF), a known AR antagonist, inhibited the DHT-dependent increase in FRET. Also, they established that deletion of the FQNLF motif within N-terminal domain was necessary for full FRET in response to DHT. In terms of prostate cancer-linked mutant forms of AR found in hormone-refractory cancer (874Y, 877A, 877S), FRET was used to show non-AR

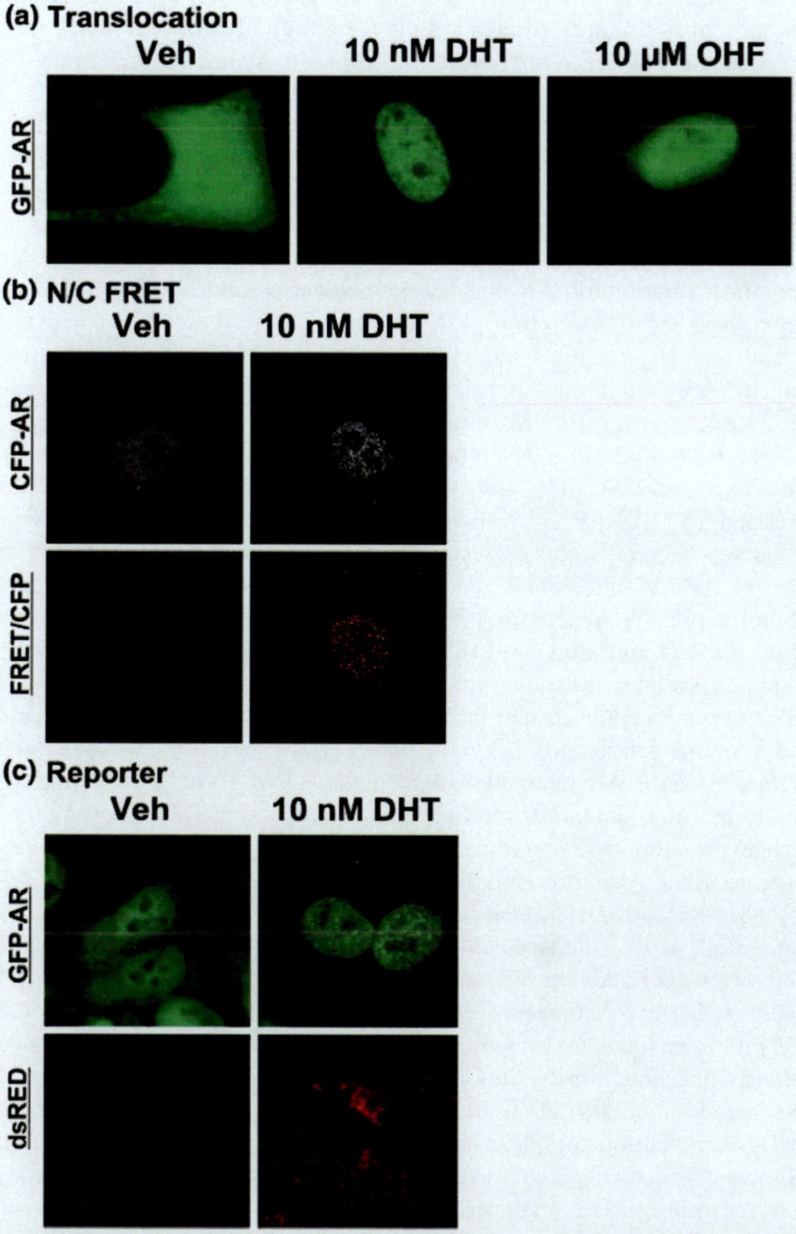

Fig. 1 Screening methods using imaging for studying AR biology. Many AR studies with imaging have used primarily 3 methods for discerning the biology. Translocation studies (**a**) look at effect on the movement of AR from the cytoplasm to the nucleus but say nothing about the conformation or reporter output. N-terminal/c-terminal FRET (**b**) illustrates the effects of a compound (or siRNA) on the conformation of the receptor. Finally the use of a reporter gene (**c**) describes the actual transcriptional activity of the receptor. These combined approaches have yielded much valuable information about the effectors of AR-mediated transcription

ligands (progesterone, estradiol) altered intramolecular AR interactions in these more promiscuous mutants. Similar results were found [28] when FRET was used to show that the FQNLF motif, located in the X domain, was necessary for AR conformational changes. Also, utilizing a multi-modal approach, this group combined FRET reporting of AR conformation with simultaneous quantification of AR molecular mobility via Fluorescence Recover After Photobleaching (FRAP). Using this technique, the authors showed a loss of FRET when AR is bound to the DNA, suggesting that binding to DNA induced yet another conformational change to the molecule. They further showed a reduced FRET signal in the immobile fraction of AR located in nuclear speckles (sites that partially overlap with active transcription [45]. The use of FRET combined with translocation and mobility analyses has shown not only agonist/antagonist activity of ligands, but also mutation-specific effects, and conformational changes AR occupies while moving through the nucleus.

Further FRAP studies on AR [46] focused on various mutants that included a DNA-binding (A573D [47] and two ligand-specificity altering substitutions (W714C and T877A) that are responsive to bicalutamide and OHF, respectively. FRAP curves showed a faster recovery time for the A573D mutation in the presence of R1881, and W714C and T877A reveals wild-type like kinetics and immobile fraction. Treatment with bicalutamide or OHF causes an increase of the immobile fraction and slows diffusion rate of W714C and T877A, respectively, which also correlates with the formation of subnuclear hyperspeckles. These mutations in the receptor change the structure of AR thus allowing the receptor to become hormone refractory.

Single cell-based AR interactions with target DNA were tested using a novel model system that contains multiple repeats of the MMTV promoter [48]. Through expression of a tetracycline-inducible GFP-AR [49], the authors first demonstrated that AR differentially translocates in a ligand dependent fashion, with R1881>RU486>DHT>OHF>Vehicle and that translocation data did not correlate well with standard transcriptional output from various luciferase reporters. However, AR localization to the MMTV promoter array positively correlated with mRNA transcription determined by FISH. FRAP of AR at the MMTV promoter locus under various ligands showed differential recovery times for agonists and antagonists, similar to GR and PR, and ER in another steroid receptor-based model system [50]. Ligand-dependent recruitment of the BRM chromatin remodeling complex in the presence of agonistic compounds was also shown. Taken together, use of a fluorescent microscopy-based assay allowed for multiplexed analyses that covered a wide range of mechanistic steps involved in the activation of AR. The final section will discuss using some of the approaches discussed above in the context of personalized medicine, specifically in a proof of concept test to treat in the context of androgen insensitivity syndrome (AIS).

2.4 High-Throughput Imaging for Characterizing Pathological AR Dysfunction Moving Towards Personalized Medicine

A major goal of biomedical research is personalized medicine and patient-specific care. This requires a deep understanding of the disease attributes that a specific patient presents, i.e. a mutation, progression, responsiveness. High throughput microscopy has been used to study responsiveness of pharmacological compounds in cell models [26] and in primary cultures from patients [27]. These manuscripts detailed the development and proof of concept applications that use HTM to characterize complex biological responses using a cell-by-cell imaging approach. In the first report, wild-type and mutant (T877A, the LnCaP), and F764L (an AIS mutation) forms of AR were tested for ligand effects in a monolayer cell culture model. All three responded normally to R1881 in terms of translocation. The assay was enhanced through the use of image analysis tools, which automatically segment nuclei and take measurements based on fluorescent signal (Fig. 2). This translocation assay was combined with a subnuclear pattern assay (Hyperspeckling), and a transcriptional reporter assay using transient expression of a probasin proximal promoter regulating expression of a dsRED2 reporter gene. With this automated system, the researchers were able to generate dose response curves for nuclear translocation, hyperspeckling, and reporter accumulation. EC50 values for many ligands including R1881, Mibolerone, estrogen, and progesterone were then established. Interestingly, the cells with the highest levels of GFP-AR had the lowest amount of reporter accumulation suggesting that over expression of AR can actually lead to failed androgen responsiveness. IC50 s for various antagonists (bicalutamide, vinclozolin, decursin) were also calculated based on translocation, hyperspeckling and reporter output. As the cell cycle has been shown to be linked to gene expression, Szafran and colleagues also demonstrated differential ligand responsiveness throughout the cell cycle. AR translocation in response to R1881 was most sensitive in G1, with the lowest sensitivity during S phase. Hyperspeckling, however, was most highly detected in G2, followed by G1, with minor hyperspeckling occurring in S phase. This study demonstrated the strength of high throughput imaging in characterizing multiple AR actions simultaneously; more importantly, however, this work showed how single cell data could be used to mine data from heterogeneous cell populations' values that would be completely missed by standard biochemical approaches.

As a step closer to patient studies, a follow-up manuscript [27] examined primary genital skin fibroblasts from both healthy individuals and patients who have either partial or complete androgen insensitivity syndrome (AIS). It was previously known that these AIS patients harbored different AR mutations: F764L and P766S (complete AIS), and R840C (partial AIS). In addition, it was previously determined that these mutations result in different levels of AR dysfunction in response to the endogenous androgen DHT (dihydroxytestosterone). Through the use of HTM, the authors were able to demonstrate a strong correlation between nuclear hyperspeckling and the transcriptional output in all wild-type and mutant

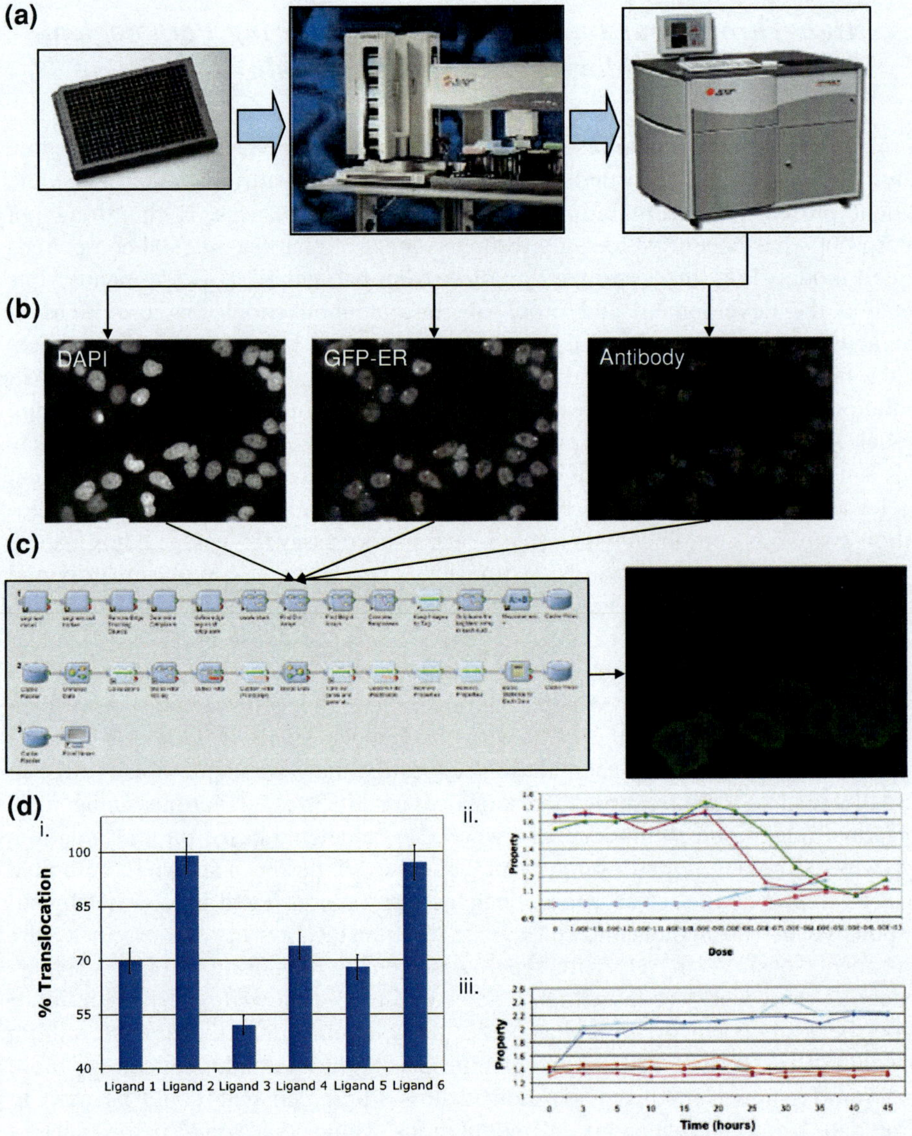

Fig. 2 Scheme for advanced multiplex NR screening. Assay workflow for a multiplex high content screen. **a** Cells are seeded in a multiwell plate made with optically sensitive glass (or high quality plastic). Cells are then treated/fixed/immunolabeled and/or stained robotically (a Beckman robot is shown here). Following fixation, the cells are imaged on an automated fluorescence microscopy platform (e.g., high throughput microscope). **b** Autofocus-based multi-channel fluorescent images are acquired from one or multiple fields of each well. **c** Images are analyzed through an automated analysis platform (PipelinePilot shown here) that performs background subtraction, then creates cell and subcellular segmentation (masks); masks are then examined for up to hundreds of imaging features (intensity, texture, statistics, etc.) that can define a systems level view of the biological responses occurring at the single cell level. **d** Example outputs from image analysis: (i) straightforward translocation measurements, (ii) dose-response curves, and (iii) kinetic analysis

strains. Whereas all AIS mutations resulted in either a moderate to profound transcriptional dysfunction in the presence of DHT, each mutation had a distinct phenotype response to the panel of ligands tested. For example, at concentrations of DHT that failed to produce significant hyperspeckling or transcriptional activity from the F764L mutated receptor, near normal levels of nuclear translocation of the receptor were observed. Furthermore, use of high levels of mibolerone, a synthetic androgen, with the F764L mutation was able to induce not only nuclear translocation, but also significant hyperspeckling and transcriptional activity. In comparison, the other complete AIS associated mutation P766S did not demonstrate a similar response or ligand preference. These results demonstrate not only the diversity of the AR response that can be appreciated when examining samples obtained from both normal individuals and patients with a similar diagnosis using an image based approach, but also the type of highly enriched data that will be necessary as personalized medicine continues to move forward.

3 Estrogen Receptor

3.1 Basic ER Biology

Estrogen receptor-α (ER) is Type I class steroid receptor and a founding member of the nuclear receptor superfamily. Primarily, ER functions as a transcription factor that facilitates regulation of hormone-dependent genes. Similar to other nuclear receptors, ER protein has five domains (from N to C): the AF-1 domain, the DNA binding domain (DBD), the hinge region, the ligand-binding domain (LBD), the AF-2 domain (within the LBD) [51], and the F-domain [52]. The two AF domains within ER have different functions. AF-1 is a ligand-independent domain acted upon by kinase signaling and interacts with many coactivators. The AF-2 domain is ligand-dependent through which ER recruits coregulators to the transcriptional apparatus [53]. Some cell types require both transactivation domains to acquire full activity, while others do not [54], adding another level of complexity to ER-mediated transcription. Unlike other classical steroid receptors, ER is a chiefly nuclear resident protein (>90%) under control conditions [55]. The natural ligand for ER is 17β-estradiol (E2). Upon E2 binding, ER is released from the chaperone heat shock proteins [56], dimerizes with another ligand-bound ER, and binds to estrogen response elements (ERE) throughout the genome. This event recruits cofactors causing alterations to the chromatin environment [57], allowing recruitment of transcriptional machinery and RNA polymerase II (Pol II), inducing target genes such as progesterone receptor, c-fos [58], and cyclin D1 [59]. ER is expressed in the female reproductive (breast, uterus, and ovary), skeletal [60], cardiovascular [61], and nervous [62] systems.

ER works through three mechanisms to activate transcription: (1) ER/ERE direct activation, (2) SP-1/AP-1 enhancers driving indirect activation of transcription [58], and (3) non-genomic signaling from kinase cascades [63]. These pathways can be activated in ligand-dependent and -independent ways while both require post-translational modifications (PTMs). ER can be highly modified by PTMs including methylation [64], acetylation [65], and phosphorylation [66] causing diverse ER signaling effects. Kinase cascades play an important role in cancer progression with certain ER phospho-sites being implicated in tamoxifen resistance [67].

Tamoxifen is one of the first compounds referred to as a selective estrogen receptor modulators (SERM), as it possesses either agonist or antagonist effects that depend upon tissue/phosphorylation context (e.g., repressive effects in breast tissue but agonistic effects in the uterus [68] and bone). Since its discovery, tamoxifen has been the chief treatment for ER-positive breast cancers and continues, today, despite an efficacy of only 50% in patients [69]. Tumors, almost invariably, develop resistance to the drug through various mechanisms: metabolic drug disposition [70], SERM reversal to agonist activity [71], overexpression of cofactors such as SRC-1 and HER2/neu [72], activation of the EGF signaling pathway enhancing tamoxifen agonism [73], and spontaneous mutations to the F-domain [74]. New SERMs have become available in recent years including raloxifene and lasofoxifene. As none of the new SERMs have exhibited efficacy better than tamoxifen, there continues to be an urgent need for continued drug screening with more sensitive screening applications.

SERM activity is mediated by structural changes within ER that recruit distinct groups of transcriptional coregulators. Significant research has been devoted to mechanisms of cancer progression driven by coregulator action. Upon interaction of ligand-bound ER with EREs, coactivators such as CBP [75], steroid receptor coactivators (SRC-1, SRC-2, SRC-3) [76], and PRMT1 [77] form multi-protein complexes that lead to decondensation of chromatin (via histone acetyltransferase recruitment), and create a protein bridge allowing recruitment of Pol II and subsequent transcription. Tamoxifen-bound ER has been shown to recruit nuclear receptor corepressor (NCOR) and silencing mediator of retinoid and thyroid receptors (SMRT) [78], which in turn recruit histone deacetylases and demethylases condensing the chromatin and inhibiting transcription. Significant effort has been devoted to studying ER interactions with its environment (chromatin/CoR) that affect ER by both conventional and microscopy-based approaches. The following sections will outline this area of study.

3.2 ER Dynamics and Chromatin Remodeling by Microscopy

As noted above, an important aspect of nuclear receptor biology is subcellular localization and trafficking. Many biochemical endpoint assays have been used to study ER translocation (cell fractionation assays [79], ER mobility, and ER-mediated chromatin remodeling. Due its flexibility and multi-parametric nature, fluorescence microscopy has provided informative windows into ER biology that have begun to supplant classic biochemical assays.

FRAP is a key means to look at mobility of proteins within living cells. Proteins fused with fluorescent tags are bleached in a specific region of a cell using a now commonly accessible laser scanning confocal microscope. The rate at which the bleached region regains fluorescence is attributed to the mobility of the tagged protein as it diffuses to return fluorescence to the targeted region. Study of ER mobility led to the first observation that nuclear proteins can have differential dynamics based upon a variety of ligand conditions. Stenoien et al. [80] showed that in HeLa cells unliganded ER has a very rapid recovery time (<1 s). Addition of estradiol or tamoxifen increases this recovery to about six seconds, an effect attributed to ER interactions with DNA and regulator proteins, and trafficking through the dense chromatin environment. Interestingly, treatment with ICI 182,780 (ICI, also known as Fulvestrant), a ligand that induces degradation of the receptor [81], caused the receptor to be irreversibly immobilized, ($t_{1/2}$=>5 min). Similar to ER, the coactivator SRC-1 took seconds to recover under estradiol and tamoxifen conditions. Unlike ER, SRC-1 recovery was not effected by ICI. Inhibition of the proteasome (through treatment with MG132) was also able to immobilize ER. Further experiments showed that helix 12 (amino acids 534–554) of ER was necessary for ICI-mediated immobilization. Irreversible binding of ER to chromatin is thus perceived to be the dominant mechanism through which ICI conveys full antagonism. While the standard single cell-based FRAP approach has analyzed AR and ER extensively, quantitative measurements are made upon the entire nuclear pool of receptor; in recent years, new tools have allowed visualization of ER bound to DNA and/or interacting with CoRs (see below).

In the past decade, a select few groups [49, 82, 83] worldwide have developed the technology to study transcriptional mechanisms at the single cell level. Pioneering efforts in this direction began in the mid-90s in the Belmont lab [84]. With the goal of determining changes in chromatin structure within the nucleus of a cell, Robinett et al. [82] integrated an extrachromosomal locus harboring lac operator repeats that could be visualized by its cognate DNA binding protein. This group has championed the now wide-spread use of an integrated cassette of 256 *lac* operator repeats, and their visualization by expression of a GFP-tagged *lac* repressor. These early, large scale chromatin alteration studies led to use of the lacO-lacR system in a variety of applications, including the first engineered cell line that contained a visible and regulated transcriptional locus expressing a fluorescent reporter gene [85]. During the same period, the Hager lab [83, 86, 87] reported a spontaneous, multi-copy integration of the MMTV viral DNA in a clonal variant of mouse mammary tumor cells (C127), which facilitated monitoring GR binding to GRE/ARE/PRE's (mentioned above, [88] found within the MMTV promoter, which has also been used to study AR and progesterone receptor [49, 88]. When GFP-fusions of the glucocorticoid receptor were expressed, they all showed ligand-induced targeting and colocalization of mRNA transcripts [87]. Importantly, when FRAP experiments were performed in this single cell model system, they revealed that NR-DNA complexes are much more dynamic than previously thought from biochemical studies [87]. Similarly, FRAP studies revealed GFP-ER exhibited a marked range in mobility based upon ligand and proteasome activity [80]; further, using a modified lac array system, ligand dependent NR-CoR interactions were also shown to be remarkably dynamic [89], quite unlike the previous models based upon in vitro studies suggesting long-lived stability of NR-CoR complexes. A series of additional transcription array studies further emphasized the dynamic nature of gene regulators at transcriptional loci, including several papers using the MMTV array system [90], a prolactin gene array system [50] (discussed below), and a NFkB/HIV promoter model [91]. While the above model systems possess intrinsically rich and minable mechanistic content, their use as tools in high throughput approaches has been limited due to challenges in automated image acquisition and quantitative analyses.

An improvement to the study of ERα transcription at a single chromosomal locus came with the creation of a multi-copy integration of the mammalian prolactin promoter and enhancer region, which includes an amplified region containing additional ERE/Pit1 synergy elements [50]. This super enhancer controls the expression of a peroxisome-targeted dsRED2 transcriptional reporter gene, and was integrated $\sim$ 100x into the genome of HeLa cells. Expression of transient GFP-ER in this cell line allows visualization of promoter occupancy with physiologically relevant transcriptional responses to ligands. Upon addition of estradiol, a large, diffuse foci appears within the cells as opposed to treatment with tamoxifen, which causes smaller, brighter foci to form. This system allowed for visualization of ER at a known genomic locus, with other coregulators, forming a type of *visual ChIP*. Some proteins were constitutively at the locus, while others (SRC-1, BRG1, SRC-3) were recruited by ER ligands. Time-lapse imaging showed rapid loading of ER followed by increasing array size. RNA fluorescence in situ hybridization (RNA FISH, a method for measure amounts of mRNA [92] confirmed rapid ($\sim$ 15 min) and active (>5-fold) induction of mRNA synthesis at the ER-occupied prolactin array. Chromatin marks (e.g., acetylated H3 and H4) also appear at the PRL array, providing further validation of the array model. FRAP of the GFP-ER loaded array showed rapid recovery after E2 ($\sim$ 6 s) or tam ($\sim$ 4 s) treatments, with almost no recovery after ICI treatment. The creation of a multi-copy ER-regulated locus has allowed a visual ChIP view of the defined steps of ER-controlled transcription activation, including quantitative time-lapse studies that monitor transcriptional output from ligand or growth factor stimulation [93]. In the next section we will discuss how these same methods and systems can be used to further study mediators of ER action, including transcriptional coregulators.

3.3 Using High-Throughput Microscopy to Study ER-Coregulator Interactions

Since their discovery of NR CoR's in the mid-90s, it is difficult to separate the study of ER in the absence of CoR's. The interactions of ER and the members of the p160 family of coactivators (SRC-1, SRC-2, SRC-3; SRCs) have been widely studied using biochemical methods (immunoprecipitation-mass spectrometry,

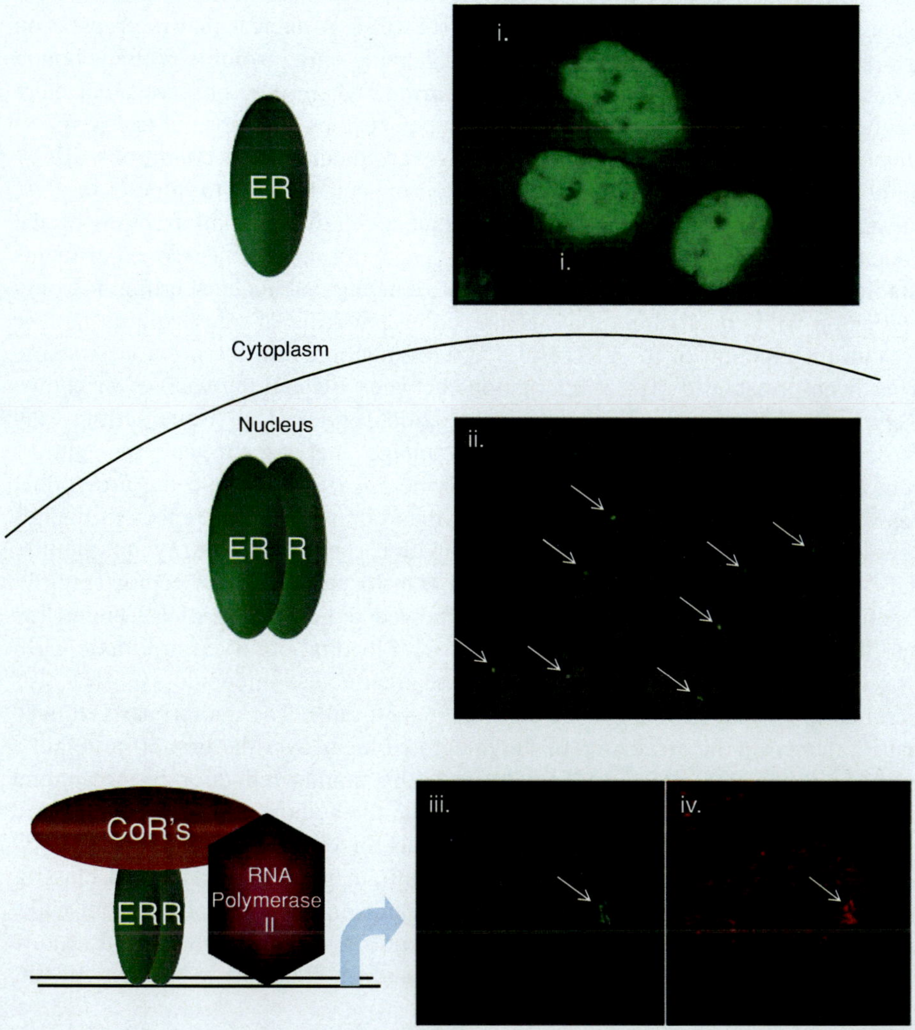

Fig. 3 Visualizing ER biology by HCA. Fluorescence microscopy visualization of multiple mechanistic steps in ER activation of transcription. Bioengineered cell line harboring a visible mammalian transcriptional unit and expressing GFP-ERα [50]. Unliganded GFP-ERα (**i**), is readily visible in a diffuse pattern primarily within nuclei [93]. Upon treatment with 17β-estradiol, ER rapidly (minutes) targets the EREs within the integrated reporter gene locus, and in a hyperspeckled pattern throughput the nucleuoplasm (**ii**), once loaded at the promoter locus (**iii**), ER recruits the transcriptional machinery (various coregulators and modifying enzymes) including RNA polymerase II (**iv**) and initiates transcription

IP-MS) but these represent single endpoint assays that cannot distinguish the patterns of gene regulation from cell-to-cell.

The use of imaging to study ERα and coregulator interactions began with a non-automated approach in an article by Stenoien et al. [93], where the authors used GFP-tagged ER in MCF-7 cells to study hyperspeckling under different ligands and colocalization of the coregulator SRC-1. A nuclear matrix preparation stripping away of soluble proteins and DNA leaving only insoluble proteins bound to nuclear structural proteins [94] was performed where they observed that there was only a small correlation between ER hyperspeckles and those of transcription sites (marked by RNA polymerase II). However, under agonist conditions SRC-1 did correlate with the ER foci indicating their expected ability to interact in vivo. Subsequent studies using FRET showed that a relatively small fraction of the colocalizing nuclear pools of ER and SRC-1 actually interact. These experiments established the interconnectivity between dynamic subnuclear trafficking and interaction with coactivators that are preceding initiation of transcription.

With the creation of the PRL-HeLa system mentioned in the previous section, it has been possible to dissect interactions between ER and the vast set of known coregulators, in terms of nuclear localization, protein-DNA interactions and transcription initiation [55]. Using robust image analysis software the authors were able to quantify loading of RNA polymerase II (polII) onto the arrays that was more highly loaded with E2 treatment than tamoxifen. Differences in ligands were also seen in hyperspeckling (agreeing with earlier reports), array area (ability of E2 to open the chromatin), and nuclear translocation of the receptor (Fig. 3). Kinetic analyses of promoter occupancy showed rapid loading of E2-bound ER onto the PRL array (<10 min), compatible with loading observed in kinetic ChIP assays [95] but more sensitive to low dose treatments. Interestingly, 4HT was recruited at a reduced rate compared to E2 ($\sim$30 min). The authors also showed that E2 increased the array area of the integrated locus over the first 30 min, but a reduction in the area after 5 h of treatment with a similar reduction in the amount of PolII loading. Using the PRL-HeLa cell line, the authors also screened a small library of known endocrine disrupting chemicals for xenoestrogen effects. The cell line was capable of distinguishing agonist from antagonist using a SVM classification strategy that separated unknown compounds into agonist or antagonist-like groups [55]. These findings emphasize the utility of this cell line for future screening of endocrine disrupting compounds and small molecule effectors of ER.

4 Conclusions

High throughput microscopy combined with high content analysis affords immense opportunities to study nuclear receptor biology. All steps of nuclear receptor-mediated transcription can be studied intensely using the methods described in this chapter. We anticipate the NR field will move forward with increasingly common multi-endpoint studies as better software and more flexible assays are developed. One bottleneck to high throughput image-based assays is the onerous demand for increased data storage and CPU-intensive processing; in the future, these challenges will continue to be solved by investing in bioinformatic resources.

Fluorescent techniques have shed light on mechanistic principles governing AR action and have led to discovery of new families of ligands. At the same time, the use of high throughput microscopy is moving towards applications in personalized medicine. Similarly, the use of high throughput microscopy has led to the discovery of many new effectors of ER biology and entire families of compounds that can bind to ER and modulate its activity. These methods have not only discovered new ligand binding partners but also shed light on the dynamics of the receptor and its interactions with the large pool of coregulators. Future studies using higher resolution microscopy with increased throughput will lead to incredible systems biology-based advances in the understanding of how the sex steroid receptors function.

Acknowledgments The authors thank Dr. Fabio Stossi for critically reviewing the manuscript.This work was funded by National Institutes of Health (NIH) grant 5R01DK055622 and support from the John S. Dunn Gulf Coast Consortium for Chemical Genomics (MAM). Additional funding was provided by NIH 1F32DK85979 (SMH), NIEHS Grand Opportunity Grant (1RC2ES018789-01, MAM), and the Keck Center NLM Training Program in Biomedical Informatics of the Gulf Coast Consortia (NLM Grant No. T15LM007093). SCCPR U54 HD-007495, P30 DK-56338, P30 CA-125123, and the Dan L. Duncan Cancer Center of Baylor College of Medicine supported imaging resources.

References

1. Vogl C, Flatt T, Fuhrmann B, Hofmann E, Wallner B, Stiefvater R, Kovarik P, Strobl B, Muller M (2010) Transcriptome analysis reveals a major impact of JAK protein tyrosine kinase 2 (Tyk2) on the expression of interferon-responsive and metabolic genes. BMC Genomics 11(8):199
2. Lee J, Budanov AV, Park EJ, Birse R, Kim TE, Perkins GA, Ocorr K, Ellisman MH, Bodmer R, Bier E, Karin M (2010) Sestrin as a feedback inhibitor of TOR that prevents age-related pathologies. Science 327:1223–1228
3. Valley C, Solodin NM, Powers GL, Ellison SJ, Alarid ET (2008) Temporal variation in estrogen receptor-alpha protein turnover in the presence of estrogen. J Mol Endocrinol 40:23–24
4. Rider C, Hartig PC, Cardon MC, Wilson VS (2009) Comparison of chemical binding to recombinant fathead minnow and humna eatrogen receptors alpha in whole cell and cell-free binding assays. Environ Toxicol Chem 28:2175–2181
5. Kudwa A, Michopoulos V, Gatewood JD, Rissman EF (2006) Roles of estrogen receptor alpha and beta in differentiation of mouse sexual behavior. Neuroscience 138:921–928
6. Bahar R et al (2006) Increased cell-to-cell variation in gene expression in ageing mouse heart. Nature 441:1011–1014
7. Blake WJ, Kaern M, Cantor CR, Collins JJ (2003) Noise in eukaryotic gene expression. Nature 422:633–637
8. Elowitz MB, Levine AJ, Siggia ED, Swain PS (2002) Stochastic gene expression in a single cell. Science 297:1183–1186
9. Hoffman M, Chang HH, Huang S, Ingber DE, Loeffler M, Galle J (2008) Noise-driven stem cell and progenitor population dynamics. PLoS One 3:e2922
10. Chang H, Hemberg M, Barahona M, Ingber DE, Huang S (2008) Transcriptome-wide noise controls lineage choice in mammalian progenitor cells. Nature 453:544–547

11. Ansel J, Bottin H, Rodriguez-Beltran C, Damon C, Nagarajan M, Fehrmann S, Francois J, Yvert G (2008) Cell-to-cell stochastic variation in gene expression is a complex genetic trait. PloS Genetics 4:e1000049
12. Lehner B (2008) Selection to minimise noise in living systems and its implications for the evolution of gene expression. Mol Syst Biol 4:170
13. van Vliet J, Oates NA, Whitelaw E (2007) Epigenetic mechanisms in the context of complex diseases. Cell Mol Life Sci 64:1531–1538
14. Rakyan V, Whitelaw E (2003) Transgenerational epigenetic inheritance. Curr Biol 13:R6
15. Lorincz M, Schubeler D, Hutchinson SR, Dickerson DR, Groudine M (2002) DNA methylation density influences the stability of an epigenetic imprint and Dnmt3a/b-independent de novo methylation. Mol Cell Biol 22:7572–7580
16. Slack M, Martinez ED, Wu LF, Altshuler SJ (2008) Characterizing heterogeneous cellular responses to perturbations. PNAS 105:19306–19311
17. Loo L, Lin HJ, Steininger RJ, Wang Y, Wu LF, Altshuler SJ (2009) An approach for extensibly profiling the molecular states of cellular subpopulations. Nat Methods 6:759–765
18. Loo L, Wu LF, Altschuler SJ (2007) Image-based multivariate profiling of drug responses from single cells. Nat Methods 4:445–453
19. Hartig S, Newberg JY, Bolt MJ, Szafran AT, Marcelli M, Mancini MA (2011) Homeostatic levels of SRC-2 and SRC-3 promote early human adipogenesis. J Cell Biol 192:55–67
20. Creyghton M, Cheng AW, Welstead GG, Kooistra T, Carey BW, Steine EJ, Hanna J, Lodato MA, Frampton GM, Sharp PA, Boyer LA, Young RA, Jaenisch R (2010) Histone H3K27Ac separates active from poised enhancers and predicts developmental state. PNAS 107:21931–21936
21. Johnson R, Huang W, Jadhav A, Austin CP, Inglese J, Martinez ED (2008) A quantitative high-throughput screen identifies potential epigenetic modulators of gene expression. Anal Biochem 375:237–248
22. Schacke H, Docke WD, Asadullah K (2002) Mechanisms involved in the side effects of glucocorticoids. Pharmaclogical Ther 96:23–43
23. Gerber A, Masuno K, Diamond MI (2009) Discovery of selective glucocorticoid receptorglucocorticoid receptor modulators by multiplexed reporter screening. PNAS 106:4929–4934
24. Quigley C, DeBellis A, Marschke KB, el-Awady MK, Wilson EM, French FS (1995) Androgen receptor defects: historical, clinical, and molecular perspectives. Endocr Rev 16:546
25. Marcelli M, Stenoien DL, Szafran AT, Simeoni S, Agoulnik IU, Weigel NL, Moran T, Mikic I, Price JH, Mancini MA (2006) Quantifying effects of ligands on androgen receptor nuclear translocation, intranuclear dynamics, and solubility. J Cell Biochem 98:770–788
26. Szafran A, Szwarc M, Marcelli M, Mancini MA (2008) Androgen receptor functional analyses by high throughput imaging: determination of ligand, cell cycle, and mutation-specific effects. PLoS One 3:e3605
27. Szafran A, Hartig S, Sun H, Uray IP, Szwarc M, Shen Y, Mediwala SN, Bell J, McPhaul MJ, Mancini MA, Marcelli M (2009) Androgen receptor mutations associated with androgen insensitivity syndrome: a high content analysis approach leading to personalized medicine. PLoS One 4:e8179
28. Van Royen M, Cunha SM, Brink MC, Mattern KA, Nigg AL, Dubbink HJ, Verschure PJ, Trapman J, Houtsmuller AB (2007) Compartmentalization of androgen receptor protein–protein interactions in living cells. J Cell Biol 177:63–72
29. Poukka H, Karvonen U, Janne OA, Palvimo JJ (2000) Covalent modification of the androgen receptor by small ubiquitin-like modifier 1 (SUMO-1). PNAS 97:14145–14150
30. La Spada A, Wilson EM, Lubahn DB, Harding AE, Fischbeeck KH (1991) Androgen receptor gene mutations in X-linked spinal and bulbar muscular atrophy. Nature 352:77–79
31. McManamny P, Chy HS, Finkelstein DI, Craythorn RG, Crack PJ, Kola I, Cheema SS, Horne MK, Wreford NG, O'Bryan MK, De Kretser DM, Morrison JR (2002) A mouse model for spinal and bulbar muscular atrophy. Hum Mol Genet 11:2103–2111

32. Fischbeck K, Lieberman A, Bailey CK, Abel A, Merry DE (1999) Androgen receptor mutation in Kennedy's disease. Philos Trans R Soc Lond B Biol Sci 354:1075–1078
33. Finsterer J (2010) Perspectives of Kennedy's disease. J Neurological Sci 298:1–10
34. Stenoien D, Cummings CJ, Adams HP, Mancini MG, Patel K, DeMartino GN, Marcelli M, Weigel NL, Mancini MA (1999) Polyglutamine-expanded androgen receptors form aggregates that sequester heat shock proteins, proteasome components and SRC-1, and are suppressed by the HDJ-2 chaperone. Hum Mol Genet 8:731–741
35. Szebenyi G, Morfini GA, Babcock A, Gould M, Selkoe K, Stenoien DL, Young M, Faber PW, MacDonald ME, McPhaul MJ, Brady ST (2003) Neuropathogenic forms of huntingtin and androgen receptor inhibit fast axonal transport. Neuron 40:41–52
36. Lieberman A, Fischbeck KH (2000) Triplet repeat expansion in neuromuscular disease. Muscle Nerve 23:843–850
37. Chen C, Welsbie DS, Tran C, Baek SH, Chen R, Vessella R, Rosenfeld MG, Sawyers CL (2004) Molecular determinants of resistance to antiandrogen therapy. Nat Med 10:33–39
38. Mahajna J, Dotan N, Zaidman BZ, Petrova RD, Wasser SP (2009) Pharmacological values of medicinal mushrooms for prostate cancer therapy: the case of ganoderma lucidum. Nutr Cancer 61:16–26
39. Cohen M, Rokhlin OW (2009) Mechanisms of prostate cancer cell survival after inhibition of AR expression. J Cell Biochem 106:363–371
40. Schaufele F, Carbonell X, Guerbadot M, Borngraeber S, Chapman MS, Ma AAK, Miner JN, Diamond MI (2005) The structural basis of androgen receptor activation: intramolecular and intermolecular amino-carboxy interactions. Proc Natl Acad Sci USA 102:9802–9807
41. Jones J, An WF, Diamond MI (2009) AR Inhibitors identified by high-throughput microscopy detection of conformational change and subcellular localization. ACS Chem Biol 4:199–208
42. Schaufele F, Carbonell X, Guerbadot M, Borngraeber S, Chapman MS, Ma AAK, Miner JN, Diamond MI (2005) The structural basis of androgen receptor activation: intramolecular and intermolecular amino-carboxy interactions. PNAS 102:9802–9807
43. Jones J, An WF, Diamond MI (2009) AR Inhibitors identified by high-throughput microscopy detection of conformational change and subcellular localization. ACS Chem Biol 4:199–208
44. Hamza M, Pott S, Vega VB, Thomsen JS, Kandhadayar GS, Ng PW, Chiu KP, Pettersson S, Wei CL, Ruan Y, Liu ET (2009) De novo identification of PPARgamma/RXR binding sites and direct targets during adipogenesis. PLoS One 4:e4907
45. Grand M, van der Kraan I, de Jong L, van Driel R (1997) Nuclear distribution of transcription factors in relation to sites of transcription and RNA Polymerase II. J Cell Sci 110:1781–1791
46. Farla P, Hersmus R, Trapman J, Houtsmuller AB (2006) Antiandrogens prevent stable DNA-binding of the androgen receptor. J Cell Sci 118:4187–4198
47. Bruggenwirth H, Boehmer AL, Lobaccaro JM, Chiche L, Sultan C, Trapman J, Brinkmann AO (1998) Substitution of Ala564 in the first zinc cluster of the deoxyribonucleic (DNA)-binding domain of androgen receptor by Asp, Asn, or Leu exerts differential effects on DNA binding. Endocrinology 139:103–110
48. Hager G, McNally JG, Misteli T (2009) Transcription Dynamics. Mol Cell 35:741–753
49. Klokk T, Kurys P, Elbi C, Nagaich AK, Henderwanto A, Slagsvold T, Chang C, Hager GL, Saatcioglu F (2007) Ligand-specific dynamics of the androgen receptor at its response element in living cells. Mol Cell Biol 27:1823–1843
50. Sharp Z, Mancini MG, Hinojos CA, Dai F, Berno V, Szafran AT, Smith KP, Lele TP, Ingber DE, Mancini MA (2006) Estrogen-receptor-alpha exchange and chromatin dynamics are ligand- and domain-dependent. J Cell Sci 119:4101–4116
51. Kumar V, Green S, Stack G, Berry M, Jin JR, Chambon P (1987) Functional domains of the human estrogen receptor. Cell 51:941–951
52. Yang J, Singleton DW, Shaughnessy EA, Khan SA (2008) The F-domain of estrogen receptor-alpha inhibits ligand induced receptor dimerization. Mol Cell Endocrinol 295: 94–100

53. Chen D, Riedl T, Washbrook E, Pace PE, Coombes RC, Egly JM, Ali S (2000) Activation of estrogen receptor alpha by S118 phosphorylation involves a ligand-dependent interaction with TFIIH and participation of CDK7. Mol Cell 6:127–137
54. McDonnell D, Norris JD (2002) Connections and regulation of the human estrogen receptor. Science 296:1642–1644
55. Ashcroft F, Newberg JY, Jones ED, Mikic I, Mancini MA (2011) High content imaging-based assay to classify estrogen receptor-a ligands based on defined mechanistic outcomes. Gene 477:42–52
56. Schlatter L, Howard KJ, Parker MG, Distelhorst CW (1992) Caomparison of the 90-kilodalton heat shock protein interaction with in vitro translated glucocorticoid and estrogen receptor. Mol Endocrinol 6:132–140
57. Nye A, Rajendran RR, Stenoien DL, Mancini MA, Katzenellenbogen BS, Belmont AS (2002) Alteration of large-scale chromatin structure by estrogen receptor. Mol Cell Biol 22:3437–3449
58. Duan R, Porter W, Safe S (1998) Estrogen-induced c-fos protooncogene expression in MCF-7 human breast cancer cells: role of estrogen receptor Sp1 complex formation. Endocrinology 139:1981–1990
59. Castro-Rivera E, Samudio I, Safe S (2001) Estrogen regulation of cyclin D1 gene expression in ZR-75 breast cancer cells involves multiple enhancer elements. J Biol Chem 276:30853–30861
60. Korach K (1994) Insights from the study of animals lacking functional estrogen receptor. Science 266:1524–1527
61. Subbiah M (1998) Mechanisms of cardioprotection by estrogens. Proc Soc Exp Biol Med 217:23–29
62. Toran-Allerand C (1996) The estrogen/neurotrophin connection during neural development: is co=localization of estrogen receptor with the neurotrophins and their receptors biologically relevant? Dev Neurosci 18:36–48
63. Marino M, Distefano E, Trentalance A, Smith CL (2001) Estradiol-induced IP(3) mediates the estrogen activity expressed in human cells. Mol Cell Endocrinol 182:19–26
64. Zhou Q, Shaw PG, Davidson NE (2009) Epigenetics meets estrogen receptor: regulation of estrogen receptor by direct lysine methylation. Endocr Relat Cancer 16:319–323
65. Kim M, Woo EM, Chong YT, Homenko DR, Kraus WL (2006) Acetylation of estrogen receptor alpha by p300 at lysines 266 and 268 enhances the deoxyribonucleic acid binding and transactivation activities of the receptor. Mol Endocrinol 20:1479–1493
66. Le Goff P, Montano MM, Schondin DJ, Katzenellenbogen BS (1994) Phosphorylation of the human estrogen receptor. Identification of hormone-regulated sites and examination of their influence on transcriptional activity. J Biol Chem 269:4458–4466
67. Sarwar N, Kim JS, Jiang J, Peston D, Sinnet HD, Madden P, Gee JM, Nicholson RI, Lykkesfeldt AE, Shousha S, Coombes RC, Ali S (2006) Phosphorylation of ERalpha ar serine 118 in primary breast cancer and in tamoxifen-resistant tumours is indicative of a complex role for ERalpha phosphorylation in breast cancer progression. Endocr Relat Cancer 13:851–861
68. Gielen S, Santegoets LA, Hanifi-Moghaddam P, Burger CW, Blok LJ (2008) Signaling by estrogen and tamoxifen in the human endometrium. J Steroid Biochem Mol Biol 109:219–223
69. Osborne C (1998) Tamoxifen in the treatment of breast cancerbreast cancer. New England J Med 339:1609–1618
70. Osborne C, Wiebe VJ, McGuire WL, Ciocca DR, DeGregorio MW (1992) Tamoxifen and the isomers of 4-hydroxytamoxifen in tamoxife-resistant tumors from breast cancer patients. J Clin Oncol 10:304–310
71. Legault-Possion S, Jolivet J, Poisson R, Beretta-Piccoli M, Band PR (1979) Tamoxifen-induced tumor stimulartion and withdrawal response. Cancer Treat Rep 63:1839–1841
72. Fleming F, Hill AD, McDermott EW, O'Higgins NJ, Young LS (2004) Differential recruitment of coregulator proteins steroid receptor coactivator-1 and silencing mediator for

retinoid and thyroid receptors to the estrogen receptor-estrogen response element by beta-estradiol and 4-hydroxytamoxifen in human breast cancer. J Clin Endocrinol Metab 89:375–383
73. Shou J, Massarweh S, Osborne CK, Wakeling AE, Ali S, Weiss H, Schiff R (2004) Mechanisms of tamoxifen resistance: increased estrogen receptor-HER2/neu cross-talk in ER/HER2-positive breast cancerbreast cancer. J Natl Cancer Inst 96:926–935
74. Herynk M, Hopp T, Cui Y, Niu A, Corona-Rodriguez A, Fuqua SA (2010) A hypersensitive estrogen receptor alpha mutation that alters dynamic protein interactions. Breast Cancer Res Treat 122:381–393
75. Smith C, Onate SA, Tsai MJ, O'Malley BW (1996) CREB binding protein acts synergistically with steroid receptor coactivator-1 to enhance steroid receptor-dependent transcription. PNAS 93:8884–8888
76. Webb P, Nguyen P, Shinsako J, Anderson C, Feng W, Nguyen MP, Chen D, Huang SM, Subramanian S, McKinerney E, Katzenellenbogen BS, Stallcup MR, Kushner PJ (1998) Estrogen activation function 1 works by binding p160 coactivators. Mol Endocrinol 12:1605–1618
77. Klinge C, Jernigan SC, Mattingly KA, Risinger KE, Zhang J (2004) EstrogenEstrogen response element-dependent regulation of transcriptional activation of estrogen receptor alpha and beta by coactivators and corepressors. J Mol Endocrinol 33:387–410
78. Varlakhanova N, Snyder C, Jose S, Hahm JB, Privalsky ML (2010) Estrogen receptors recruit SMRT and N-CoR corepressors through newly recognized contacts between the corepressor N terminus and the receptor DNA binding domain. Mol Cell Biol 30:1434–1445
79. Lazier C, Richman J, Lonergan K (1984) The effect of molybdate on the intracellular distribution of estrogen receptor in mammary tumors. Breast Cancer Res Treat 4:19–26
80. Stenoien D, Patel K, Mancini MG, Dutertre M, Smith CL, O'Malley BW, Mancini MA (2001) FRAP reveals that mobility of oestrogen receptor-alpha is ligand- and proteasome-dependent. Nat Cell Biol 3:15–23
81. Wardell S, Marks JR, McDonnell DP (2011) The turnover of estrogen receptor a by the selective estrogen receptor degrader (SERD) fulvestrantis a saturable process that is not required for antagonist efficiency. Biochem Pharmacol 82:122–130
82. Robinett C, Straight A, Li G, Willhelm C, Sudlow G, Murray A, Belmont AS (1996) In vivo localization of DNA sequences and visualization of large-scale chromatin organization using lac operator/repressor recognition. J Biol Chem 135:1685–1700
83. Stavreva D, Wiench M, John S, Conway-Campbell BL, McKenna MA, Pooley JR, Johnson TA, Voss TC, Lightman SL, Hager GL (2009) Ultradian hormone stimulation induces glucocorticoid receptor-mediated pulses of gene transcription. Nat Cell Biol 11:1093–1102
84. Chuang C, Belmont AS (2007) Moving chromatin within the interphase nucleus-controlled transitions? Semin Cell Dev Biol 18:698–706
85. Tsukamoto T, Hashiguchi N, Janicki SM, Tumbar T, Belmont AS, Spector DL (2000) Visualization of gene activity in living cells. Nat Cell Biol 2:871–878
86. Htun H, Barsony J, Renyi I, Gould DL, Hager GL (1996) Visualization of glucocorticoid receptor translocation and intranuclear organization in living cells with a green fluorescent protein chimera. PNAS 93:4845–4850
87. McNally J, Muller WG, Walker D, Wolford R, Hager GL (2000) The glucocorticoid receptor: rapid exchange with regulatory sites in living cells. Science 287:1262–1265
88. Rayasam G, Elbi C, Walker DA, Wolford R, Fletcher TM, Edwards DP, Hager GL (2005) Ligand-specific dynamics of the progesterone receptor in living cells and during chromatin remodeling in vitro. Mol Cell Biol 25:2406–2418
89. Stenoien D, Nye AC, Mancini MG, Patel K, Dutertre M, O'Malley BW, Smith CL, Belmont AS, Mancini MA (2001) Ligand-mediated assembly and real-time cellular dynamics of estrogen receptor alpha-coactivator complexes in living cells. Mol Cell Biol 21:4404–4412
90. Becker M, Baumann C, John S, Walker DA, Vigneron M, McNally JG, Hager GL (2002) Dynamic behavior of transcription factors on a natural promoter in living cells. EMBO Rep 3:1188–1194

91. Bosisio D, Marazzi I, Agresti A, Shimizu N, Bianchi ME, Natoli G (2006) A hyper-dynamic equilibrium between promoter-bound and nucleoplasmic dimers controls NF-kappaB-dependent gene activity. EMBO J 25:798–810
92. van Raamsdonk C, Tilghman SM (2001) Optimizing the detection of nascent transcripts by RNA fluorescence in situ hybridization. Nucleic Acids Res 29:E42
93. Stenoien D, Mancini MG, Patel K, Allegretto EA, Smith CL, Mancini MA (2000) Subnuclear trafficking of estrogen receptor-alpha and steroid receptor coactivator-1. Mol Endocrinol 14:518–534
94. Nickerson J (2001) Experimental observation of a nuclear matrix. J Cell Sci 114:463–474
95. Metivier R, Penot G, Hubner MR, Reid G, Brand H, Kos M, Gannon F (2003) Estrogen-alpha directs ordered, cyclical, and combinatorial recruitment of cofactors on a natural target promoter. Cell 115:751–763

Micropatterned Surfaces as Tools for the Study of the Rapid Non-genomic Actions of Steroid Receptors

Andrew C. B. Cato, Emmanuel Oppong and Sylwia Sekula-Neuner

Abstract Steroid hormones control several developmental and physiological processes by binding to intracellular receptors that, in turn, interact with DNA to alter gene expression. These processes typically take at least 30 to 60 min for an increase in mRNA expression to be observed. In contrast, other regulatory actions of steroid hormones such as increases in activity of mitogen activated protein kinases are manifested within seconds to a few minutes and are far too rapid to be due to changes at the genomic level. Because these effects are not impaired by inhibitors of mRNA transcription, they are referred to non-genomic or rapid actions to distinguish them from the classical genomic effects at the transcriptional level. The non-genomic effects are thought to occur at the plasma membrane but have proven difficult to analyse in detail because of technical problems arising from capturing the receptors at the membrane due to their dynamic behaviour, subcellular sizes and complexity of action. Here we describe a novel technique for studying the non-genomic action of steroid hormones making use of dip-pen nanolithography (DPN) for patterning supported lipid bilayers containing haptenated lipids onto glass surfaces. Mast cells have been chosen for these studies because of the crucial role they play in allergic reactions and because the

A. C. B. Cato (✉) · E. Oppong
Institute of Toxicology and Genetics,
Karlsruhe Institute of Technology, Hermann-von-Helmholtz-Platz 1,
76344 Eggenstein-Leopoldshafen, Germany
e-mail: andrew.cato@kit.edu

E. Oppong
e-mail: emmanuel.oppong@kit.edu

S. Sekula-Neuner
Institute of Nanotechnology, Karlsruhe Nano-Micro Facility,
Karlsruhe Institute of Technology, Hermann-von-Helmholtz-Platz 1,
76344 Eggenstein-Leopoldshafen, Germany
e-mail: Sylwia.Sekula-Neuner@kit.edu

G. Castoria and A. Migliaccio (eds.), *Advances in Rapid Sex-Steroid Action*,
DOI: 10.1007/978-1-4614-1764-4_15,

non-genomic action of steroid hormones have been reported as one of the means whereby allergy is regulated in these cells. Since mast cells express IgE receptors on their surfaces, they are treated with an anti-IgE antibody and allowed to settle on the patterned surfaces. The IgE receptor is then cross-linked through interaction with the haptenated lipids and this leads to the recruitment of different signalling molecules including steroid receptors to the patterned lipids. The DPN approach allows a nano-scale characterisation of the activating events afforded by the lipid bilayer. The patterns enable quantitative evaluation of co-localised cellular components and the steroid receptors to be assessed. This assay also allows visualisation and analysis of the interacting proteins to be made on a single cell level as well as receptor-proximal events triggered by allergens and regulation by steroid receptors to be measured. This method could be adapted for studying the rapid action of steroid hormones in other cell types.

Keywords Dip-pen nanolithography · Non-nuclear action · Glucocorticoid receptor · Mast cells · Single cell analysis

Contents

1 Introduction

Steroid hormones are small lipophilic molecules that mediate a variety of physiological responses varying from the control of carbohydrate metabolism to the mediation of stress response. They are also important for proper embryonic development as well as acquisition of secondary sexual characteristics [1]. These hormones function by binding to an inactive intracellular receptor such as the glucocorticoid or androgen receptors that are localized in the cytoplasm. Upon hormone binding they are translocated to the nucleus where they bind to hormone response elements to alter the expression of hormone regulated genes [1]. Nuclear translocation of the hormone bound receptor usually takes between 10 and 30 min [2–4] and changes in gene transcription are observed after about 120 min [1, 5, 6]. This mechanism is referred to as genomic action of steroid hormones and has been well defined for the almost all members of the steroid receptor family [1].

Increasing evidence suggests that the variety of responses seen in cells after hormone treatment cannot all be explained by genomic mechanisms. Some responses are too rapid to be explained by transcriptional activation and protein synthesis and are therefore referred to as non-genomic mechanism [7]. Almost all members of the steroid receptor family have now been reported to act via a rapid non-genomic mechanism [7–11] but the mechanisms involved are not fully understood [12, 13]. Nonetheless, the plasma cell membrane remains the unanimously accepted site for the rapid non-genomic action of steroid hormones.

2 Membrane Receptors

Some studies postulate the existence of novel membrane bound receptors for the rapid action of steroid hormones. For example membrane glucocorticoid receptors (mGR) in amphibian neuronal membranes and in rodent lymphoma cells have been described but the origin and function of these receptors are still unexplained [12]. Reports of novel membrane progesterone receptors that held great promises as pharmaceutical targets in the treatment of gynaecological and obstetrical disorders have been discarded [14]. Another example of a G protein coupled receptor proposed to mediate the rapid effect of oestrogen has received very little support [14, 15].

Several studies now show that the rapid non-genomic action of steroid hormones occur through membrane bound classical intracellular receptors and this has initiated a number of studies on this novel action of steroid receptors.

2.1 Classical Intracellular Steroid Receptors as Membrane-Bound Steroid Receptor

Initial studies to demonstrate that the rapid non-genomic action of steroid hormone is mediated by the classical intracellular receptors were carried out with fluorescently labelled steroids attached to bulky proteins that prevented their transport across the plasma membrane, so that the steroid complexes remained on the cell surface. The membrane-bound hormone binding entities were then confirmed as classical intracellular receptors by the use of antibodies directed against different regions of the steroid receptor. For example, oestrogen-BSA conjugates were used to analyse the oestrogen-mediated rapid release of prolactin in GH3/B6 rat pituitary cells [16]. In these studies, the membrane localised binding was identified as ERα after the use of antibodies that recognised different parts of the ERα [16].

Studies using total internal reflection fluorescence microscopy where excitation of fluorophores is limited to within 70–100 nm of the cell surface showed the presence of the androgen receptor at the membrane of Sertoli cells [17]. However not a larger number of sites of the steroid receptors have been identified at the plasma membrane. In an earlier work only 20% of oestrogen binding sites have, for example, been estimated at the plasma membrane of MCF7 human breast cancer cells. The other sites include the nucleus (45%), cytosol (10%) and other organelles [18]. The low number of sites and dynamics of association with the plasma membrane have made it very difficult to come up with a unified mode of action for the rapid non-genomic effects of steroid hormones compared to the genomic effects. So far several different mechanisms have been put forward to describe the rapid action of steroid hormones and a few examples are listed below.

2.1.1 Mechanisms of Rapid Non-genomic Action of Steroid Receptors

1. Steroid receptors such as the androgen and oestrogen receptors (AR and ER) are reported to occur in caveolae. Caveolae, also known as plasmalemmal vesicles, are 50- to 100-nm diameter flask-shaped sub compartments of the plasma membrane. They contain an important structural component caveolin, a 22-kD transmembrane phosphoprotein that forms a scaffold onto which many classes of signalling molecules can assemble to generate pre-assembled signalling complexes [19]. Steroid receptors such as ER and AR are reported to interact with caveolin [20, 21] but it is not clear whether this interaction is necessary for the rapid non-genomic acid of the receptors.
2. The most studied pathway for the rapid action of steroid hormones is the activation of the Ras/Raf-1/ERK pathway by oestrogen. Different mechanisms have been proposed to explain the initial processes that trigger this pathway:

- ERα is reported to bind to insulin like growth factor-1 (IGF-1) receptor to stimulate phosphorylation of this receptor in a ligand-specific fashion [22]. The phosphorylated IGF-1 receptor transmits signals that activate ERK1 and ERK2.
- Oestrogen activates human colon carcinoma-derived Caco-2 cell growth through a rapid and reversible stimulation of intermediates in the signal transduction pathway of the c-Src-related tyrosine kinases c-Src and c-Yes, as well as of ERK1 and ERK2 [23]. In the human breast cancer cell line MCF-7, estradiol triggers a rapid increase in the active form of p21ras, rapid tyrosine phosphorylation of Shc and p190, and association of p190 with the guanosine triphosphatase (GTPase) activating protein (GAP) for p21ras, p21ras-GAP [24]. Both Shc and p190 are substrates of activated Src, and once phosphorylated they interact with other proteins and stimulate p21ras [24]. ERα interacts with Src [24], and this interaction may be responsible for the activation of ERK1 and ERK2.
- ERα-mediated activation of ERK1 and ERK2 is reported to occur through interaction of the receptor with Shc, a downstream target of Src [25].
- Activation of ERK1 and ERK2 by oestrogen increases the expression of the prolactin gene in cultured rat lactotroph and somatolactotroph cell lines.

The mechanism by which ERK1 and ERK2 is activated by the hormone is not quite clear, but it is independent of the activation of c-Src family of tyrosine kinases [26]. Rapid and transient tyrosine phosphorylation of c-Raf-1 has been implicated in this action [26].

3. It has been shown that methylation of an arginine residue at position 260 of the ER allows it to interact with the p85 subunit of phosphatidyl-inositol 3-kinase (PI3K) and Src at the plasma membrane to mediate the rapid action of oestrogen [27]. In another study tyrosine phosphorylation of the ER at position 537 is reported to be responsible for it to interact with the SH2 domain of Src [28].
4. In yet another report, it is thought that the affinity of the ER for Src is through allosteric modification brought about by the adaptor protein MNAR (modulator of non-genomic action of oestrogen receptor) [29].
5. ERα interacts with the WD-repeat protein striatin and targets it to the cell membrane and serves as a scaffold for an ERα-Gα1 complex. Destruction of this complex blocks the rapid non-genomic action of ERα [30].
6. ERα associates with microtubules through the microtubule-binding protein haematopoietin PBX-interaction protein (HPIP) and also helps in the recruitment and activation of the p85 subunit of PI3 kinase and Src in a ligand dependent manner [31].
7. Recently, a cDNA of an alternatively spliced variant of ERα, termed ER-α36 has been cloned [32]. The predicted protein possesses three potential myristoylation sites located near the N-terminus that are thought to anchor the receptor into the plasma membrane. These findings thus predict that ER-α36 functions very differently from ERα in response to oestrogen signalling. It is proposed that ER-α36 is predominantly associated with the plasma membrane where it transduces both oestrogen- and antiestrogen-dependent activation of the mitogen-activated protein kinase/extracellular signal-regulated kinase signalling pathway and stimulates cell growth [32].

2.1.2 Physiologic Significance of the Rapid Action of Steroid Hormones

In terms of its physiological significance several studies have shown that the rapid non-genomic action of steroid receptors function together with the genomic response to enhance the physiological action of steroid receptors [12]. It is well recognised that important effects of sex steroid hormones such as apoptosis protection, cyclin D1 up regulation and bone protective effects may occur through activation of non-genomic pathways [33].

Since the rapid non-genomic action of steroids defines a novel mechanism of steroid hormone action, several pharmaceutical companies were interested in ligands that apparently bind the steroid receptors with a bias towards activation of the non-genomic pathway over the classical genomic response. The exact physiological role of the rapid action of steroids is however not known since it seems to be intertwined with the classical genomic action.

So far the rapid action of steroids has been reported in diverse cells and tissues including breast, prostate, bone, the cardiovascular system and in the immune system. One of the important cells in the immune system that responds to the rapid action of steroid hormones that we have chosen for our studies is the mast cell.

3 Rapid Action of Steroids in Mast Cells

We use mast cells as a model to study the rapid non-genomic action of steroids because they play very important roles in allergy. Allergies have become progressively more common over the past two decades in response to rapid changes in the environment and people's lifestyle. Nearly one in three Europeans suffers, or will suffer, from an allergic disorder. In the adult population, 70% of those affected attest that allergies limit their daily activities. The European Federation of Allergy and Airways Diseases Associations (EFA) claims that asthma is responsible for 9 billion lost working days in the European Union. The social cost-in terms of health care and absenteeism, for example—is estimated at € 45 billion/year.

Mast cells express high affinity IgE receptors (FcεRI) organized as α, β and γ chains on their surfaces. When bound to IgE, the receptors are aggregated by allergens that initiate biochemical events leading to the release of inflammatory mediators [34]. Many of the mediators include histamine, numerous specific proteases and tumour necrosis factor-α (TNF-α). On activation, they also rapidly synthesise bioactive metabolites of arachidonic acid, prostagladins and leukotrienes. A programme of gene expression is activated leading to de novo synthesis of several cytokines and chemokines [34].

At the molecular level, the first demonstrable response after cross-linking and the activation of FcεRI is the rapid activation of cytoplasmic protein kinases and effector pathways that control mast cell responses. One such kinase is Lyn that is converted from an inactive to an active state before it phosphorylates specific motifs on the β- and γ-chains of the FcεRI complex (Fig. 1). In the activated state, Lyn recruits Syk to the receptor γ-chain to further activate the signal transduction pathway [34] that ends up in the production of the inflammatory mediators. Steroid receptors such as glucocorticoid (GR), progesterone receptor [35], oestrogen receptor (ER) and androgen receptor (AR) are all expressed in mast cells. A number of them (e.g. GR, ER and PR) have been implicated in the regulation of mast cells action through rapid non-genomic pathways. For example while the GR and PR [36] are reported to inhibit mast cell action, ER activates this pathway [11, 36]. Since the activation of mast cells occurs primarily at the plasma membrane, we have developed a system to study the non-genomic action of the steroid receptors at the cell membrane using dip-pen nanolithography (DPN) as indicated in Fig. 1.

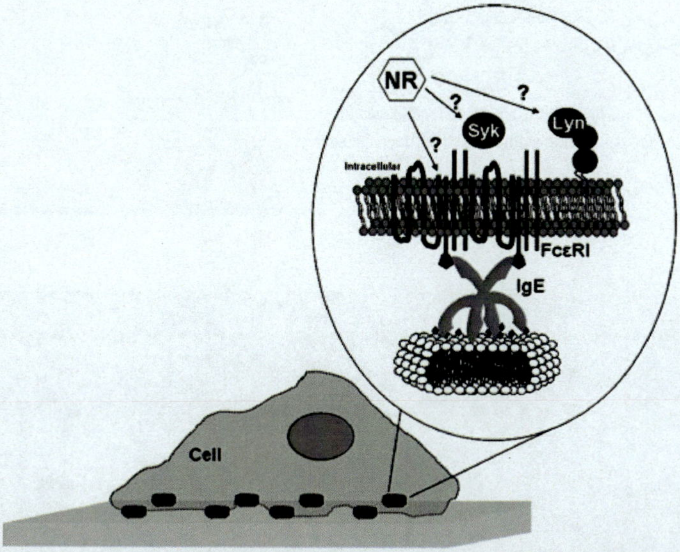

Fig. 1 Schematic diagram of a lipid patterned surface carrying the allergen DNP. Crosslinking the IgE receptor (FcεRI) at the lipid rafts in the membrane (represented by the dots) will lead to the rapid recruitment of the kinases Lyn and Syk to phosphorylate and activate the cell. Steroid receptors (NR) could be rapidly recruited to these lipid rafts to interfere or enhance the signalling process by interacting directly with Lyn, Syk, the IgE receptors or other signalling molecules at the lipid rafts

4 Dip-Pen Nanolithography to Study Events at the IgE Receptor

The technique we are using in this work is dip-pen nanolithography (DPN) that is based on Atomic Force Microscopy (AFM) principle invented by the group of Chad Mirkin [37] for patterning a wide variety of compounds onto surfaces. This has enabled the study of many fundamental phenomena in surface chemistry [38]. DPN is a method of chemical deposition that employs an atomic force microscope (AFM) probe "pen" that has been coated with a molecular "ink" compound. This probe, upon contact with a surface, deposits the ink by diffusion through a water meniscus that forms under ambient conditions between the tip and the substrate. Through control of various conditions such as ambient humidity and writing speed, this method allows the generation of complex patterns with features as small as 15 nm, depending on the ink composition used. Since its initial demonstration, patterns from a wide variety of compounds have been written or templated using this technique including polymers, colloidal nanoparticles and biomolecules.

Biomimetic membrane patterns formed by DPN have recently been used as substrates for the selective adhesion and activation of T-cells [39]. We have now adapted this technique for our analysis of mast cells using as ink the

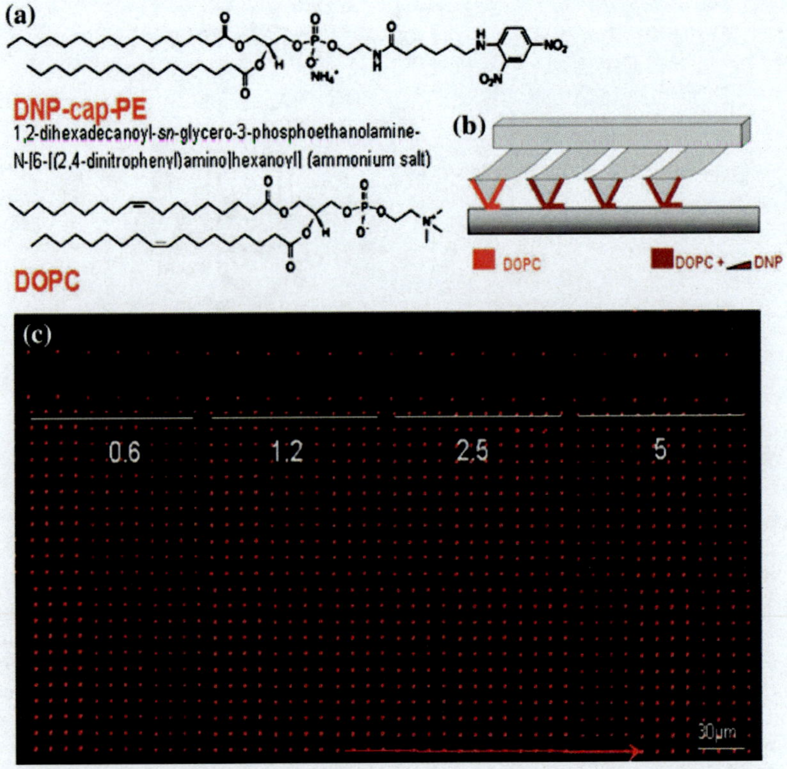

Fig. 2 Multiplexed lithography of phospholipids with allergenic headgroups. **a** Chemical structures of DOPC carrier lipid and allergenic phospholipid DNP-cap-PE. **b** Schematic illustration of the multiplexed patterning of different lipid mixtures. **c** Fluorescence image of nanoarrays composed of DOPC and increasing amounts of DNP phospholipid with the rhodamine labelled lipid admixture

phospholipid 1,2-Dioleoyl-sn-Glycero-3-phosphocholine (DOPC) as a main carrier. In preliminary studies, we can show that the bioactive lipid with the allergenic head group 1,2-dipalmitoyl-*sn*-glycero-3-phosphoethanolamine-N-[6-[(2,4-dinitrophenyl)amino]-hexanoyl] (DNP-cap-PE) when mixed with DOPC can be co-patterned onto glass surfaces (Fig. 2). In these experiments we used fluorophore-labelled 1,2-dioleoyl-sn-glycero-3-phosphoethanolamine-N-(lissamine rhodamine B sulfonyl) (18:1 lissamine rhodamine/PE) (Avanti Polar Lipids, Alabaster, AL, USA) for visualisation of the pattern. DPN was performed with commercially available instrumentation (DPN 5000, Nanoink Inc., USA). Tip coating and writing were carried out using a commercially available ink wells MW-6 and one-dimensional tip arrays of the M type. The inkwells were filled with a chloroform solution of the phospholipid ink (3 μl, 10 mM, doped with 1 mol% of the fluorophore-labelled lipid). The solvent was allowed to evaporate for 30 min before coating the tips. Tips were inked by placing them in contact with the inkwell and increasing the humidity to 70% for at least 30 min. Excess ink was

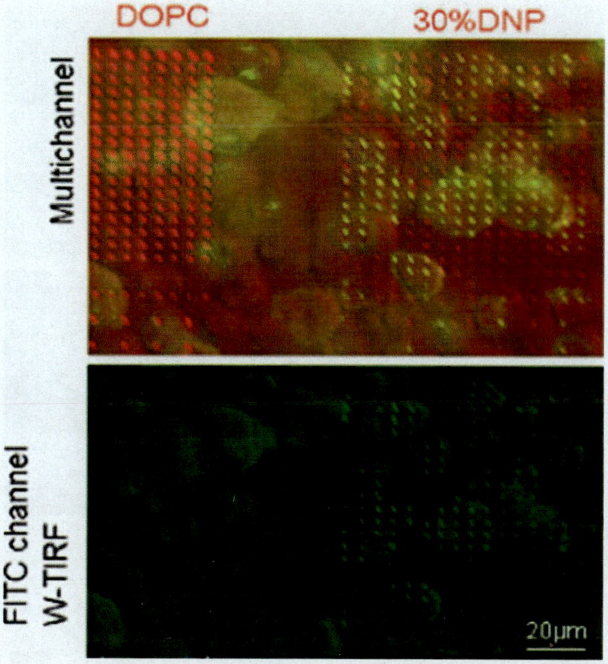

Fig. 3 RBL-2H3 mast cells FcεRI receptor (labelled green with Alexa 488-IgE antibody) clustering on DNP patterns labelled red with rhodamine. Antibody-receptor clusters (green) are co-localized (in yellow) over the 30% patterned DNP ligand but not over the DOPC control

removed from freshly coated tips by writing at high humidity (>65%) on a sacrificial substrate for ~10 min. Patterning of the dot arrays was done at 35% humidity, 23°C, with writing speed 10 μm/s. Glass substrates were plasma treated with oxygen (20 sccm, 100 mTorr, 30 s). Oxygen plasma treatment decreases the contact angle of water, making the substrate more hydrophilic and better suitable for the lithography.

RBL-2H3 mast cells were treated with Alexa Fluor® 488-labelled Monoclonal Antibody to IgE (In vitrogen for Alexa 488 and Sigma for IgE antibody). The labelled antibody was used to sensitise the mast cells to make them visible in live cell imaging. The cells were then place over the pattern and it can clearly be seen that they bind the surface containing the 30% DNP (evident by the yellow dot) and not the area containing only the DOPC (Fig. 3).

With no haptenated lipid present, the cells remained rounded and mostly detached from the patterned surface. When the bilayers contain DOPC and DNP, the cells flatten and spread out. Clustering of IgE receptor on mast cells initiates signal transduction that leads to degranulation and release of chemical mediators. This process is accompanied by polymerisation of cytoskeletal actin leading to spread of the rounded cell and ruffling caused by extension of lamellipodia. The clear morphological changes allow us to establish that the receptors clustered by the haptenated lipid stimulate a cellular response. In cases where this process is not yet clearly visible, the cell activation could be detected via staining with phosphotyrosine antibody. One of the very early events following cross-linking of the

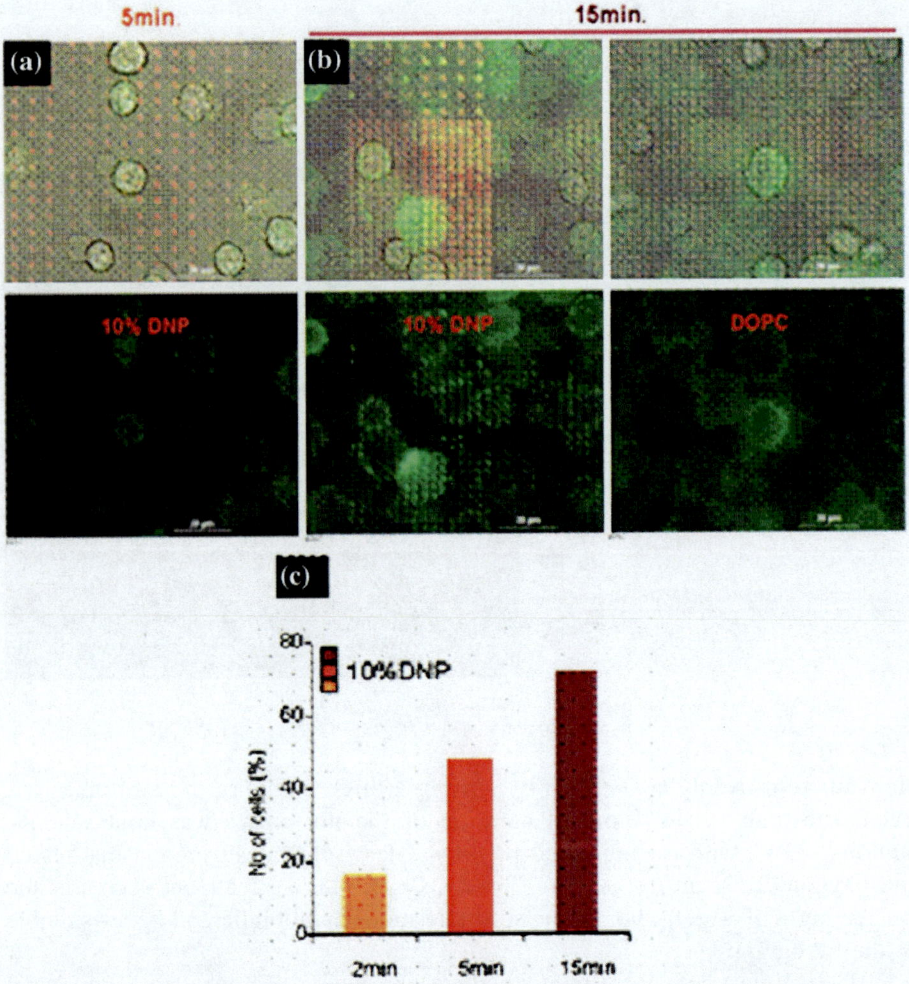

Fig. 4 Activation of mast cells on DNP-lipid patterns. **a** RBL 2H3 cells show micrometer-scale concentration of phosphorylated tyrosine, which appears as early as 5 min. **b** At 15 min, the phosphorylated tyrosine signal reaches a maximum. Cells on the DOPC pattern show no detectable tyrosine phoshorylation. **c** Plot of the percentage of activated cells on DNP arrays over time

IgE receptor is tyrosine phosphorylation brought about by the recruitment of various kinases to the cross-linked receptor. Our preliminary quantification of the phosphorylation events showed that approx. 2 min after cross-linking nearly 18% of the cells were activated in terms of positive phosphotyrosine signal rising to 45% at 5 min time point. The system is therefore set for analysing the rapid action of steroid hormones triggered after activation of the cells by allergenic hapten (Fig. 4).

5 Questions to be Answered

How are the steroid receptor recruited to the plasma membrane?

We will use the above-described approaches to find out how fluorescently-labelled GR and ER are recruited to the lipid rafts following activation of these receptors. Upon hormone treatment it is thought that the steroid receptors present in an inactive state in complexes with molecular chaperones dissociate and are transported into the nucleus. Since the receptors could also be transported to the plasma membrane, we would like to know how this is brought about and to determine the dynamics of this recruitment. In this connection, we would use photobleaching experiments to measure the recovery of fluorescence after the ablation of the signal (FRAP) to determine the kinetics of the recovery. This would give an idea as to the dynamics of recruitment and the mobility of the receptors.

What molecules interact with the steroid receptors at the plasma membrane?

To analyse protein–protein interaction, the bimolecular fluorescence complementation (BiFC) would be used. This assay is based on the splitting of the yellow florescence protein (YFP) into two parts (C-terminal part of YFP: YC and N-terminal part of YFP, YN). These two parts do not spontaneously re-associate and do not fluoresce. Fusing the YN and YC to two potentially interacting proteins will lead to fluorescence only when they interact. Using the BiFC assay with the steroid receptor as prey and members of the signalling molecules of the mast cells (e.g. Lyn, Fyn or Syk) as bait will determine the in vivo interacting partners of the receptor. Mutant receptors will also be analysed to identify the domains and sequences needed for their recruitment and action at the lipid raft.

6 Conclusions

We have described here a novel method to elucidate the early processes underlying the rapid non-genomic action of steroid receptors using mast cells as model. This is to be accomplished using the technique of dip-pen nanolithography (DPN) for the direct patterning of model allergens such as haptenated lipids onto surfaces in order to activate the signalling cascade. Mast cells will be allowed to settle on these patterned surfaces and to make contact with the hapten through their surface expressed IgE receptor. This approach will allow recruitment of signalling molecules including steroid receptors to the lipid domains collectively referred to as lipid rafts to be visualised and analysed at the single cell level. It will also allow receptor-proximal events triggered by antigenic IgE receptor cross-linking and interference or enhancement by steroid receptors to be measured. Through the use of fluorescently labelled lipids and IgE or steroid receptor, FcεRI clustering and subsequent events can be measured in living cells in "real time". Time course experiments of tyrosine phosphorylation of the mast cells will be used as a read-out for the activation of the cells. Alternatively, measurements of the intracellular Ca^{2+} levels of the cell could be used as a measure of the degree of activation.

Rapid action of steroids has so far proven difficult to analyse in any great depths because of technical problems arising from capturing the receptors at the plasma membrane. With the use of the latest developments in DPN, these problems could now be overcome. It would make it possible for molecular interactions of the steroid receptors with cellular signalling components to be assessed with great precision. Above all, this would generate knowledge that could be further explored at the level of identification of specific ligands for this pathway for the determination of the physiological relevance of the rapid action of steroids.

Acknowledgments his work was financed in part by funds from the DFG (SPP 1394) to A.C.B.C. and S.S.N. would like to acknowledge DFG-CFN for financial support.

References

1. Cato AC, Ponta H, Herrlich P (1992) Regulation of gene expression by steroid hormones. Prog Nucleic Acid Res Mol Biol 43:1–36
2. Nishi M, Kawata M (2006) Brain corticosteroid receptor dynamics and trafficking: Implications from live cell imaging. Neuroscientist 12:119–133
3. Nishi M, Takenaka N, Morita N, Ito T, Ozawa H, Kawata M (1999) Real-time imaging of glucocorticoid receptor dynamics in living neurons and glial cells in comparison with non-neural cells. Eur J Neurosci 11:1927–1936
4. Rose JD, Moore FL (1999) A neurobehavioral model for rapid actions of corticosterone on sensorimotor integration. Steroids 64:92–99
5. Cullinan WE, Herman JP, Battaglia DF, Akil H, Watson SJ (1995) Pattern and time course of immediate early gene expression in rat brain following acute stress. Neuroscience 64: 477–505
6. Kovacs KJ, Sawchenko PE (1996) Regulation of stress-induced transcriptional changes in the hypothalamic neurosecretory neuronsneurons. J Mol Neurosci 7:125–133
7. Croxtall JD, Choudhury Q, Flower RJ (2000) Glucocorticoids act within minutes to inhibit recruitment of signalling factors to activated EGF receptors through a receptor-dependent, transcription-independent mechanism. Br J Pharmacol 130:289–298
8. Blackmore PF (2008) ProgesteroneProgesterone metabolites rapidly stimulate calcium influx in human platelets by a src-dependent pathway. Steroids 73:738–750
9. Levin ER (2008) Rapid signaling by steroid receptors. Am J Physiol Regul Integr Comp Physiol 295:R1425–R1430
10. Peterziel H, Mink S, Schonert A, Becker M, Klocker H, Cato AC (1999) Rapid signalling by androgen receptor in prostate cancer cells. Oncogene 18:6322–6329
11. Zaitsu M, Narita S, Lambert KC, Grady JJ, Estes DM, Curran EM, Brooks EG, Watson CS, Goldblum RM, Midoro-Horiuti T (2007) Oestraddiol activates mast cellsmast cells via a non-genomic oestrogen receptor-alpha and calcium influx. Mol Immunol 44:1977–1985
12. Cato AC, Nestl A, Mink S (2002) Rapid actions of steroid receptors in cellular signaling pathways. Sci STKE 2002:re9
13. Stahn C, Buttgereit F (2008) Genomic and nongenomic effects of glucocorticoids. Nat Clin Pract Rheumatol 4:525–533
14. Fernandes MS, Brosens JJ, Gellersen B (2008) Honey, we need to talk about the membrane progestin receptors. Steroids 73:942–952
15. Langer G, Bader B, Meoli L, Isensee J, Delbeck M, Noppinger PR, Otto C (2010) A critical review of fundamental controversies in the field of GPR30 research. Steroids 75(8–9): 603–610

16. Pappas TC, Gametchu B, Watson CS (1995) Membrane oestrogen receptors identified by multiple antibody labeling and impeded-ligand binding. FASEB J 9:404–410
17. Cheng J, Watkins SC, Walker WH (2007) Testosterone activates mitogen-activated protein kinase via Src kinaseSrc kinase and the epidermal growth factor receptor in sertoli cells. Endocrinology 148:2066–2074
18. Marquez DC, Pietras RJ (2001) Membrane-associated binding sites for oestrogen contribute to growth regulation of human breast cancerbreast cancer cells. Oncogene 20:5420–5430
19. Okamoto T, Schlegel A, Scherer PE, Lisanti MP (1998) Caveolins, a family of scaffolding proteins for organizing "preassembled signaling complexes" at the plasma membrane. J Biol Chem 273:5419–5422
20. Lu ML, Schneider MC, Zheng Y, Zhang X, Richie JP (2001) Caveolin-1 interacts with androgen receptor A positive modulator of androgen receptor mediated transactivation. J Biol Chem 276:13442–13451
21. Schlegel A, Wang C, Katzenellenbogen BS, Pestell RG, Lisanti MP (1999) Caveolin-1 potentiates oestrogen receptor alpha (ERalpha) signaling. Caveolin-1 drives ligand-independent nuclear translocation and activation of ERalpha. J Biol Chem 274:33551–33556
22. Kahlert S, Nuedling S, van Eickels M, Vetter H, Meyer R, Grohe C (2000) Oestrogen receptor alpha rapidly activates the IGF-1 receptor pathway. J Biol Chem 275:18447–18453
23. Di Domenico M, Castoria G, Bilancio A, Migliaccio A, Auricchio F (1996) Oestraddiol activation of human colon carcinoma-derived Caco-2 cell growth. Cancer Res 56:4516–4521
24. Migliaccio A, Di Domenico M, Castoria G, de Falco A, Bontempo P, Nola E, Auricchio F (1996) Tyrosine kinase/p21ras/MAP-kinase pathway activation by oestraddiol-receptor complex in MCF-7 cells. EMBO J 15:1292–1300
25. Song RX, McPherson RA, Adam L, Bao Y, Shupnik M, Kumar R, Santen RJ (2002) Linkage of rapid oestrogen action to MAPK activation by ERalpha-Shc association and Shc pathway activation. Mol Endocrinol 16:116–127
26. Watters JJ, Chun TY, Kim YN, Bertics PJ, Gorski J (2000) Oestrogen modulation of prolactin gene expression requires an intact mitogen-activated protein kinase signal transduction signal transduction pathway in cultured rat pituitary cells. Mol Endocrinol 14:1872–1881
27. Le Romancer M, Treilleux I, Leconte N, Robin-Lespinasse Y, Sentis S, Bouchekioua-Bouzaghou K, Goddard S, Gobert-Gosse S, Corbo L (2008) Regulation of oestrogen rapid signaling through arginine methylationarginine methylation by PRMT1. Mol Cell 31:212–221
28. Castoria G, Migliaccio A, Giovannelli P, Auricchio F (2009) Cell proliferation regulated by oestradiol receptor: therapeutic implications. Steroids 75(8–9):524–527
29. Wong CW, McNally C, Nickbarg E, Komm BS, Cheskis BJ (2002) Oestrogen receptor-interacting protein that modulates its nongenomic activity-crosstalk with Src/Erk phosphorylation cascade. Proc Natl Acad Sci U S A 99:14783–14788
30. Lu Q, Pallas DC, Surks HK, Baur WE, Mendelsohn ME, Karas RH (2004) Striatin assembles a membrane signaling complex necessary for rapid, nongenomic activation of endothelial NO synthase by oestrogen receptor alpha. Proc Nat Acad Sci U S A 101:17126–17131
31. Manavathi B, Acconcia F, Rayala SK, Kumar R (2006) An inherent role of microtubule network in the action of nuclear receptor. Proc Nat Acad Sci U S A 103:15981–15986
32. Wang Z, Zhang X, Shen P, Loggie BW, Chang Y, Deuel TF (2006) A variant of oestrogen receptor-{alpha}, hER-{alpha}36: transduction of oestrogen- and antioestrogen-dependent membrane-initiated mitogenic signaling. Proc Natl Acad Sci U S A 103:9063–9068
33. Migliaccio A, Castoria G, Di Domenico M, de Falco A, Bilancio A, Lombardi M, Bottero D, Varricchio L, Nanayakkara M, Rotondi A, Auricchio F (2002) Sex steroid hormones act as growth factorsgrowth factors. J Steroid Biochem Mol Biol 83:31–35
34. Turner H, Kinet JP (1999) Signalling through the high-affinity IgE receptor Fc epsilonRI. Nature 402:B24–B30
35. Harrell JM, Murphy PJ, Morishima Y, Chen H, Mansfield JF, Galigniana MD, Pratt WB (2004) Evidence for glucocorticoid receptor transport on microtubules by dynein. J Biol Chem 279:54647–54654

36. Zhou J, Liu DF, Liu C, Kang ZM, Shen XH, Chen YZ, Xu T, Jiang CL (2008) Glucocorticoids inhibit degranulation of mast cells in allergic asthma via nongenomic mechanism. Allergy 63:1177–1185
37. Piner RD, Zhu J, Xu F, Hong S, Mirkin CA (1999) "Dip-Pen" nanolithography. Science 283:661–663
38. Mirkin CA (2007) The power of the pen: development of massively parallel dip-pen nanolithography. ACS Nano 1:79–83
39. Sekula S, Fuchs J, Weg-Remers S, Nagel P, Schuppler S, Fragala J, Theilacker N, Franzreb M, Wingren C, Ellmark P et al (2008) Multiplexed lipid dip-pen nanolithography on sub-cellular scales for the templating of functional proteins and cell culture. Small 4:1785–1793

Index

G. Castoria and A. Migliaccio (eds.), *Advances in Rapid Sex-Steroid Action*,
DOI: 10.1007/978-1-4614-1764-4,